Understanding
Clinical Negotiation

Understanding Clinical Negotiation

Richard L. Kravitz, MD, MSPH
Distinguished Professor, UC Davis Department of Internal Medicine
Director, UC Center Sacramento
Sacramento, California

Richard L. Street, Jr, PhD
Professor, Department of Communication, Texas A&M University
Professor, Department of Medicine, Baylor College of Medicine
College Station, Texas

Mc
Graw
Hill

New York Chicago San Francisco Athens London Madrid Mexico City
New Delhi Milan Singapore Sydney Toronto

Understanding Clinical Negotiation

1 2 3 4 5 6 7 8 9   LCR   26 25 24 23 22 21

ISBN 978-1-260-46249-4
MHID 1-260-46249-8

This book was set in Chaparral Pro by MPS Limited.
The editor was Kay Conerly.
The production supervisor was Catherine Saggese.
Project management was provided by Jyoti Shaw and Poonam Bisht of MPS Limited.
The cover designer was W2 Design.

Library of Congress Cataloging-in-Publication Data

Names: Kravitz, Richard, author. | Street, R. L., Jr. (Richard L.), author.

Title: Understanding clinical negotiation / Richard L. Kravitz, Richard L.
    Street, Jr.
Description: New York : McGraw Hill, [2021] | Includes bibliographical
    references and index. | Summary: "This book argues that
    knowing what patients want and working with them toward mutually defined
    goals is the essence of good patient care. Skillful clinical negotiation
    can also augment the rewards, and help overcome the challenges, of
    clinical practice"— Provided by publisher.
Identifiers: LCCN 2021019253 (print) | LCCN 2021019254 (ebook) | ISBN
    9781260462494 (paperback) | ISBN 9781260462500 (ebook)
Subjects: MESH: Patient-Centered Care | Professional-Patient Relations |
    Patient Acceptance of Health Care | Clinical Decision-Making—methods |
    Negotiating
Classification: LCC R727.3 (print) | LCC R727.3 (ebook) | NLM W 84.7 |
    DDC 610.69/6—dc23
LC record available at https://lccn.loc.gov/2021019253
LC ebook record available at https://lccn.loc.gov/2021019254

McGraw Hill books are available at special quantity discounts to use as premiums and sales promotions, or for use in corporate training programs. To contact a representative, please visit the Contact Us pages at www.mhprofessional.com.

Photo images in Figure 5-3 are reproduced with permission from TriStar Pictures/Entertainment Pictures/Alamy Stock Photo; Deborah Feingold/Corbis/Getty Images.

Photo images in Figure 9-1 are reproduced with permission from Image Source/Getty Images; Cecilie_Arcurs/Getty Images; Ajr_images/Getty Images.

Contents

Contributor

Stephen G. Henry, MD, MSc
Associate Professor in General Medicine
UC Davis Medical Center
Sacramento, California

Preface

"Understanding Clinical Negotiation" means finding and holding common ground with patients. The requisite skills are fundamental to patient-centered care. Thus, this book is addressed mainly to practicing generalist physicians, nurse practitioners, and physicians' assistants, as well as students and post-graduate trainees aspiring to become accomplished clinicians.

Caring for patients can be uniquely rewarding but also uniquely challenging. It is not getting any easier. Over the past half-century, the number of available diagnostic and therapeutic technologies has increased greatly. At the same time, the information environment has changed dramatically. Both clinicians and patients are exposed to a tidal wave of health-related information of widely varying quality. Meanwhile, practice environments have grown increasingly complex, so that patients do not always know who is in charge of their care, where they can go for after-hours emergencies, and how much it will cost. There are times, therefore, when patients and clinicians find themselves at a loss. Ginned up by direct-to-consumer advertising, the internet, and text messages from concerned relatives, patients approach the clinical encounter with more specific and more exacting expectations than in the past. In trying to provide high-value care, maintain patient safety, preserve patient satisfaction, and restrain costs, it is the rare clinician who does not sometimes feel overwhelmed, as the current literature on physician burnout amply testifies. This book argues that knowing what patients want and working with them toward mutually defined goals is the essence of good patient care. Skillful clinical negotiation can also augment the rewards, and help overcome the challenges, of clinical practice.

How this Book Came to Be

While the actual writing of this book began in 2019, its genesis is much longer. For almost 40 years, one author (RLK) has taught and practiced general internal medicine at teaching hospitals while developing a research program focused on patients as agents for their own quality of care.[1] Working with patients and performing patient-centered research not only is intensely gratifying but has produced gratifying synergies; many research ideas (and almost all of the good ones) emerged directly from issues, challenges, or questions arising in the care of patients in the clinic and on the wards. Over roughly the same period, the other author (RLS) applied the tools of communication science to examine the uniquely human endeavor of health care, while simultaneously contributing to theories and methods that help sustain the field. Although never at the same institution, RLK and RLS have collaborated on numerous projects for over two decades. Their complementary perspectives as a clinician and communication scientist contribute to what we hope is the unique character of this book.

Why Clinical Negotiation?

To some clinicians, the term "negotiation" will sound dissonant, foreign, and disconnected from more traditional framings of clinician-patient communication. After all, books with the word "negotiation" in the title are usually shelved with books on marketing, sales, and leveraged buy-outs, not with books on health and medicine. Yet we have chosen clinical negotiation as our focus for three reasons.

First, the concept of clinical negotiation has a distinguished history. To the best of our knowledge, the term was introduced in 1975 by psychiatrist Aaron Lazare and extended to general medical practice several years later by psychiatric services researcher Wayne Katon and psychiatric anthropologist Arthur Kleinman.[2,3] These pioneers in the art and science of the clinician-patient relationship meant for "negotiation" to mean nothing more—and nothing less—than a *conversation* directed at clarifying and achieving mutual goals. In this sense, clinical negotiation is the intellectual forebear and close cousin of shared decision-making.

Second, framing the clinical encounter as a negotiation not only illuminates the underlying communication processes but extends the range of our analysis. The most critical tasks of the clinician-patient encounter are, we would argue, to identify patients' most fervent aspirations, clarify goals, and develop appropriate plans. Optimally, these plans should be concordant with the patient's wishes, aligned with their interests and values, and consistent with professional knowledge. In this sense, negotiation is not merely a tool for conflict resolution but an approach to clinical care in its entirety: from defining and naming the problem, to engaging in mutual exploration of goals and means of achieving them, to agreeing on a diagnostic and therapeutic plan that is both medically sound and personally acceptable.

Finally, clinical negotiation is even more relevant to the study of clinician-patient communication today than it was in the time of Lazare, Katon, and Kleinman, for the simple reason that there is far more to negotiate *about*. Health care teams and systems are more complex. The diagnostic and therapeutic armamentarium is larger. Sub-specialization concentrates expertise but further balkanizes the profession. Patients are exposed to a confusing array of health messages appearing in traditional and social media, in direct-to-consumer advertising of prescription drugs, and in marketing materials produced by the very health care organizations from which they seek care.[4] In this evolving landscape, finding common ground through effective clinical negotiation is both more challenging and more important than ever.

What the Book is (and isn't) About

This book is about identifying, understanding, and responding to patients' wants, needs, desires and expectations in ways that leads to better outcomes for patients and more satisfying health care relationships for everyone. The primary purpose is to equip front-line generalist medical practitioners—primary care physicians, hospitalists, nurse practitioners, physician assistants, or those training for these roles—to recognize the contours of clinical negotiation and how to reach a satisfactory resolution as quickly and efficiently as possible. While our aims are pragmatic, we also hope to show how health communication research has informed our understanding of how patients think, what doctors say, and how clinicians of all stripes can more effectively guide patients and their families towards the pursuit of better health.

This book covers a lot of ground, but in our effort to keep the manuscript to a manageable size and to stay in an authorial lane defined by our joint experience and expertise, many important topics receive less attention than they deserve. Perhaps most pressingly in the current moment (when policing methods, systemic racism, and social unrest are all in the news), our coverage of health disparities, cultural competence, racism in medicine, and diversity and inclusion within the health professions is incomplete. However, we have tried to be sensitive to these issues from a stance of genuine cultural humility[5] while still emphasizing universal communication principles. In addition, while we do address the contribution of health care systems and organizations to the clinical negotiation, we focus largely on what individual practitioners can control: their relationship with patients and with other health care professionals. Even there, we do not attempt systematic coverage of the many permutations of interprofessional conflict and cooperation, focusing mainly on clinician-patient, physician-physician and nurse-physician interactions.

A Word About Language

This book is directed toward a broad audience. In referring to health professionals engaged in the diagnosis and treatment of diseases, we incline towards the term "clinician," which is meant to be respectfully inclusive of physicians, advanced practice nurses, and physicians' assistants as well as those who are training to join their ranks. Especially but not solely in Chapter 10 (Negotiating with Physician Colleagues and Other Health Care Professionals), we refer specifically to "physicians" when it seems likely that the scenario under discussion is primarily relevant to medical doctors.

Except for the partial transcripts of Chapter 8, the clinical vignettes presented throughout the book represent composites of our clinical and research experience. All names are fictitious. Regarding the use of personal pronouns, our writing style tends to alternate between he, she, and they, though not necessarily in equal parts. While we have tried to celebrate and mirror the diversity of patients, clinicians, and clinical scenarios that readers will encounter in practice, we apologize in advance for any lapses.

Uses and Organization

The book's format lends itself to several learning styles. Practitioners, trainees, and students interested in gaining a thorough introduction to clinical negotiation will benefit from reading the book from cover-to-cover, taking time after each chapter to review the bulleted summary points, answer the discussion questions (or better yet, talk about them with peers), and apply any learnings to their own interactions with patients. This approach will also work well for students training to be physicians, advanced practice nurses, physicians' assistants, or health care administrators for whom the book is employed as a text in courses covering the clinician-patient relationship, medical interviewing, health communication, or health administration. However, each chapter is relatively self-contained, so that readers drawn to particular aspects of the clinical negotiation can gainfully attend to the parts of the book that most interest them.

The book is organized into three parts. **Part 1 (Background and Rationale)** prepares readers with the fundamental vocabulary and concepts needed to adopt strategies and handle situations introduced subsequently. In two introductory chapters we define clinical negotiation and patients' expectations, desires, and requests; introduce a model for clinical negotiation; trace the origins of patients' expectations (including their hidden meanings); and examine the economic, social, and cultural forces that influence how the clinical negotiation unfolds.

Part 2 (Barriers and Strategies) covers specific structural features of the health care system that influence clinical negotiation; strategies for fostering patients' full disclosure of relevant information; methods for raising awareness of and managing emotions in clinical care; the power of empathy; and the importance of physician self-awareness and self-control. This part of the book closes with a chapter wholly devoted to our MASTerDOC strategy for undertaking successful clinical negotiation, including modifications for patients from varied cultural backgrounds and patients perceived as "difficult."

Finally, **Part 3 (Applications)** considers a wide range of applications including approaches for negotiating around tests, prescriptions, and referrals; negotiating with patients who have been prescribed controlled substances; negotiating with hospitalized patients and their families; and finally, negotiating with colleagues.

Special Features

A unique feature of this book is the combination of science and practice. The main text tilts toward practice, with just enough health communication research inserted throughout to provide support for the conclusions. Many of the lessons we hope to share are woven around specific clinical vignettes or (in Chapter 8) actual transcripts of doctor-patient interactions. Some chapters begin with a clinical vignette, some do not, but all incorporate scenarios we have encountered in research and practice. We invite readers interested in exploring the theory or practice of communication science in greater depth to read the special "Deeper Dive" sections. These textual insets explore research evidence supporting the principles described in the main text and attempt to unravel some of the more intriguing, elusive, and taken-for-granted features of communication processes and contexts. Those interested in learning even more can consult the extensive references.

Recognizing the pedagogic value of emphasizing key concepts, each chapter begins with "Clinical Take-aways" and ends with a set of summary bullet points. Learners at all levels who incorporate these "pearls" into clinical practice, teaching, or administration will have gained much of what the book has to offer. The take-aways at the beginning of each chapter emphasize actionable lessons that can be applied immediately in practice. The summary points at the end of each chapter provides a more comprehensive review.

Many readers, particularly students and trainees who are using the book as part of a course or communication skills program, may wish to review the "Questions for Discussion" included at each chapter's end. Like so many questions in health and medicine, these questions often have no clear or definite answer. They are included to stimulate readers to think more deeply about the concepts addressed in the text and to foment discussion among learners, teachers, and peers.

Conclusion

This book is meant to equip clinicians with enough background to confidently apply new communication skills in the office and on the hospital wards. Readers will find plenty of practical pointers, but they will also learn the scientific underpinnings of the various approaches. Understanding the theoretical and empirical basis of effective clinical negotiation takes more effort than memorizing a list of rules, but we believe that assimilating the principles will lead to deeper, more sustained learning and more flexible, effective practice.

We hope this book helps you become an even more skillful and caring clinical negotiator than you are already.

Richard L. Kravitz, MD, MSPH
Richard L. Street, Jr., PhD

References

1. Kravitz RL. Beyond gatekeeping: enlisting patients as agents for quality and cost-containment. In: Springer; 2008.
2. Katon W, Kleinman A. Doctor-patient negotiation and other social science strategies in patient care. In: *The Relevance of Social Science for Medicine.* Springer; 1981:253-279.
3. Lazare A, Eisenthal S, Wasserman L. The customer approach to patienthood. Attending to patient requests in a walk-in clinic. *Arch Gen Psychiatry.* 1975;32(5):553-558.
4. Larson RJ, Schwartz LM, Woloshin S, Welch HG. Advertising by academic medical centers. *Archives of Internal Medicine.* 2005;165(6):645-651.
5. Tervalon M, Murray-Garcia J. Cultural humility versus cultural competence: A critical distinction in defining physician training outcomes in multicultural education. *Journal of Health Care for the Poor and Underserved.* 1998;9(2):117-125.

About the Authors

Richard L. Kravitz, MD, MSPH is Distinguished Professor of Internal Medicine at UC Davis and Director of the University of California Center, Sacramento. A general internist, he sees patients and supervises trainees in both outpatient and inpatient settings. He has led studies examining patients' expectations and requests for care, direct-to-consumer advertising of prescriptions drugs, and aligning care with patient's individual needs, values and preferences. The author or co-author of over 300 academic papers, he has twice won Academy Health's Article-of-the-Year award and was the 2013 recipient of the George Engel Award for Outstanding Research Contributing to the Theory, Practice and Teaching of Effective Health Care Communication and Related Skills.

Richard L. Street, Jr. PhD is Professor of Communication at Texas A&M University and Professor of Medicine at Baylor College of Medicine. His research focuses on clinician-patient communication, pathways linking communication to improved health outcomes, and strategies for increasing patient involvement in care. His research and teaching awards include Outstanding Health Communication Scholar from the International Communication Association, L. Donohew Health Communication Scholar Award from the University of Kentucky, TAMU Distinguished Achievement Awards in Teaching and Research, and 2012 George L. Engel award from the American Academy on Communication in Healthcare.

Acknowledgments

Although we take full responsibility for its contents, a book like this is a collective undertaking. We are grateful to the many people who have helped to bring about this work, whether knowingly or not. Among these are our patients; our students, trainees, and colleagues at UC Davis, Texas A&M University and Baylor College of Medicine; two professional societies (Society of General Internal Medicine and Academy of Communication in Health Care); and the many communication researchers on whose shoulders we stand.

The authors gratefully acknowledge the contributions of colleagues who generously provided feedback on parts of the book: Andrew Auerbach, Lauren Bloom, Kevin Burnham, Paul Duberstein, Ronald Epstein, Tonya Fancher, Ishani Ganguli, Jodi Halpern, Dana Hinojosa, Marianne Matthias, Kelley Skeff, and Steven Woloshin. Special thanks are due to Robert Bell, a longtime colleague at UC Davis whose work inspired and helped to shape the initial contours of this book.

Finally, this work could not have been completed without the loving support of our wives (Helaina Laks Kravitz, MD, published author, voracious reader, and a gentle but persistent critic; and Nancy James Street, award winning teacher, invaluable colleague, and a much appreciated—and needed—proponent of imagination and creativity). We are also grateful for the inspiration of our adult children (David, Aaron, and Joshua Kravitz; Rachel Crowder, Joshua Street, Jonathan Street, and Madeline West), who represent the next generation and our hopes for the future.

PART I

Background and Rationale

CHAPTER 1

Clinical Negotiation and the Search for Common Ground

Clinical Take-Aways

- The aim of clinical negotiation is for the clinician and patient to find common ground, bridging the clinician's professionalism and experience with the patient's goals and values.
- Well-executed clinical negotiation facilitates patient empowerment, shared decision-making, and patient-centered care.
- Many forces conspire against successful clinical negotiation; becoming an expert clinical negotiator is a career-long journey.
- Clinicians should:
  - View clinical negotiation as a fundamental clinical skill.
  - Approach each clinical encounter in a spirit of curiosity.
  - Privilege patients' goals and values without abandoning their own claim to expertise.

SECTION 1.1: INTRODUCTION

After a few years in practice, clinicians find that some encounters with patients are routine. The patient's symptoms are few and easily categorized. The diagnosis is straightforward. The clinician and patient know and trust each other. The intended treatment is firmly established by evidence and reinforced by professional experience. The patient accepts the diagnosis, adheres to therapy, and makes a full recovery. Good feelings abound.

Other clinical encounters are more fraught. Symptoms are prolonged, distressing, or not readily mapped to an accepted medical ontology. The patient and clinician don't know each other, don't trust each other, or both. The diagnosis is elusive. An endless series of diagnostic studies and consultations leads nowhere. Confusion and uncertainty push the patient's tolerance and the clinician's equanimity to the brink.

Between these extremes resides the majority of clinical encounters.

Mr. Vaughan is a 34-year-old construction worker seeing his new internist. He is generally in good health but requests referrals to cardiology because "there is heart disease in my family" and to dermatology because of mild-moderate acne.

Ms. Carluchi is a 45-year-old nurse with intermittent low back pain, worse over the past week following a particularly demanding shift at the hospital. The pain is moderately severe, located to the right of the midline, and without radiation to the extremities. Neurological examination is benign. She asks for time off work and wonders whether an "MRI might show what's really going on so we don't have to keep guessing."

Mr. Gonzalez, 85 years of age, is a retired agricultural foreman who recently immigrated from Mexico to live with his son, daughter-in-law, and granddaughter. His son, a math teacher at the local community college, is worried about the patient's declining cognitive function and possible depression. The patient has been offered antidepressant medication in the past but has adamantly refused.

In each of these situations, the physician's immediate reaction may be one of resistance or defensiveness. A cardiology referral in the absence of heart disease? A magnetic resonance imaging procedure for uncomplicated acute-on-chronic low back pain? Both requests are out-of-step with best practice, and both may represent low-value care. Refusal to consider effective care for a serious mental health condition? With that kind of attitude, maybe the patient should see someone else!

Such situations are not only common, their outcomes can vary markedly depending on the clinician's skill in defining, framing, and communicating about the problem. Do it right and the patient gets appropriate care even as the patient-clinician relationship is strengthened. Do it wrong and clinicians can jeopardize the patient-clinician relationship, their professional self-worth, and even their patients' health.

This book is about identifying, understanding, and responding to patients' wants, needs, desires, and expectations in ways that lead to better outcomes for patients and more satisfying health care relationships for all. The primary purpose is to equip front-line medical practitioners, students, and trainees—be they current or future physicians, nurse practitioners, or physician assistants—to recognize the contours of clinical negotiation and reach a satisfactory resolution as quickly and efficiently as possible. While our aims are fundamentally pragmatic, we also hope to show how 40 years of scientific research in health communication have informed our understanding of how patients think, what doctors say, and how clinicians of all stripes can more effectively guide patients and their families towards the pursuit of better health.

SECTION 1.2: DEFINING CLINICAL NEGOTIATION

The idea that doctors and patients can and should engage in a continuous effort to understand each other seems commonplace now, but it represents a break with tradition. Beginning in the early 1970s, the authoritarian model of the doctor-patient relationship was gradually supplanted by a more egalitarian approach in which patients assumed a more active role in their own care. It is probably no coincidence that this medical-cultural revolution coincided with other sweeping social movements of that period, including civil rights, women's rights, consumer rights, and the anti-war movement. In earlier decades, physicians prescribed and patients complied—or at least pretended to. Now, on the heels of a slow evolution toward empowerment of the disenfranchised, the paternalistic model of medical practice suddenly seems not just quaint but genuinely regressive. Many patients have rightly demanded that they no longer be passive subjects of physicians' attention. Instead, they are active partners in their own care. Inevitably, they are also negotiators. And so are the health professionals entrusted with their care.

The word negotiation carries connotative baggage. Of the numerous books in print with "negotiation" in the title, most focus on business transactions, and many describe a zero-sum game in which the goal is to emerge the winner. These books exhort the reader to "never split the difference," to "bargain for advantage," and to learn "101 ways to win every time." And, of course, when there are winners, there are also losers. However appropriate this competitive worldview might be for entrepreneurs and real estate moguls, it doesn't apply to healing relationships. Unlike two business executives, patients and health care professionals generally share the same basic goal: to achieve the best possible health outcomes for the patient. When the parties differ, it usually has to do with the definition of the problem, the value assigned to different health outcomes, or the means available to achieve the ultimate goal of improved health. Addressing gaps in communication around these issues is a major aim of this book.

In this book, we use the term "clinical negotiation" to refer to a *discussion between patient and health care professional that is aimed at reaching agreement.* These discussions may focus on the interpretation of symptoms, the meaning of illness, the pace or process of diagnostic testing, the choice of therapy, or the implications of prognosis. Agreement on these points can pave the way to healing. Disagreement, when unresolved, can distort clinical information gathering, derail the diagnostic process, interrupt adherence to beneficial treatment, disrupt continuity of care, and detract from patient satisfaction. Borrowing from Moira Stewart's pathbreaking work on patient-centered care [1], we view reaching clinical agreement as the process of *finding common ground.* The metaphor of common ground is useful because it implies that reaching clinical agreement is not an all-or-nothing process. Areas of agreement (common ground) and areas of disagreement (disputed territory) can co-exist within the same healing relationship. In the terminology of the field of negotiation, we conceive of the clinical negotiation as being integrative, not distributive.

Deeper Dive 1.1: Distributive versus Integrative Negotiations

Negotiation gets a bad rap, so much so that some of our clinician-colleagues have claimed that "negotiation" plays no role in their practice of medicine or nursing. This objection reflects the assumption that "negotiation" is a cut-throat social process characterized by the selfish pursuit of personal interests at the expense of the other side. Under this rubric, negotiation is a zero-sum game in which one individual's gains are another's losses. Winning is achieved through exertion of power, force of personality, and even chicanery.

To be sure, negotiations can take on the characteristics of battle. For example, in negotiations between corporate management and the representatives of a labor union, every dollar "won" by one side is a dollar "lost" by the other. Every extra vacation day conceded is a day of productive labor lost. The stakes are high, with each side exercising every tool of persuasion and coercion at their expense (for example, labor strikes and management lockouts). Negotiation experts, drawing upon the classic work of Walton and McKersie, refer to such situations as *distributive negotiations*.[42]

By contrast, in clinical negotiations, the objective is to integrate the interests of clinician and patient. In such *integrative negotiations*, the parties seek out a win-win course of action that targets optimal fulfillment of patient preferences and evidence-based practice. The goals of clinician and patient are similar (if not always precisely congruent), organized around providing the best health care possible to the patient. Integration of interests is possible because at least some of the resources the patient needs are not fixed. For example, the provider "gives" compassionate care—she does not "give up" compassionate care. The tools of coercion and deception that often creep into distributive negotiation are replaced by a desire to cultivate a relationship characterized by open communication that enables pursuit of mutual interests.

The purpose of this book is to equip clinicians with the evidence-based knowledge and skills for finding as much common ground with their patients as possible. This aim is based on the premise that clinical negotiation is a core clinical skill that materially influences

patients' health and thus represents a key dimension of clinical competence. Furthermore, skill in clinical negotiation is the underlying competency needed to make shared decision-making, patient empowerment, and patient-centered care possible.

SECTION 1.3: HEALTH GOALS, VALUES, AND AGENDAS

Finding common ground means discovering shared goals, shared values, and shared agendas.[2] Health *goals* are the aims of care. What are we really trying to achieve? Is it a clear diagnosis, an accurate prognosis, clinical cure, alleviation of symptoms, improved function, avoidance of harm, palliation of distress, or something else? While it might seem obvious that most patients go to the doctor because they want to get "better," there is substantial variation in how patients with the same condition define success, as well as considerable discordance between patients and clinicians.[3,4] In a recent study, we asked 87 chronic pain patients and their physicians to prioritize their goals of care. Altogether, 48% of patients ranked reducing pain intensity as their top priority, whereas 22% ranked finding a diagnosis as most important. Physicians ranked improving function as the top priority for 41% of patients and reducing medication side effects as most important for 26%.[5]

Values are the weights patients and clinicians place on *processes* and *outcomes* of care. Consider, for example, two 65-year-old men considering whether to undergo prostate specific antigen (PSA) screening for prostate cancer. Both have been counseled that if the PSA is high, the next step would be prostate biopsy, and if that were positive for cancer, the patient would need to consider radical surgery, radiation therapy, hormonal therapy, or so-called "active surveillance" (monitoring the patient closely to decide when, if ever, to invoke surgery, radiation, or hormones).

> *Mr. Gruella values his independence, enjoys travelling overseas, just remarried 3 years ago and has an active sex life, and worries about the impact prostate cancer treatment could have on his quality of life. He is willing to forego a small reduction in his risk of death by prostate cancer in order to avoid the side effects of prostate cancer treatment. Therefore, he chooses not to undergo PSA screening.*
>
> *Mr. Connelly had a friend die of prostate cancer 4 years ago; he remains agonized by memories of his friend's final days. He is willing to do whatever he can to avoid a similar fate. He knows that the benefits of PSA screening are probably small and that prostate cancer treatment can lead to erectile dysfunction and urinary incontinence. Nevertheless, he reasons that if there's a test available that can reduce his chances of dying of prostate cancer, he'll take it.*

Mr. Gruella and Mr. Connelly share similar clinical characteristics but differ in the way they think about the tradeoffs between quantity and quality of life. Such differences in values can be powerful drivers of patients' preferences.

Clinicians can gain insight into patients' values in two ways. In the context of a long-standing patient-clinician relationship, values can emerge organically as the pattern of choices patients make. Most seasoned practitioners can recall patients who "don't like to take medicines," who "tend to worry if they don't get definitive testing to quell their fears," or who "will do anything to avoid surgery." Absent such continuity, however, there is no substitute for sensitive but direct questioning. **Asking questions like "what worries you most about your condition?" or "what is most important to you?" can help clarify patients' values and set the stage for more focused conversations about diagnostic and therapeutic options.**

Process of care refers to the interactions, interventions, prescriptions, referrals, and procedures that are delivered to the patient—essentially anything a health care provider does to or for the patient. Outcomes of care refers to all of the health benefits and harms that may result from illness or its treatment. Because the number of important clinical questions will always overwhelm the capacity of the clinical research enterprise to address them, data linking processes to outcomes are often elusive. In addition, processes are linked to outcomes probabilistically. Executing a particular diagnostic or therapeutic strategy may influence the *likelihood* of achieving a particular outcome (e.g., freedom from metastatic prostate cancer), but even perfect implementation can never guarantee a specific result.

Agendas refer to what the patient and clinician want to accomplish during a given encounter such as an office visit, emergency department visit, or hospital stay. **Numerous studies suggest that patients frequently come to the clinical encounter with specific agendas but that these agendas may not be communicated to the treating clinician unless directly solicited.**[6–8] Given that clinicians frequently interrupt their patients within 15-30 seconds of initial presentation,[9,10] it is not surprising that unspoken agendas abound.

It is important to acknowledge that **clinicians have their own agendas**, usually tied to the goal of efficiently diagnosing the patient's complaint, ruling out serious illness, and offering a treatment plan consistent with evidence and experience. While some aspects of the clinician's agenda are readily transparent to patients, others remain obscure. Medical students and residents learning to conduct a medical interview are taught to solicit the patient's agenda, identify clinical priorities, and address the patient's concerns (e.g., "I'm worried that I'm losing my hair, I need a certification form to obtain a home health aide, and my motorized wheelchair doesn't work") without neglecting important medical needs ("Your blood pressure is 170/103"). However, clinicians are not typically taught whether and how to disclose factors that are surely germane to the patient's care (e.g., that they are running behind and cannot permit the patient to continue to monopolize their time; that they may have financial incentives to recommend [or withhold] certain approaches to diagnosis and therapy; that they are ill or sleep-deprived and may not be in the best position to undertake a complex procedure; or that they are about to finish residency and won't be available to the patient any more).

Patients' goals, values, and agendas are not always readily apparent; they need to be discovered. Fortunately, the process of discovery can be extremely rewarding. The main requirements are a healthy sense of curiosity, a systematic approach, and patience. **Curiosity is underrated as a quality of mind to be cultivated by clinicians at all levels of experience**. Why is this patient here? Why now? What about the patient's circumstances could have triggered or exacerbated the present illness? What has been the patient's experience with previous health care providers? From the patient's perspective, where did they go right or wrong? What does the patient think about the nature of the problem? What were they hoping the clinician might do? How committed are they to a particular course of action? Even the most seemingly trivial symptoms can provoke catastrophizing in a patient whose life circumstances, vicarious experience, or informational environment are configured in such a way as to foment health-related worry. In contrast, other patients manifest enormous capacity for ignoring or denying potentially serious symptoms. Being curious is the first and most important step in developing a rich, accurate understanding of the patient.

But curiosity alone is insufficient. **Understanding patients' goals, values, and agendas requires a systematic approach that begins with practiced silence**. Ask the patient what brings them in today. Then give them time to answer. The urge to interrupt is often overwhelming, as the clinician seeks to clarify vague references, pursue a diagnostic hypothesis, or shut down rambling or incoherent discourse. Clinicians fear that the patient will go on forever. But research has shown that only **the rare patient will talk for more than three minutes if allowed to speak uninterrupted**; the average patient takes much less.[10] Being quiet while the patient tells their story requires patience and a suspension of judgment. But it is often worth it in the end.

Deeper Dive 1.2: The Interrupting Clinician

Ever since Beckman and Frankel documented the high prevalence of physician interruptions in clinical visits (a finding that would be of little surprise to most patients), considerable attention has been given to the importance of giving patients "conversational space" for sharing their concerns. Beckman and Frankel's study, which has been cited nearly 1300 times, has been widely interpreted as evidence that "doctors don't listen."[9] An interruption can indicate poor listening, as when the interruption changes the topic of conversation. It can also be seen by patients as an exertion of power and control and, worse, as rude. Patient-centered doctors don't interrupt!

But are things really this simple? In recent years, some medical communication experts have called for a more nuanced treatment of interruptions in clinical dialogues. To be sure, an interruption can be thoughtless and rude—a "sharp knife," to quote Larry Mauksch, a professor of family medicine.[43] But it can also be thoughtful ("Wow! How did that make you feel?"), seek patient elaboration ("Is that a sharp or dull pain you are experiencing?"), and even show compassion ("I can only imagine what you're going through"). It is doubtful that patients even "hear" such interruptions as such, because they help the patient to share their experience more fully. Furthermore, Mauksch reminds us that patients might sometimes need to be interrupted as they tell their story because there could be other clinically relevant stories that are not being told by the patient that the doctor needs to hear.

Health services researchers need to examine the effects of different forms of interruptions on clinical communication. For example, Florian Menz and Ali Al-Roubaie have recently developed a classification system that groups physician interruptions into two broad groups—*supportive* and *nonsupportive*—that are composed of more refined subcategories.[44] One of their findings is that nonsupportive interruptions which are intended to shorten the medical visit actually lengthen it. We anticipate that some forms of interruptions will enhance patient satisfaction, the medical interview process, and overall quality of care, whereas other forms will prove to be detrimental.

SECTION 1.4: BARRIERS TO FINDING COMMON GROUND

The premise of this book is that negotiation is a useful approach whenever patients and clinicians diverge in how they understand the clinical problem or how they feel the problem should be addressed. Such divergence in perspectives plays out on a spectrum, bracketed by misunderstandings on one end and overt disagreements on the other. Over 40 years ago, Katon and Kleinman[11] developed a useful taxonomy of misunderstandings (Table 1-1).

At this point in the 21st century, Katon and Kleinman's taxonomy seems accurate but incomplete. As we will discuss in Chapter 3, modern clinical practice creates many more opportunities for misunderstanding. Not only are the diagnostic and therapeutic options more numerous, the complexity of health care systems has multiplied. Misunderstandings can now arise not only in how problems are conceptualized, what diagnostic pathways are to be pursued, and which treatments are to be entertained but also how the health system is to be navigated.

At the other end of the spectrum are overt disagreements. Here the patient and clinician have defined the problem using a common vocabulary, but they

Table 1-1 **A Taxonomy of Semantic Misunderstandings in Clinical Settings**[11]

Category	Example
Using different terms	"Cardiac problem" versus "heart problem"
Using the same term but meaning different things	"Low blood" as shorthand for anemia versus hypotension
Using the same terms for the same phenomena but with different etiological concepts	Hypertension caused by increased vascular resistance versus life stress
Using the same terms and referents but with different implications	Among Puerto Ricans in the 1970s, a diagnosis of "ulcer" was thought to predispose to cancer[12]
Using the same terms and referents but with different emotive meanings	Mental illness is just another problem for the physician but may be a deeply stigmatizing label for the patient

disagree on the way forward. For example, a patient with hypertension acknowledges the cardiovascular risks conveyed by uncontrolled blood pressure but is still reluctant to add a second blood pressure medication. The patient with headache understands that serious neurological disease is unlikely but still requests magnetic resonance imaging of the brain. Or a patient with rotator cuff tendinopathy rejects physical therapy because "last time it made the pain worse."

Trying to distinguish between misunderstanding and disagreement is important, because misunderstandings can often be resolved through careful listening, respectful questioning, and education, whereas disagreements generally require some form of negotiation and compromise. Gaining a full appreciation of the patient's mental representation of illness—which is to say, their understanding of the clinical problem—requires time and effort. But the payoff can be large. Once the clinician understands that the patient with hypertension saw her mother stroke out shortly after addition of a second anti-hypertensive; that the patient with headache knew someone at church with a brain tumor; and that the patient with tendinopathy embarked on a program of PT last time that was "too much, too soon," the doctor can adjust the approach to fit the patient's specific concerns.

We further examine misunderstandings, disagreements, and other ways communication can fail in Chapter 4.

The biggest pitfall for clinicians is taking what patients say at face value or guessing at what they mean. For example, a patient recently seen in our General Medicine clinic wasted no time in demanding, "I need something stronger for this pain." Our immediate assumption was that he wanted more opioids for his chronic back pain. But as the patient's story unfolded, it became clear that his main concern was being able to continue to keep his job. The patient worked at a car wash and was required to stand for long periods of time. We arranged for physical therapy, ordered a functional back brace, and recommended a soft standing mat to be placed underfoot while working. He left the office satisfied with his care, and he continued to take low-dose opioids without incident.

SECTION 1.5: WHY FINDING COMMON GROUND IS HARD

We assume that patients and clinicians can almost always find common ground and that doing so will advance the healer's charge to "cure sometimes, relieve often, and care always." But that doesn't mean that the task is easy or that there will always be 100% agreement. The clinical landscape is complex, marked by tangled jungles of symptoms and signs, deep forests of unconscious motives, and inevitably, sharp chasms of separation between the patient confronting illness and the clinician peering in from the outside, seeking to help. In navigating this landscape, it is best to bring a map.

Patients come to medical encounters bearing a complex mix of hopes, expectations, and desires. Often, these anticipations are refracted, amplified, or interpreted by friends or loved ones who may accompany patients to visits and assist with their care. Of course, if patients are hospitalized, the clinical encounter comes to them. Either way, the moment the clinician enters the room is not the first time the patient or caregiver has thought about what might be causing the problem (diagnosis); how it might evolve over time and affect their future, near or far (prognosis); how it might be treated; and what help they might need to cope. These pre-visit ruminations can be amorphous but are powerful and sometimes surprisingly specific.

At the moment of the encounter, clinicians bring their own collection of predispositions, assumptions, needs, and goals. As detailed in Table 1-2, the clinician's approach to a given patient will be influenced by numerous personal, professional, circumstantial, historical, and environmental factors.

Most physicians (and other primary care practitioners and PCPs-in-training to whom this book is also addressed) have pursued a career in the health professions because they want to help healthy people stay healthy and help sick people get well. If they are lucky, every doctor has experienced the satisfaction that comes from reversing an acute asthma attack, controlling a patient's blood pressure, or successfully treating depression. But that doesn't mean there aren't other, ancillary motives, including earning the gratitude of patients, the esteem of colleagues, and a fine living besides.

Seeing the world through the patient's eyes is a noble but challenging endeavor.[23,24] **To a large extent, patients and clinicians inhabit different worlds.**[25] For clinicians, the personal experience of serious illness narrows the emotional divide. An alternative to becoming sick oneself is to cultivate empathy, "imagining *how* it feels to experience something in contrast to imagining that something *is* the case."[26] What is it like to have a vague sense of abdominal unease for months? What if that unease is experienced around the time of

Table 1-2 **Influences on Clinicians' Styles of Care**

Broad Category	Specific Influence	Example
Personal	Demographics	On average, women physicians adopt a more patient-centered communication style than men.[13]
	Personality	Personality trait "openness" is associated with higher patient satisfaction.[14]
Professional	Specialty training	Primary care physicians achieve higher participatory decision-making style ratings than subspecialty physicians.[15]
	US/Canadian versus international medical school	International graduates fall short on a few selected process measures but are more likely to practice in rural underserved areas and overall quality is similar.[16,17]
Practice setting	Method of payment	Fee-for-service payment associated with greater patient-physician trust than capitation or salary.[18]
	Group size	Small group practices achieve low rates of hospital admission.[19]
	Panel size	Using a team model may increase primary care capacity per physician by up to 50%.[20]
Situational	Duration and quality of prior clinician-patient relationship	Increased continuity associated with increased provision of preventive care and reduced hospitalizations.[21]
	Time pressure	Adverse working conditions (including time pressure) associated with physician burnout but no clear association with quality of care.[22]

the anniversary of a parent's death from colon cancer? By asking such questions, thinking about them, and offering reflections that indicate an interest in, if not a full understanding of, patients' explicit concerns as well as inner state, the clinician can create an atmosphere of trust that lends comfort to the patient while maximizing the likelihood that diagnostically useful information will be revealed.

SECTION 1.6: SOCIAL AND CULTURAL DIMENSIONS OF CLINICAL NEGOTIATION

Any rational approach to the clinical negotiation has to start with an uncomfortable fact: social relationships are, at least in part, determined by the relative power of the involved parties. And power is not distributed equally between clinician and patient.

Viewing the clinical encounter through this lens is jarring to many health professionals, as they rarely think of their day-to-day encounters with patients in terms of exercising power. Patients come to the office or the hospital with a problem to be solved, and clinicians are there to solve it as expeditiously and compassionately as possible. Nevertheless, the thoughts, attitudes, and behaviors of both clinicians and patients are mutually influenced. In other words, each exerts power over the other. Patients influence doctors to talk or to listen, to feel emotional commitment (or sometimes, revulsion),[27] and to prescribe treatments that align with patients' wishes. But ultimately, clinicians hold most of the cards. Using one classic framework,[28] clinicians command power based on their medical expertise, the specialized information they alone have access to, the formal privileges society affords them, their identification with a trusted profession, and their ability to grant or deny access to desired resources (such as prescriptions, referrals, diagnostic studies, durable medical equipment, and disability benefits, to name a few). Patients, of course, enter the clinical setting with their own sources of power, a point that is often overlooked in health services research.

Deeper Dive 1.3: The Bases of Patient Power

There is an inherent power differential in the provider-patient relationship, as noted, but it would be wrong to assume that patients enter the clinical negotiation powerless. The primary source of a patient's power is information—what they know about their health circumstances. Some patients take the time to "study up" on their symptoms, diagnoses, and treatments. Providers who sincerely support the health consumerism movement hold such patients in high esteem. Unfortunately, other patients come misinformed, but do not realize that the website they read before their visit is incomplete or inaccurate. Most pediatricians, for example, have dealt with parents who are convinced that vaccines are unsafe and ineffective.

Patients also have power by virtue of the formal privileges afforded to them under the law. This includes the power to reject any examination, medical test, or treatment plan that the physician may suggest. Even if the doctor knows best, the patient's "no" prevails.

Expertise is a great source of power. While physicians generally outmatch their patients in terms of medical expertise, some patients have expert power by virtue of their own careers in health care. These could include patients who work as physicians, nurses, or in a bioscience-based career. A "meeting of the minds" in such situations is usually facilitated by the patient's expertise.

In our experience, patients seldom attempt to use coercion or reward to elevate their power in clinical negotiations. Although coercion has been reported—for example, by patients who misuse controlled substances, suffer from a mental illness, or are just generally frustrated by "the system" in which care is being delivered—such encounters are fortunately infrequent. Patient power through the control of rewards is possible in theory, but in practice there are few rewards that patients control beyond affecting the esteem of their providers through words and actions.

Referent power is also unlikely to be of much relevance in most clinical encounters. This basis of power would flow from a physician's self-defining identification with the patient and/or a group from which the patient comes. However, the high status society ascribes to physicians generally undermines the referential power of patients.

To summarize, the basis of power for many patients derives from the experience of their own bodies; from medical knowledge garnered through dialog, media exposure, and research; from active participation in the medical encounter; and from their right to reject clinicians' recommendations. There is a growing recognition of the need for doctors to empower patients through information and education.[45] Empowered patients understand their health needs, have developed the skills to manage their health, and thus have increased control over their lives. Empowering patients through access to reliable information should be a goal of every clinician and can be expected to facilitate successful clinical negotiation.

Patient autonomy—the idea that competent adults should have control over medical decisions that affect their bodies—dominates Western biomedical ethics. Yet it is a steep climb from principle to practice. As Stimson (1978) pointed out, one frequently hears the doctor say, "Now I want you take these tablets three times a day," but rarely does one hear the ostensibly "autonomous" patient say, "Now I want you to examine me and prescribe something appropriate." Yet numerous studies suggest that redistributing power from clinician to patient can have significant benefits. **Patients who are more assertive, who ask more questions, who command more conversational space in the clinical encounter tend to be more adherent to therapy, to be more satisfied with care, and to experience greater functional (and perhaps even physiological) improvement**.[29,30] However, a patient's propensity to engage assertively with their provider is itself a function of many factors, including dispositional, socio-logical, and situational variables.

Patient dispositional factors include relatively fixed dimensions of personal-ity, including conscientiousness, agreeableness, and extraversion, all of which have been shown to predict adherence to therapy. (The relationship of adherence to outcomes is, as we discuss in Chapter 7, more complicated than many real-ize: doing exactly what the doctor says may not always be good for you.) Another dispositional factor is neuroticism, defined as the tendency to experience strong or frequent negative emotion, which has a negative relationship to adherence.[31] Sociological factors include gender, race/ethnicity, and socioeconomic status, especially educational attainment. **The interplay of these factors, with each other and with the treating clinician, are complex.** Women tend to offer more information and ask more questions than men, but physicians (especially men) tend to give shorter and less technical answers to women's questions.[32] African-Americans have lower trust in the health care system than their white counterparts, but this may be partially offset when they are matched with cul-turally attuned physicians.[33] Working-class patients face gaps of income, class, education, status, and even vocabulary, yet these gaps can be narrowed via a patient-centered approach.[34] Finally, situational factors are often underesti-mated. These include the urgency and complexity of the clinical problem; the cur-rent clinic backlog; the time of day; and the availability of resources such as health coaches, pharmacy support, and home nursing.

In our increasingly diverse society, an additional driver of the power differential between clinicians and patients is language. About 15% of US citizens over age 18 speak a language other than English at home (Figure 1-1). Patients with limited English proficiency are less likely to have a usual source of care, to receive needed preventive care, and to adhere to therapy.[35,36] Trained med-ical interpreters and bilingual providers improve outcomes.[37] However, whether interpreters can facilitate active negotiation by patients with limited English proficiency is an unanswered question requiring further study. Therefore, by necessity, most of what we talk about in this book applies most directly to patient-clinician dyads matched by language.

Beyond language, culture itself is a strong influence on the process and outcomes of clinical negotiation. There are strong cultural influences on how patients think about symptoms, how they formulate ideas about what is wrong, and how they articulate their concerns to providers. Patients develop mental representations of illness along multiple dimensions, including the degree of health threat, their abil-ity to cope with that threat, and their own life context (particularly life stress).[38] However, these illness representations have strong culture antecedents.[39] Becoming expert in the disparate cultural interpretations of illness in our diverse society is a daunting task. **Fortunately, it is not necessary for medical practitioners to become amateur cultural anthropologists.** In fact, doing so might be dan-gerous, in that it can lead to stereotyping ("this Latino patient must be seeing a

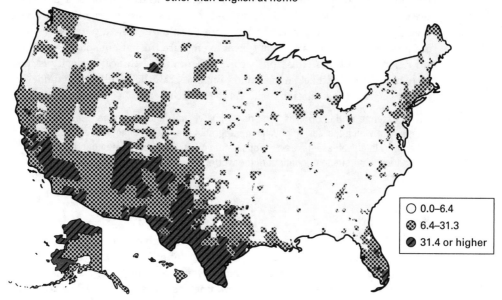

The geography of American linguistic diversity

% of U.S. citizens age 18 and older speaking a language
other than English at home

Figure 1-1. American linguistic diversity.
(*Source:* US Census via Chicago Tribune https://www.chicagotribune.com/nation-world/ct-us-citizens-english-speakers-20180521-story.html)

curandero," "that Chinese patient probably thinks he has too much feng [wind]").
Physicians must instead solicit and attend to patients' own views of illness causation, manifestations, prognosis, and implications. Part of the process of clinical negotiation is to reconcile the patient's views, culturally shaped or otherwise, with the biomedical or biopsychosocial models embraced by most clinicians.

Lay concepts and folk beliefs aside, there is an additional issue that is especially salient in the United States: **culturally based mistrust in the health care system**. (Culture is only one of many antecedents to mistrust of the health care system, and we take up more of them in Chapter 7.) Mistrust may arise from direct personal experience here or in the patient's country of origin or from cultural memory of historical mistreatment. For example, older Russian immigrants raised in the Soviet system may believe they need to exaggerate their symptoms to receive conscientious care. In contrast, African-Americans are not only aware of the troubled and often violent history of race relations in the United States, many are traumatized by memories of Tuskegee, Henrietta Lacks, and other abuses.

Front-line clinicians are in no position to breach every social, linguistic, and cultural barrier that threatens the clinician-patient relationship.

But clinicians are equipped with a powerful tool: the ability to listen with curious intent. By asking patients to express their own ideas about problem causation, to describe the illness experience, and to lay out their hopes for treatment, the clinician can lay the groundwork for successful negotiation. As we will emphasize relentlessly in this book, **you can't negotiate what you don't understand.** The clinician doesn't have to embrace the patient's ideas, just hear and reflect upon them. This approach of open-minded clinical curiosity is indirectly linked to what Ezekiel and Linda Emanuel call the "deliberative model" of the physician-patient relationship.[40] As they conclude:

> The essence of doctoring is a fabric of knowledge, understanding, teaching, and action, in which the caring physician integrates the patient's medical condition and health-related values, makes a recommendation on the appropriate course of action, and tries to persuade the patient of the worthiness of this approach and the values it realizes.

SECTION 1.7: THE ETHICS OF CLINICAL NEGOTIATION

In framing the clinical negotiation as a process in which patient and clinician seek common ground, we are deliberately eschewing definitions of negotiation that are purely transactional (as in business) or adversarial (as in big-power diplomacy). **In the ideal clinical negotiation, the two parties advance towards a common goal.** The advance may be steadfast or hesitant, direct or meandering. But underneath the slips and misunderstandings, the ambiguities and misinterpretations, is the shared purpose of healing.

Nevertheless, it is easy for the clinical negotiation to veer off track. Here we discuss two ways this can happen, each with important implications for the ethics of the clinician-patient relationship. The issues are best illustrated with a case:

> Mr. George Willis is a 64-year-old man with type 2 diabetes. His glycated hemoglobin is 10.6% on three oral agents. Dr. Linda Fredericks has made multiple attempts to persuade him to begin insulin injections, all to no avail. She referred Mr. Willis to an endocrinologist (which required substantial effort due to insurance issues), but he didn't keep the appointment. Finally Dr. Fredericks tells the patient that she really can't help him if he doesn't start insulin. Mr. Willis says he'll think about it. He never returns to the clinic.

In this scenario, Dr. Fredericks exhibits considerable patience, but in the end, she exercises her medical authority in an attempt to persuade the patient to accept a therapy he clearly is not ready for. While there is no way to be sure, there are two ways this scenario might have gone differently. First, Dr. Fredericks could have inquired about the patient's reasons for resisting the idea of insulin. It is not uncommon for patients to have witnessed friends or relatives start insulin and then soon thereafter develop kidney failure, blindness, or stroke. They are interpreting insulin as the *cause* of their associate's demise rather than a *consequence* of poorly controlled diabetes. Second, Dr. Fredericks could have tried to address the non clinical factors that may have contributed to the patient's resistance. For example, Mr. Willis may have been worried about out-of-pocket costs, whether he could handle the injections, what the presence of needles in the house would mean for the safety of his grandchildren, or whether this might be the nail in the coffin of his long-suffering marriage. A combination of intensive diabetic teaching by a nurse specialist, a home visit by a nurse or pharmacist, and perhaps a family meeting might have helped address these concerns.

The problem with an authoritarian or coercive approach to clinical care is twofold. First, as in this example, it simply may not work. Medical outpatients spend more than 99% of their time at home and work and relatively little in physicians' offices. Physicians can prescribe all they want, but patients are the ultimate arbiters of the therapies that are actually followed. Second, authoritarian coercion conflicts with the ethical principle of autonomy. The idea that adults with decision-making capacity should steer their own destiny is now so thoroughly woven into our political, social, and legal discourse as to be virtually beyond question.

On the other hand, what if Dr. Fredericks had simply acquiesced to Mr. Willis' preferences to continue managing his diabetes with oral agents, with no attempts at persuasion? Though this clinical indulgence would at least superficially seem to respect patient autonomy, it would violate *beneficence*, the obligation of health care professionals to act in ways that benefit the patient. The definition of benefit, of course, can and should be negotiated with the patient. But when patients' stated preferences are clearly counter to any reasonable definition of benefit, physicians have no obligation to acquiesce. After all, the medical profession has made a grand bargain with society: doctors receive subsidized training, prestige, financial security, and a monopoly on certain kinds of examinations and procedures. In return, society expects physicians to apply their specialized knowledge for the benefit of patients and the public. **To simply collapse in the face of patients' preferences when those preferences are clearly counter to the patient's own interests would be to abdicate this responsibility.**[41]

SECTION 1.8: A MODEL FOR UNDERSTANDING CLINICAL NEGOTIATION

Social processes, such as those found in clinical negotiations, are influenced by a myriad of factors. An understanding of such influences is aided by developing a model that isolates key variables and their relationships. A model can be thought of as a simplified representation of something. Figure 1-2 depicts a model that reflects our current understanding of clinical negotiation—a model that has guided our research and been shaped by our studies. We will return to this model from time to time in the chapters that follow.

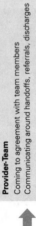

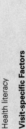
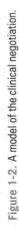

PROVIDER FACTORS

General Factors
Medical training and experience
Communication skills
Personality (openness, extroversion,
   neuroticism, etc.)
Control preferences

Visit-specific Factors
Preparation for visit
Length and quality of relationship
Trust in patient

PATIENT FACTORS

General Factors
Trust in medical insitututions
Personality (openness, extroversion,
   neuroticism, etc.)
Communication skills
Control preferences
Social-cultural background
Health literacy

Visit-specific Factors
Preparation for visit
Nature of presenting problem
Expectations and initial agenda
Trust in physician
Illness perceptions

THE CLINICAL NEGOTIATION

Provider-Patient
Eliciting the patient's agenda
History building
Physical examination
Developing a shared model of illness
Working towards consensus on a treatment plan
Supporting patient engagement (including requests for
   information and action)
Confirming shared understanding
Transcending barriers to agreement
   Cultural barriers
   Literacy barriers
   Difficult behaviors (e.g., substance abusing patients)

Provider-Team
Coming to agreement with team members
Communicating around handoffs, referrals, discharges

CONTEXTUAL FACTORS

Nature of patient's health (acute, chronic, end-of-life)
Time pressures (situational demands for efficiency)
Third-party interference/facilitation (spouses, family
   members,caretakers)
Health plan restrictions

OUTCOMES

Patient
Better self-management skills
Enhanced understanding
Improved satisfaction and
   adherence Improved health

Provider
Improved visit-specific and
   professional satisfaction
Less burnout

Relationship
Mutual respect and trust
Increased openness

Figure 1-2. A model of the clinical negotiation.

As shown in the model, clinician-patient interactions concerned with seeking a shared understanding of the patient's health circumstances are shaped by three broad categories of variables, *clinician factors*, *patient factors*, **and** *context factors*. Clinicians differ markedly in terms of communication skills and training, personality, and control preferences. Clinicians who are confident in their communication skills, open to new experience, and prefer sharing responsibility for decisions with their patients will be better at finding common ground.

The model also identifies clinician factors that exert influence at the time of the clinical encounter itself, including time pressure, duration of the patient-clinician relationship, and pre-existing trust. The most diligent of clinicians may, on some days, be so overwhelmed with personal and professional responsibilities that their preparation for the visit is less than optimal. Clinical negotiations are facilitated by the length of the relationship the clinician has with the patient and the quality of that relationship. And higher levels of trust, which are sometimes formed instantly but must often be earned over time, can facilitate the search for agreement with patients.

Clinical negotiations are also influenced by what patients bring to their visits. General factors that shape how patients generally interact with clinicians include their sociocultural background, trust in medical institutions, patient personality, health literacy, and interpersonal communication skills.

Visit-specific patient factors include the extent to which the patient has prepared for the visit by making careful observations of his or her symptoms (including reflecting upon the chronology of the present illness), becoming informed about diagnoses and treatments, and developing a preliminary agenda for the visit. Even prepared patients vary in how much they trust the health care system and in the specific assumptions they make about the cause of their condition, the controllability (versus curability) of the condition, and timeline to recovery. Finding agreement will be easier if the patient has realistic perceptions of their illness.

The focal point of the model is the top center box, labeled *Clinical Negotiation*. As indicated in the model, **clinicians may need to contend with at least two different negotiations for any given patient.** First, the clinician will be negotiating with the patient, seeking to come to an agreement about what to believe and do. Second, in those cases in which the patient is being treated by a team of health care professionals, the clinician will need to come to an understanding ("get on the same page") with other team members. (See Chapter 10 for more on this.)

With regard to the clinician-patient negotiation, the clinician will first need to elicit the patient's agenda. Although patients typically present with a complaint and are eager to state what they want out of the visit, this is not always the case. Every clinician has stories about patients with agendas that are hidden or submerged—at least until near the end of the visit. **Patient agendas themselves may need to be negotiated.** The patient may have formulated an agenda based on a misinterpretation of their symptoms, a misreading of Internet information, or (unfortunately) a correct reading of Internet *mis*information. Before discussion of treatment plans commences, the clinician and patient need to come to a shared understanding of the illness and mutual commitment to undertake a specific diagnostic and treatment plan.

The process just described is not easy. Potential barriers to success include socio cultural gaps; economic obstacles; shortfalls in health literacy; or difficult patient behaviors such as substance abuse, doctor shopping, and abusive behavior stemming from mental illness.

When the patient and clinician have come to a shared understanding of next steps, that understanding needs to be conveyed to other team members. These members may be responsible for carrying out important aspects of the treatment plan, for example. In particular, there is a growing body of literature on how difficult clinician-team negotiations can be with regard to patient handoffs, referrals to specialists, and hospital discharges. Negotiation among team members is the subject of Chapter 10.

The clinical negotiation occurs in a context that can facilitate or impede the development of shared understanding. Some clinical settings are resource-rich, others less so. Some have ready access to specialized expertise and teams of health professionals, others are more isolated. Some allow for a leisurely dispensing of medical advice (think concierge care), others are more time-pressured. Third parties, including the patient's spouse, other family members, and caretakers, can be a great source of assistance to the clinician or a source of exasperation. A spouse, for example, can be "the enforcer" who ensures patient adherence or complicates the negotiation by introducing expectations not owned by the patient. Finally, the patient's health plan may restrict the treatment options available to the patient in ways that can frustrate the patient and discourage the clinician.

In the model we specify that the clinical negotiation has real consequences for valued outcomes affecting *patients*, *clinicians*, and *relationships*. Coming to shared agreement can leave the patient with a treatment plan that they support, greater ability to self-manage their medical condition, better understanding of their medical condition, and elevated satisfaction with the care they receive, culminating in improved health. Effective negotiations may leave the clinician satisfied with the visit and their chosen profession, decreasing the risk of burnout. The well-conducted clinical negotiation is also relationship building. The clinician and patient conclude the visit with increased mutual respect, trust, and openness.which lays the foundation for future success.

SECTION 1.9. ORGANIZATION OF THIS BOOK

As discussed in the Preface, the 10 chapters of this book are organized into three parts. **Part 1 (Background and Rationale)** covers the core terms and concepts needed to understand how clinicians and patients come to a shared understanding and plan for managing the patient's health. In this chapter we have introduced the notion that integrative negotiations are a fundamental aspect of clinician-patient communication. In the next chapter, we develop further the ideas introduced in this initial chapter, with a focus on how patient expectations develop, how they are translated into a visit agenda, and the role that requests play in the process. We will be revisiting the general and visit-specific patient factors introduced above as we explore their explicit, implicit, and sometimes hidden expectations for physician behavior.

Part 2 (Barriers and Strategies) focuses on barriers that clinicians and patients often confront as they seek to come to a shared understanding. As noted in the model (Figure 1-2), these take on different forms. In the third chapter, we note that these barriers can flow from organizational characteristics and other structures that provide the context in which care is negotiated; the resources available to the clinician, especially time; and the nature and duration of the clinical relationship between negotiating parties. In chapter 4, we observe that effective clinical negotiations require the complete and honest exchange of information. Unfortunately, free exchange of information cannot be taken for granted. Where trust is lacking, or when clinicians communicate in a judgmental manner, patients may elect to disclose incompletely and sometimes even deceptively. Clinicians need to be aware of what they can do to reduce patient reticence. They also need to be armed with strategies for dealing with patients' omissions of fact, evasiveness, and outright lies. Depending on their health circumstances, patients can enter the clinical negotiation feeling weak, vulnerable, uncertain, and even powerless. Clinicians need to be adept at helping patients to name, explore, and manage their emotions. Empathy is key here. Clinicians also need to be aware of their own emotional states and how these can influence their interactions with the patient and their professional and personal well-being. These are the topics of Chapter 5. In Chapter 6, we advance a seven-step strategy for clinical negotiation that is systematic, evidence-based, and effective.

Part 3 (Applications) applies the model of Section 1.8 to four challenging circumstances that clinicians confront on a near-daily basis. Chapter 7 draws heavily on our own research, as well as the studies of other health services researchers, to examine the nature of patients' requests for treatments, tests, and referrals. When such requests are warranted, negotiations are usually quick and focus on achieving an understanding of the nature, objectives, and potential outcomes of decisions made. We therefore focus much of our attention in this chapter on those difficult situations in which requests cannot be justified on medical grounds and lay out strategies for "getting to no" that preserve the clinician-patient relationship. In our experience, the most consistently difficult clinical negotiations involve patients who are taking controlled substances, which is the topic of Chapter 8, co-written with our colleague Dr. Stephen G. Henry. Here the clinician needs to balance patients' genuine need for symptom relief against the potential for misuse of, and addiction to, these medications. Chapter 9 explores clinician-patient negotiations in hospital settings. Hospitals can be very strange and threatening places that leave many patients feeling vulnerable, frightened, and stressed. Often the patient has no history with the clinicians charged with their care and may be further confused by the ever-changing array of people providing their care over the course of the three-shift, 24-hour day. Clinicians in these situations need to be adept at "cultivating trust on the fly" as they discuss such sensitive, emotionally laden issues as do-not-resuscitate (DNR) orders, informed consent, transfers and discharges, and end-of-life palliative care. The final chapter of the book examines the neglected topic of clinician negotiations with other clinicians. Increasingly, patient care is becoming a team sport. Multiple clinicians must come to agreements about who will be primarily responsible for coordinating the patient's care, what each clinician will be charged with doing, when and where the services provided will be delivered, and with what intended outcomes. Channels of communication (face to face, electronically mediated exchanges) need to be selected deliberately to ensure coordination and continuity of care. Mutual respect and professionalism must reign.

SUMMARY POINTS:

- The purpose of clinical negotiation is to find common ground.
- Finding common ground means discovering shared *goals*, shared *values*, and shared *agendas*.
- Goals are what patients seek in the long run, values are priorities for processes and outcomes of care, and agendas are what we hope to accomplish in the short term.
- Two parties can have trouble finding common ground owing to misunderstandings (which are remediable through active listening and clear communication) and disagreements (which require negotiation).
- Although, in a diverse society, social and cultural barriers can impede effective clinical negotiation, physicians can permeate these barriers by approaching each encounter with curious intent: asking patients to express their own ideas about problem causation, to describe the illness experience, and to lay out their hopes for treatment.
- The ethical practice of medicine is a tightrope between allegiance to beneficence and autonomy. Physicians and other clinicians must strive to help patients achieve their goals without abdicating their professionalism. Clinicians must strive to understand their patients' interests, but they are not obligated to perform services that subvert those interests, no matter how much the patient pleads.
- All models are false, but a model for clinical negotiation that includes patient, clinician, and contextual factors can be useful.

QUESTIONS FOR DISCUSSION:

1. What are the similarities and distinctions among patients' goals, values, and agendas?

2. Consider these two non clinical situations. Which is an instance of misunderstanding versus disagreement? If you were the grocery clerk, how would you seek to resolve the matter in each case?

   a. A customer misreads the pricing sticker on a package of toilet paper (in short supply during the early days of the COVID-19 pandemic) and questions the check-out clerk when he rings up $3.96 instead of $3.69.

   b. A customer sees the clerk ring up a package of toilet paper for $3.96 and accuses the store of price gouging.

3. In Table 2-1, 68% of patients seen in primary care considered it necessary for the doctor to "listen to my heart." What value do patients see in the physical examination? Why might auscultation of the heart and lungs have been especially valued? Given that the study producing these data was performed in the early 1990s, how do you think the results might differ today? How might they differ in 2030?

4. Jacqueline Solvang is a 37-year-old woman with intermittent abdominal pain and diarrhea for 11 years. Basic lab work has always been normal; she carries a diagnosis of irritable bowel syndrome. Her 67-year-old-uncle was just diagnosed with colon cancer. She presents to her primary care physician (PCP) requesting a colonoscopy. What might Jacqueline be thinking about the cause and prognosis of her symptoms? What communication options are available to the PCP?

5. Under what circumstances is there a tension between beneficence and autonomy? How can this tension be reconciled? Is the clinician always obligated to accede to the patient's well-considered requests? Why or why not?

6. Despite the inclusion of dozens of variables, the model proposed in Figure 1-1 is "simple" in that it does not consider interaction or effect modification. For example, the forces affecting clinical negotiation may be different if the clinician is male and the patient female than if the clinician is female and the patient male; both may differ from gender-concordant encounters or from cis/trans pairings. In what ways do you think the proposed model is an accurate representation of the clinical world you are familiar with? In what ways is the model too simple?

References

1. Stewart M, Brown JB, Donner A, et al. The impact of patient-centered care on outcomes. *J Fam Pract*. 2000;49(9):796-804.
2. Kravitz RL. Patients' expectations for medical care: an expanded formulation based on review of the literature. *Med Care Res Rev*. 1996;53(1):3-27.

3. Heisler M, Vijan S, Anderson RM, Ubel PA, Bernstein SJ, Hofer TP. When do patients and their physicians agree on diabetes treatment goals and strategies, and what difference does it make? *J Gen Intern Med*. 2003;18(11):893-902.

4. Nagl M, Farin E. Congruence or discrepancy? Comparing patients' health valuations and physicians' treatment goals for rehabilitation for patients with chronic conditions. *Int J Rehabil Res*. 2012;35(1):26-35.

5. Henry SG, Bell RA, Fenton JJ, Kravitz RL. Goals of chronic pain management: do patients and primary care physicians agree and does it matter? *Clin J Pain*. 2017;33(11):955-961.

6. Bell RA, Kravitz RL, Thom D, Krupat E, Azari R. Unsaid but not forgotten: patients' unvoiced desires in office visits. *Arch Intern Med*. 2001;161(16):1977-1984.

7. Kravitz RL, Callahan EJ, Paterniti D, Antonius D, Dunham M, Lewis CE. Prevalence and sources of patients' unmet expectations for care. *Ann Intern Med*. 1996;125(9):730-737.

8. McKinley RK, Middleton JF. What do patients want from doctors? Content analysis of written patient agendas for the consultation. *Br J Gen Pract*. 1999;49(447):796-800.

9. Beckman HB, Frankel RM. The effect of physician behavior on the collection of data. *Ann Intern Med*. 1984;101(5):692-696.

10. Marvel MK, Epstein RM, Flowers K, Beckman HB. Soliciting the patient's agenda: have we improved? *JAMA*. 1999;281(3):283-287.

11. Katon W, Kleinman A. Doctor-patient negotiation and other social science strategies in patient care. In: *The relevance of social science for medicine*. Springer; 1981:253-279.

12. Harwood A, Kleinman A. Ethnicity and clinical care: selected issues in treating Puerto Rican patients. *Hosp Physician*. 1981;17(9):113-118.

13. Roter DL, Hall JA. Physician gender and patient-centered communication: a critical review of empirical research. *Annu Rev Public Health*. 2004;25:497-519.

14. Duberstein P, Meldrum S, Fiscella K, Shields CG, Epstein RM. Influences on patients' ratings of physicians: Physicians demographics and personality. *Patient Educ Couns*. 2007;65(2):270-274.

15. Kaplan SH, Greenfield S, Gandek B, Rogers WH, Ware JE. Characteristics of physicians with participatory decision-making styles. *Ann Intern Med*. 1996;124(5):497-504.

16. Cadieux G, Tamblyn R, Dauphinee D, Libman M. Predictors of inappropriate antibiotic prescribing among primary care physicians. *Can Med Assoc J*. 2007;177(8):877-883.

17. Norcini JJ, Boulet JR, Dauphinee WD, Opalek A, Krantz ID, Anderson ST. Evaluating the quality of care provided by graduates of international medical schools. *Health Affairs*. 2010;29(8):1461-1468.

18. Kao AC, Green DC, Zaslavsky AM, Koplan JP, Cleary PD. The relationship between method of physician payment and patient trust. *JAMA*. 1998;280(19):1708-1714.

19. Casalino LP, Pesko MF, Ryan AM, et al. Small primary care physician practices have low rates of preventable hospital admissions. *Health Affairs*. 2014;33(9):1680-1688.

20. Altschuler J, Margolius D, Bodenheimer T, Grumbach K. Estimating a reasonable patient panel size for primary care physicians with team-based task delegation. *Ann Fam Med*. 2012;10(5):396-400.

21. Cabana MD, Jee SH. Does continuity of care improve patient outcomes? *J Fam Pract*. 2004;53(12):974-981.

22. Linzer M, Manwell LB, Williams ES, et al. Working conditions in primary care: physician reactions and care quality. *Ann Intern Med*. 2009;151(1):28-36.

23. Heymann J, Heymann M. *Equal partners: A physician's call for a new spirit of medicine*. University of Pennsylvania Press; 2000.

24. Gerteis M, Edgman-Levitan S, Daley J, Delbanco TL. Through the Patient's Eyes: Understanding and Promoting Patient-Centered Care. *J Healthc Qual*. 1997;19(3):43.

25. Trillin AS. Of dragons and garden peas: a cancer patient talks to doctors. *New Engl J Med*. 1981;304(12):699-701.

26. Halpern J. *From detached concern to empathy: humanizing medical practice*. Oxford University Press; 2001.

27. Groves JE. Taking care of the hateful patient. *N Engl J Med*. 1978;298(16):883-887.

28. French JRP, Raven B. The bases of social power. In: Studies in Social Power. Cartwright DP, ed. *Ann Arbor*. 1959:150–167.

29. Street RL Jr, Makoul G, Arora NK, Epstein RM. How does communication heal? Pathways linking clinician-patient communication to health outcomes. *Patient Educ Couns*. 2009;74(3):295-301.

30. Greenfield S, Kaplan S, Ware JE Jr. Expanding patient involvement in care. Effects on patient outcomes. *Ann Intern Med*. 1985;102(4):520-528.

31. Kohli R. A systematic review to evaluate the association between medication adherence and personality traits. *Value in Health*. 2017;20(9):A686.

32. Beisecker AE. Patient power in doctor-patient communication: What do we know? *J Health Commun*. 1990;2(2):105-122.

33. Cooper LA, Roter DL, Johnson RL, Ford DE, Steinwachs DM, Powe NR. Patient-centered communication, ratings of care, and concordance of patient and physician race. *Ann Intern Med*. 2003;139(11):907-915.

34. Waitzkin H. Doctor-patient communication. *JAMA*. 1984;252(17):2441-2446.

35. Flores G. Language barriers to health care in the United States. *N Engl J Med*. 2006;355(3):229-231.

36. Woloshin S, Bickell NA, Schwartz LM, Gany F, Welch HG. Language barriers in medicine in the United States. *JAMA*. 1995;273(9):724-728.

37. Flores G. The impact of medical interpreter services on the quality of health care: a systematic review. *Med Care Res Rev*. 2005;62(3):255-299.

38. Cameron L, Leventhal EA, Leventhal H. Symptom representations and affect as determinants of care seeking in a community-dwelling, adult sample population. *Health Psychol*. 1993;12(3):171-179.

39. Kleinman A, Eisenberg L, Good B. Culture, illness, and care: clinical lessons from anthropologic and cross-cultural research. *Ann Intern Med*. 1978;88(2):251-258.

40. Emanuel EJ, Emanuel LL. Four models of the physician-patient relationship. *JAMA*. 1992;267(16):2221-2226.

41. Kravitz RL, Halpern J. Direct-to-Consumer Drug Ads, Patient Autonomy, and the Responsible Exercise of Power. *Virtual Mentor*. 2006;8(6):407-411.

42. Walton RE, McKersie RB. *A behavioral theory of labor negotiations: An analysis of a social interaction system*. Cornell University Press; 1991.

43. Mauksch LB. Questioning a taboo: physicians' interruptions during interactions with patients. *JAMA*. 2017;317(10):1021-1022.

44. Menz F, Al-Roubaie A. Interruptions, status and gender in medical interviews: the harder you brake, the longer it takes. *Discourse Soc*. 2008;19(5):645-666.

45. Anderson RM, Funnell MM. Patient empowerment: myths and misconceptions. *Patient Educ Couns*. 2010;79(3):277-282.

CHAPTER 2

The Nature of Patients' Expectations and Requests

Clinical Take-Aways

- Patients approach the clinical encounter hoping for an explanation for what is wrong, reassurance, advice on what to do, or a humanely delivered prognosis.
- Each encounter is an opportunity for clinicians to set patients' expectations anew.
- Clinicians should:
  - Ask patients how they were hoping the clinician or clinic might help with their concerns.
  - Ask patients how they imagine any requested services might be helpful.
  - Try to focus on the patient's underlying concerns, not (just) the specific request.
  - Be prepared to negotiate over services where the expected net benefits are marginal or negative.

SECTION 2.1: DEFINING PATIENTS' EXPECTATIONS

Mr. A, a 32-year-old professor and running enthusiast, developed acute lower back pain while getting out of his car one Friday morning. Ibuprofen and bed rest over the weekend offered modest relief, but when the patient was seen on Monday, he continued to have moderate pain with activity, sometimes with radiation down the posterolateral aspect of the right thigh. Physical examination showed mild paraspinous muscle tenderness but no bony tenderness or neurologic findings. The patient's gait was essentially unaffected. The preliminary impression was mechanical lower back pain accompanied by possible irritation of the S1 nerve root. Heat, analgesics, and progressive graded exercise were suggested, but the patient "couldn't wait around" and insisted on having a magnetic resonance imagining (MRI) scan and evaluation by a spine specialist. A preauthorization request was initially rejected by the Accountable Care Organization (ACO), but Dr. M (his primary care physician) obtained permission to proceed after speaking with the ACO's medical director. The MRI showed some facet arthropathy and a very mild lateral disc bulge at L5-S1. After reviewing the scan, the orthopedist prescribed heat, analgesics, and progressive graded exercise, and the patient improved rapidly over the next 4 weeks.

To talk sensibly about Mr. A's story, we need to agree on terms. **The academic literature has struggled to generate a common vocabulary for describing patients' hopes, aspirations, goals, values, needs, wants, desires, expectancies, entitlements, requests, and demands.** Our jumbled lexicon has arguably impeded research, teaching, and practice.

The first step towards definitional clarity is to distinguish between patients' *internal experiences* and the way patients *communicate* (or elect not to communicate) with clinicians.[1-3] On the verge of a clinical encounter, patients experience hopes and desires; these can take on shades of *need* (if the patient feels the object of desire is essential to their well-being) or *entitlement* (if the patient feels the object of desire is something they are owed as a matter of fairness). *Requests* are desires that are communicated to the clinician.

In our own research on patient-clinician communication, we have adopted the term *patients' expectations* to refer broadly to the way patients think the clinical encounter should unfold. Like Brody et al. before us, we have tended to focus on perceptions of *need or necessity*, which in our view represent patients' wishes (desires) tempered to some degree by what they believe to be reasonable and fair. In fact, following Brody et al., we have often made this balancing act explicit, by cautioning survey respondents to be realistic: "Realizing that it is not possible for your doctor to do everything in a single visit, please indicate the things you think are necessary for your doctor to do today."[4,5]

In choosing this approach, we have left aside nuanced distinctions between **what is desired** (ideal expectations), **what should happen** (normative expectations), **what is predicted to happen** (expectancies), and **what is unformed**.[6] We have also ignored the observation that patients' expectations may not be fully conscious or capable of articulation. Using our less formal but more inclusive approach, patients' expectations are taken to reflect *values* rather than probabilities (which are properly called expectancies); to represent desires, wishes, or perceptions of need pertinent to a *specific encounter* rather than medical care in general; and to play out across the *structure-process-outcomes* trifecta promulgated by Donabedian.[7] The relevant dimensions are represented in the dark-shaded boxes of Figure 2-1.

In terms of the case, we can presume that Mr. A placed a high value on high-quality information, precise diagnosis, and rapid recovery (general expectations). However, he clearly had some well-formed ideas about what he hoped to obtain from his encounter with Dr. M (visit-specific expectations). He both *wanted* the MRI and spine consult (value expectations) and thought he had a pretty good

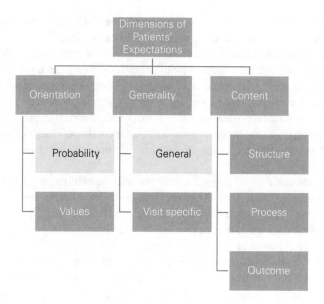

Figure 2-1. Classification of patients' expectations according to generality, orientation, and content.

chance of persuading the clinician (probability expectations). Finally, though Mr. A's ultimate goal was a rapid recovery (i.e., his clinical *outcome*), his focus was on specific care *processes* that he considered essential to accelerating his return to his usual state of health.

SECTION 2.2: SCOPE OF PATIENTS' EXPECTATIONS FOR SPECIFIC MEDICAL ENCOUNTERS

From the advent of Medicare in 1966 until the late 1990s, private practice, fee-for-service medicine was the characteristic mode of practice in the United States. Most doctors were organized into solo offices or small groups, and they received payments from insurers, often at "usual and customary rates," for the medical services they provided (e.g., office visits, hospital visits, or procedures). During this era, work on patients' expectations for office-based care focused on broad categories of care, first in the realm of psychotherapy [8,9] and later in general medicine.[4] For example, Lazare and colleagues demonstrated that among patients attending a walk-in psychiatric clinic, the most commonly endorsed needs and desires were clarification, ventilation, support, diagnosis, and help accessing community resources. Although psychiatric settings and general medical settings differ in many ways, the work of Brody and others suggests that **there is considerable overlap in the fundamental goals of help-seeking across clinical arenas. As emphasized by exponents of patient-centered care, most patients**

want to be heard, to be respected, and to have their concerns taken seriously; perhaps most of all, they want to feel cared for.[10]

The rise of managed care in the 1990s brought about payment models emphasizing shared risk, where groups of clinicians (often in primary care) accepted financial responsibility for some or all of the health care services needed by their assigned patient panel. This placed many primary care physicians into the new and often uncomfortable role of "gatekeeper," and sometimes pitted physicians and patients against one other as patients sought costly services while physicians worried about the financial consequences for themselves and members of their medical group.

As a member of a small general internal medicine faculty practice in the early 1990s, one of us (RLK) was on the front lines of the transformation ushered in by managed care. The traditional fee-for-service model was partially supplanted by a hastily negotiated capitated contract that placed our group of roughly a dozen physicians at full financial risk for the inpatient and outpatient services required by some 5000 patients. The per-member per-month payment for outpatient care was less than $30, meaning we had about $150,000 each month to cover laboratory tests, imaging studies, specialty consultations, and procedures for the 5000 patients in our care. If anything was left, we apportioned it among the faculty to help support salaries. Sometimes there was nothing left.

To meet these challenges, the group organized itself. The faculty members taking after-hours call for the group were encouraged to meet patients at the office rather than direct them to the emergency department. There were weekly utilization review committee meetings in which physicians' previously unquestioned decisions to order "big-ticket" diagnostic studies (e.g., CT scans or magnetic resonance imaging) or obtain specialty consultation were scrutinized by peers. Not infrequently, the verdict of the committee was unfavorable. It was left to the physician to explain this to his or her patient.

Not surprisingly, tensions developed, both within the medical group and between physicians and patients. Physician autonomy was being challenged, to be sure. But so were patients' expectations. In research conducted within the very clinic in which these changes were occurring, **we found that patients approached the clinical encounter not only hoping to be heard and to be cared for but also to receive *specific medical services*.**[11] As illustrated in Table 2-1, when asked just prior to an internal medicine office visit what they thought it was necessary for the doctor to do, some endorsements (indeed the most universal) would have been familiar to an earlier generation of researchers: to demonstrate respect by discussing the patient's own ideas about treatment (71%) and to provide prognostic information (69%). However, patients also expected specific medical services: 68% expected the physician to listen to their heart, 65% to listen to their lungs, 52% to order blood tests, over one-third to prescribe new medications, and almost 40% to refer to a specialist. These findings were consistent with earlier results reported by Brody et al. [4]

Table 2-1. Prevalence Of Patients' Broad and Narrow Expectations for Primary Care Visits.

General Domain	Broad Categories as Applied by Brody et al. 1989 (% endorsing; $n = 118$)	Narrow Interventions Used in Kravitz et al. 1994 (% endorsing; $n = 304$)
Technical care	Perform examination (65%)	Examine eyes, ears, nose, throat (55%)
		Listen to lungs (65%)
		Examine abdomen (54%)
		Perform rectal exam (25%)
		Examine breasts (women only) (30%)
		Listen to heart (68%)
	Tests or x-rays (48%)	Cholesterol test (38%)
		Pap test (women only) (26%)
		Blood tests (52%)
		X-rays (20%)
		EKG (electrocardiogram) (22%)
		Mammography (women only) (18%)
		Urine tests (31%)
		Exercise stress test (17%)
	Prescribe new medication (30%)	Pain pills (13%)
		Antibiotics (16%)
		Other medications (32%)
		Injection (shot) (10%)
	Recommend non drug treatment (43%)	Referral to a physical/occupational therapist (15%)
		Referral to a specialist for care of a particular problem (37%)
		Diet or exercise counseling (38%)
Non technical care (interpersonal care)	Educate about health problem (70%)	Smoking/alcohol counseling (18%)
		Provide information about whether I'm going to get better, and how fast (69%)
	Provide stress counseling (24%)	Stress counseling (40%)
	Discuss patient's own ideas about how to manage health problem (25%)	Discuss patient's own ideas about how to manage condition (71%)

Sources: Brody et al. 1989[4]; Kravitz et al. 1994[11]

Those of us who learned to elicit and respond to patients' expectations managed to traverse the era of tightly managed care with our professionalism intact. Those who didn't suffered or seethed along with our patients. Some left practice altogether. Over time, a national backlash arose, and by the mid-2000s tightly managed payment models emphasizing capitation at the level of individual physicians or small groups washed away. Nevertheless, the lessons evident during that period are true today.

Deeper Dive 2.1: Expectation, Placebo, and Nocebo Effects

Throughout history, medical practice has relied on the relationship between beliefs and outcomes.

In the modern era, a vast literature has examined the various physiological and psychological mechanisms underlying placebo, nocebo, and catastrophizing effects.[46–48] Of interest here is the important role communication plays in shaping expectations, which can in turn influence treatment effects on health, particularly patient-reported outcomes such as pain, functional well-being, mental health, and experience of symptoms.[49] Malani and Houser have summarized evidence suggesting that psychophysiological placebo effects (e.g., the ability of a placebo pill to maintain alertness relative to a caffeine-containing pill) are mediated by patient expectations, including beliefs, hope for improvement, and attitudes toward treatment.[50] Clinicians' words can shape patients' beliefs and thus their response to treatment.

For example, in one study, patients receiving acupuncture from a clinician communicating optimistically about the prospects for positive results reported greater satisfaction with their treatment 4 weeks after the initial visit. Higher satisfaction in turn predicted better patient-reported pain control and physical functioning 6 weeks after completion of treatment. Results for patients seeing acupuncturists communicating uncertainty about treatment effectiveness were not as positive.[51]

Conversely, poor communication can promote negative expectations, with detrimental consequences for health and well-being. Poor outcomes (nocebo effects) have been observed for subjective indicators like pain and observable indicators such as erectile dysfunction.[52,53] One reason minority patients may suffer from health disparities is that their interactions are characterized by less warmth, empathy, and patient engagement than interactions with majority patients, leading to less potent placebo effects.[54] While we would never suggest that clinicians should mislead patients, these and similar studies point to the therapeutic value of more positive, hopeful communication.[55]

Finally "catastrophizing" refers to a dysfunctional cognitive style where patients' fears and anxieties overwhelm more rational cognitive mechanisms, leading to magnification, rumination, and helplessness.[56] Catastrophizing is particularly problematic in the experience of pain and can contribute to poor health outcomes.[48] Catastrophizing can also significantly accentuate negative and attenuate positive expectancy effects, leading to less benefit from placebo and more harm from nocebo. In the context of pain, catastrophizing may lead to increased displays of exaggerated, observable pain behaviors, which can subsequently derail the clinician's attempts to achieve rapport and provide reassurance.[57]

SECTION 2.3: ORIGIN OF PATIENTS' EXPECTATIONS

How do patients come to carry such a large and varied plate of expectations? Certainly, patients' general expectations for careful listening; empathetic understanding; and the provision of clear-eyed but sensitive diagnostic and prognostic information are nearly universal, deeply human, and at least partially innate. However, more specific expectations are varied, culturally embedded, and almost certainly learned. But how does this learning take place? And what are the sources of knowledge that patients rely on?

One approach to these questions derives from self-regulation theory in health psychology. The basic tenet of self-regulation is that people have the learned capacity to respond to threats and to manage the attendant emotions. **New symptoms or other health concerns are a clear threat to emotional equilibrium. In response, people develop multidimensional representations of illness** which help them to make sense of what is happening and to cope with the consequences. In Leventhal's "common sense" model, these so-called *illness representations* encompass identity (how the symptoms or illness are named or described), chronology (how rapidly the symptoms appeared and evolved), consequences (perceived physical and/or social impact of the illness), causes (what produced the illness), and control (what might be required to resolve or manage the problem).[12]

The larger point here is that patients do not arrive for their medical appointments as blank slates. They have typically thought about their symptoms or health status, sometimes at length. Many have clear mental representations of illness. In some recent examples from our practice:

- A 52 year old man with mild scalp and forearm itching believes he acquired a parasite after ocean swimming in Hawaii;
- The daughter of an 83 year old woman with smelly urine (but no other symptoms) believes her mother has a urinary tract infection that may land her in the hospital;
- A 75 year old retired cardiologist with cough and upper respiratory tract symptoms is concerned about aspiration pneumonia (which he developed years ago after an alcohol binge);
- A 38 year old woman with a 1-month history of scant rectal bleeding requests a referral to surgery to "get these hemorrhoids taken care of;" and
- A 55 year old businessman "wakes up snorting" and wants a referral to the sleep lab to rule out sleep apnea.

Returning to the patient described in the opening paragraph of this chapter, we might—on careful questioning—discover that Mr. A was concerned about a structural derangement in his back. Though he is admittedly no expert in musculo-skeletal anatomy, he can readily imagine something (Connective tissue? Cartilage? Bone? Nerve?) tearing, ripping, or pulling. Maybe there's inflammation in the surrounding tissue. He can see the damage in his mind's eye, and he wonders whether – without a proper diagnosis and prompt treatment – the damage might get worse. Given this mental representation, it is no surprise that Mr. A seeks anatomic confirmation with an MRI and expert evaluation by a spine specialist.

Accepting the fundamental role of mental representations, can we derive a more specific taxonomy of the sources of patients' expectations? In one study, we proceeded on the theory that understanding the underlying sources of patients' expectations and requests could help clinicians address patients' concerns while reducing conflict and provision of low-value care.

To identify the sources of patients' expectations, we approached the problem from the back door, first identifying patients who reported that they had certain unmet expectations at a recent visit, then asking them about how they came to form those expectations in the first place. Of 688 adult patients seen at three diverse practices in Sacramento, 125 (18%) reported at least one unfulfilled expectation within eight broad categories of care (Table 2-2). Of these, 88 were successfully contacted and agreed to be interviewed.

During the interviews, we asked patients directly about the elements of care they thought their doctor had omitted. Specifically, we asked patients how they came to believe that a particular element of care was needed. Given the opportunity to interview Mr. A (and assuming that his request for an MRI was declined), we might have asked him what he thought an MRI might show. How did he think it might help? And how did he come to that opinion? Our dialog might have gone this way:

Interviewer: You mentioned on your questionnaire that you were hoping to get an MRI scan to look at your back, but apparently the doctor didn't order one. Can you tell me more about that?

Table 2-2. **Prevalence of Perceived Omissions of Care**[13]

Perceived Omission Category	Example	Number of Patients (%)
Physician preparation for visit	Failing to review chart before patient's arrival	29 (4.3)
History taking	Not asking about specific medical or lifestyle factors	33 (4.9)
Physical examination	Not listening to heart	37 (5.5)
Laboratory testing / imaging	Not ordering cholesterol test or magnetic resonance imaging	35 (5.2)
Prescription medication	Not prescribing pain medicine	24 (3.6)
Referral to specialists	Not arranging for consult with neurosurgery	33 (5.0)
Information and counseling	Not answering questions about prognosis	19 (2.8)
Other	Not completing disability paperwork	31 (4.7)
Total reporting one or more omissions		125 (18.2)

Source: Reproduced with Permission from Kravitz RL, Callahan EJ, Paterniti D, Antonius D, Dunham M, Lewis CE. Prevalence and sources of patients' unmet expectations for care. *Ann Intern Med.* 1996;125(9):730–737.

Mr. A: I've been having back pain for a while. I started to get worried when the pain started going into the back of my thigh. The pain was very bad sometimes, and I had to cut back on my workouts. I also found standing for long periods at my lab to be difficult.

Interviewer: The pain was starting to interfere with what you wanted and needed to do.

Mr. A: Yes, and I wondered what was going on. I've had several friends who developed chronic back pain. One used to play tennis and can't anymore; the other has had to limit travel for work because sitting for long periods is just too painful.

Interviewer: So how did the conversation go with Dr. S?

Mr. A: I told him about what I've been going through and he did an exam. To be honest it was all kind of quick. He tugged on a few things and tapped my reflexes. He told me I had "back strain" and suggested some home exercises. When he didn't offer an MRI, I brought it up. I told him I respected his opinion but I wanted a little more clarity. He suggested we wait another 6 weeks to see if I improved on my own. He also told me about some symptoms I should watch out for, like trouble with urinating. I went along with it, because what could I do? But I have to admit I wasn't too happy.

Interviewer: You mentioned wanting more clarity. Can you talk some more about that?

Mr. A: I'm an engineering professor. I'm a visual person. I just thought getting a clear picture of what's pressing on what would help us decide if I needed more intense treatment, I'm not sure what. Maybe an injection or even surgery. I also wanted to know how long whatever I damaged would take to heal. I certainly don't want any permanent damage, and I don't want to end up like my two friends. In my 20s I could just shake things off. Now.... When I did a Google search on back pain, I saw a bunch of ads for centers specializing in microsurgery. Apparently there are some promising techniques that require a very small incision. So an MRI just seemed like the next logical step.

Mr. A's words are revealing. His pain is troubling, not only for its severity but for the way it interferes with usual activities and for what it might portend for the future. He feels less able to recover from injury like he used to; he's not in his 20s anymore. Though his friends' medical situations may be quite different from his own, their outcomes are not reassuring. He is dispositionally inclined to seek precision (even if, as savvy physicians know, anatomic precision in back pain is often misguided).[14] And he is privy to sources of information that, for reasons both medical and commercial, extol interventionism.

SECTION 2.4 FOUR SOURCES OF PATIENTS' EXPECTATIONS

In interviews with the 88 patients, **we identified four broad categories of "sources" of patients' expectations for care** (Table 2-3). *Somatic symptoms* affected expectations of 74%. These patients described their symptoms in terms of intensity, duration, functional impairment, and perceived seriousness. *Perceived vulnerability* to illness was described by 50%, often in relation to aging, a previously diagnosed condition, a family history of illness, or personal lifestyle factors which the patient recognized as detrimental to their health. *Previous experience* with illness or with the health care system – both personal and vicarious – was important for 42%. These patients interpreted their current health situation in light of their own experience or the experiences of others they were close to. Finally, 54% of patients *acquired knowledge* from external sources, which included the media but also physicians and nurses the patient had seen in the past. When the advice of trusted health professionals was challenged, patients became suspicious. As one older woman put it, "[My prior doctor] thought it was very important once a year that I have that test where they put the dye and you ride the treadmill and then you go into nuclear medicine...[But now] suddenly I don't need it!"

Somatic Symptoms

Physical symptoms drive most ambulatory visits.[15] Symptoms can dominate a patient's experience because of their severity ("It was like a hot needle in my eye."); duration ("The pain never quits;" "I've been feeling so tired for months."); or impairment of physical, role, or social functioning ("Since this started, I haven't even felt like going to church.") But perhaps the most salient

Table 2-3. Sources of Patients' Expectations for Care

Putative Source	Percentage of Patients (n = 88)
Somatic symptoms	74
Intensity of symptoms	42
Functional impairment	14
Duration of symptoms	49
Perceived seriousness of symptoms	35
Perceived vulnerability to illness	50
Related to age	12
Related to a previously diagnosed condition	26
Related to a family history of illness	9
Related to personal lifestyle	9
Derived from remarks of medical office staff	9
Previous experience	42
With similar symptoms or illness	40
Acquired while caring for others	8
Transmitted knowledge	54
Personal education or training in health care field	7
Friends or relatives trained in health care fields	10
Statements by lay friends or relatives	8
Pronouncements by other clinicians	42
The media	7

symptom dimension with respect to clinical negotiation relates less to *experience* than to *interpretation*. **Patients who are concerned that their symptoms represent a serious underlying disorder will often perseverate upon and subsequently amplify the adverse bodily sensations they are experiencing.** In patients suitably predisposed, catastrophizing (focusing only on the "worst case") ensues. The "wicked triad" of *perseveration, amplification,* and *catastrophizing* (PAC) will not only diminish well-being but can also complicate the clinical negotiation, in two ways. First, PAC makes history-taking more challenging. Many clinicians have encountered a version of this phenomenon in encounters with chronic pain patients who calmly describe their pain as "10 on a scale of 0-10." Second, PAC cranks up the emotional tension and makes it less likely that a rational explanation will take hold.

Deeper Dive 2.2: Eliciting Patients' Expectations

We have claimed that patients' expectations are broad in scope (incorporating aspects of psychosocial care, physical examination, diagnostic investigation, and therapeutic intervention) and often quite specific. But how should expectations be elicited and measured? The answer seems obvious: just ask. But when? And how? The timing and approach might (or might not) make a big difference.

For example, presenting patients with a before-visit checklist of clinical services might generate a longer, more specific list of expectations than asking them an open-ended question about what they hope the visit might achieve. To our knowledge, only two studies have directly addressed this issue.[5,58] To summarize, more comprehensive pre-visit surveys tend to elicit more expectations than shorter questionnaires or open-ended interviews, but all three approaches have predictive validity insofar as the number of elements desired before the visit but not received predicts lower patient satisfaction. However, because most of the variance in satisfaction is captured by simply asking patients about their unmet expectations post-visit, this approach provides an expeditious method for studying patients' expectations and their consequences.

As is introduced in Section 2.3, patients also bring into consultations expectations about how the interaction with their clinician will unfold. These "communication expectations" may include topics to be discussed, questions to be addressed, and degree of patient involvement in decision-making that is desired. Although communication expectations differ by patient literacy, race/ethnicity, age, gender, and health condition,[59-61] expectations for care are also grounded in patients' personal or vicarious experiences with health care.[62] However, patient expectations are often opaque to providers. Various pre-consultation tools (e.g., Question Prompt Lists and patient activation resources) have been developed to facilitate sharing of patients' hopes, desires, and requests.[63,64] These tools allow patients to indicate what questions or concerns they would like to address in the consultation and help clinicians focus on aspects of care that are most important to the patient. None of these tools are in widespread clinical use, however, and clinicians will often do just fine by relying on a few basic communication principles: using open-ended questions, asking about the patient's questions and concerns, and avoiding unnecessary interruptions.[65]

Vulnerability

In our study, perceived vulnerability to illness emerged from several sources. Many patients voiced concerns related to aging. These concerns stemmed from heightened perceived risk of disease and a greater awareness of mortality. By the time they reach middle age, most adults have experienced health threats of one kind or another, and the majority are well past any illusions of invulnerability. **Aging creates a sense, often-enough validated by hard experience, that bodily functions can and will go wrong.** However, the effect of age on health risk perceptions appears non linear, rising throughout youth and early middle age, peaking in late middle age, and then leveling off in old age;[13] the flattening of the risk perceptions curve associated with growing older may have less to do with Medicare eligibility than with the assumption that new-onset symptoms are a normal accompaniment of aging rather than disease.[16] Attributing symptoms to old age may be, as many gerontologists point out, erroneous and potentially harmful if it results in delays in care.[17] But these attributions nevertheless offer a kind of defense against the otherwise inexorable march of age-related vulnerability.

William Faulkner famously observed that "the past is never dead; it's not even past." As a 67-year-old with heart disease told researchers, "So I feel like, having a heart condition where I take two drugs for it, that he [the doctor] automatically should listen to the heart and lungs when I go in. I don't feel like I should have to ask." The perceived vulnerability need not be reified in a personal medical diagnosis, but rather woven into family history or, increasingly, revealed through genetic testing. As a woman enrolled in our 1996 study declared, "I went in for some concerns about ovaries...I was having some lower abdominal pain...and my mother, grandmother, and great-grandmother all died of cancer." Two decades later, Klitzman quoted another woman who exemplified the promise and perils of the genetic revolution:

> There's something wrong with me that's not even physical—it's like my body or the blueprints of my body don't work well. The computer that determines the functions of my body, the central processing unit, doesn't work right. At any time, something can go wrong. It's like I'm walking with one leg. I don't have the checks and balances most people have. [18]

Patients like this will become increasingly the norm, as genetic testing permits the detection and labeling of a growing number of genomic variants.

A third source of vulnerability arises from patients' reflections upon their own health habits, which they (often rightly) have assessed as sub optimal. These patients recognize the health threats arising from smoking, excessive eating or drinking, substance abuse, psychological stress, or a sedentary lifestyle. They are not necessarily prepared to change, but they're worried enough to see the doctor.

Joe was a long-time smoker we saw in clinic recently. He had concerns about white spots in his mouth. He wondered if they might be caused by smoking. Generally prone to minimizing his symptoms, Joe was worried enough to come in. We were worried enough about pre-cancerous leukoplakia that we referred him to a head and neck specialist for biopsy. Yet when we offered help with smoking cessation, Joe was clearly pre-contemplative. "Not now, doc. I'm not ready. I have too much going on."

Finally, the experience of vulnerability may have wholly psychological roots that have nothing to do with inheritance or personal habits. Simply recalling the difficult experiences of family members can inspire specific requests for care. As one man told us, "Pneumonia killed my father...and that's why I'm going back to get a chest x-ray."

Every family has stories. Here's one: An uninsured 82-year-old-man was hospitalized at Los Angeles County-USC Medical Center in 1966 for pneumococcal pneumonia. He immigrated to the United States from Poland just before the winds of World War I picked up. The 1930 US Census lists his occupation as "huckster." (Then a term for peddler; he sold vegetables on the streets of Cleveland, Ohio.) He had a history of penicillin allergy, but this was over looked. After his first dose of intravenous penicillin, he died of anaphylaxis. His grandson (RLK) became a general internist attuned to the possibility of medical error and the importance of inquiring about allergies to antibiotics.

Previous Experience

Two out of five patients described unmet expectations that were shaped by their own personal experiences with care or by experiences acquired while assisting others. Past experience could shape expectations for both diagnosis and therapy. As one woman said:

> If you're as tired as I am and everything, a basic blood test wouldn't hurt...That's how they found out [the last time I was sick] – my blood [platelet] count was down to 5000 on the night they put me in the hospital for my spleen. It was just a simple blood test.

In one sense, this patient may have been right: because of her past history, the pre-test probability of her having a blood condition as the underlying cause of fatigue was above average. As a result, an abnormal CBC could potentially convey significant diagnostic information. However, it is fair to say that the emotional salience of her past experience was arguably stronger than a straightforward Bayesian calculus would warrant.

With respect to expectations for treatment, we have seen many patients whose attitude towards elective surgery is influenced, sometimes unduly, by their own positive or negative past experiences. Patients for whom prior surgeries went well are happy to submit to further operations. Those for whom surgery did not result in the expected cure or which caused unexpected pain or disability are far more reluctant to proceed.

Acquired Knowledge

The last source from which patients' expectations seem to emerge is knowledge they acquire from outside – from their own education and training; from conversations with friends, relatives, and health care professionals; and through instruments of popular culture such as newspapers, television, and increasingly, social media. There are approximately 1 million physicians and 2 million nurses in the United States. Assuming each has 10 friends and family members with whom they are willing to share their professional expertise, at least 30 million Americans have access to this form of unfiltered "free advice." (Of course, access to expertise of this type is relatively scant among groups under-represented in medicine and nursing) If you add in other health professionals such as dentists, optometrists, licensed vocational nurses, and physical therapists, the number is even higher. Patients can and do dip into this well of knowledge. The results are sometimes surprising, as with the veterinary technician who proclaimed, "When we have an animal with a fever we would routinely do a blood count. I'm not sure why if it's good for the animals why it wouldn't be good for me."

Clinicians' words and actions count, and not just in the present moment. All clinicians must know that each time they prescribe an antibiotic for what is likely to be a viral infection, obtain imaging for acute uncomplicated low back pain, or refer patients with stable angina to a cardiologist inclined to stent anything that's stenosed, they are not merely deviating from best practice. They are also shaping patients' mental representations of illness and expectations for care that may persist for years to come. As one older patient in our study stated, "[My prior doctor] thought it was very important once a year that I have that test where they put the dye and you ride the treadmill and then you go to nuclear medicine....[But now] suddenly I don't need it." Another patient, a 32-year-old, moderately overweight man with type 2 diabetes, arrived for his first visit at our clinic with a list of "auto-antibodies" (islet cell antibodies, glutamic acid decarboxylase antibodies, and zinc transporter 8 antibodies) he claimed his endocrinologist (based in another city) had urged him to obtain annually. (Prior testing iterations were negative.) Recognizing that the patient was younger than average for type 2 diabetes, and momentarily nonplussed, we placed the lab order, triggering charges of over $1000, with – as we later confirmed through reading and consultation with colleagues – little or no chance of clinical benefit.

Finally, **media matters**. Newspapers, television, radio, the Internet ("Dr. Google"), and social media disseminate information and disinformation. Consider just one source: direct-to-consumer (DTC) advertising of prescription drugs. These ads – virtually non existent until a little-heralded 1997 ruling by the Food and Drug Administration – are now ubiquitous; no Super Bowl would be the same without ads for Viagra® and Flomax.® A large body of research has shown that consumers read, see, or hear these ads; that they attend to them; and that they often bring them to the attention of their doctors.[19-24] We also know, from one of the few experiments of its kind, that when patients make direct-to-consumer ad-driven requests, their physicians tend to comply, no matter whether the request is unequivocally appropriate or of uncertain medical utility.[25]

Deeper Dive 2.3: Influence of Direct-to-Consumer Advertising on Prescribing

A number of investigations have demonstrated that direct-to-consumer advertising (DTCA) can influence what physicians prescribe for their patients.[66,67] Specifically, DTC advertising stimulates patients' interest in and expectations for advertised medications, leading to patients' requests. As demonstrated in at least one large randomized trial, patient requests for directly advertised medicines are powerful influences on physician prescribing.[67] In a recent study, consumers with greater exposure to DTCA for HMG-CoA-reductase inhibitors ("statins") were more likely to be diagnosed with dyslipidemia, suggesting that patients' requests not only result in accommodative behavior by clinicians but may also influence diagnosis to justify such accommodations. In this study, the marginal increase in diagnosis and treatment appeared particularly strong for people at lowest risk for cardiac events, the opposite of what one might wish when taking a public health perspective.[22]

These studies demonstrate that high exposure to advertised medications can influence patients' expectations and clinicians' behaviors. Yet it is important to view these results in context. Many other variables affect patients' treatment preferences, including social, cultural, and psychological factors. While clinicians should certainly be aware of *what* shapes patients' expectations, the more important issue from their perspective is how these expectations can be anticipated, managed, and changed as appropriate. Patients' expectations and preferences vary in their stability. Clinical negotiation can change or redirect expectations,[68] especially when using communication strategies that take into account the patient's perspective.[69]

In the genesis of patients' expectations and requests, DTC ads are not the only influential medium. Patients read newspapers (and tabloids) constantly touting new medical discoveries. They watch television programs like Dr. Oz, whose recommendations – according to a recent study – are supported by evidence 46% of the time, contradicted 15% of the time, and unconnected to any evidence 39% of the time.[26] Patients also perform Internet searches, with up to 35% of US adults reporting that they have gone online to diagnose a medical condition in themselves or someone else.[27] And increasingly, they use social media (particularly Facebook) and sometimes join health-related support groups like DailyStrength .org or Cancer Support Community.[28] While participation in online communities may be associated with benefits,[29] social media can also propagate false ideas that in turn create the capacity for harm. Before the COVID-19 pandemic stole the headlines, the United States was in the midst of a measles epidemic resulting from under vaccination of children in certain communities. One reason some parents have chosen not to vaccinate their children is the erroneous idea that vaccines cause autism, but other conspiracy theories abound.[30] Social media provides the fuel that can set health beliefs afire.

Medical misinformation can be dangerous in the best of times, but is particularly perilous during public health crises such as the (ongoing) COVID-19 outbreak. Within the first months of the pandemic, influential media outlets with only lax ties to the truth were already spreading unfounded conspiracy theories and hyping treatments with no scientific support.[31]

Physicians and other health professionals need to be aware of what patients are learning outside of the office, because these views can be hard to dislodge.

SECTION 2.5: CLINICAL NEGOTIATION IN THE LARGER SOCIETY

Patients' expectations for care do not arise in a vacuum. They are shaped (and sometimes determined) by the economic, sociocultural, and organizational context in which patients fall ill and care is delivered. Perhaps the best evidence for this conclusion is the wide variations in patterns of illness and care across developed countries. In a recent international comparison, patients in the United States are hospitalized at less than half the rate of Germans, make two-thirds fewer doctor visits than the Japanese, but obtain nearly three times as many MRI scans as Australians.[32] Even within the United States, geographic variations in practice patterns abound and have provided rich source material for health services researchers and journalists alike.[33,34]

Americans live in a regulated capitalist economy. In many areas of life, markets determine the price and quantity of available goods and services. However, the proper role of markets in health care is controversial.[35,36] Whatever the direction of the US health care system, the market orientation of the US economy as a whole cannot help but shape patients' attitudes. As mentioned above, patients are consistently exposed to advertisements touting the merits of new drugs, new devices, new genetic tests, and shiny new specialty-oriented hospitals.[37] Consumers pay attention to these ads; are motivated to discuss advertised products with their health care providers; and effectively influence clinicians to prescribe, order, or refer.[23,38,39]

As anyone who browses the business section in airport bookstores knows, "culture eats strategy for lunch." While this aphorism may oversimplify, it reflects a deep truth about the importance of cultural determinants of behavior – including health-related behaviors. **The last 60 to 70 years have seen dramatic shifts in US societal norms.** Change has occurred along multiple dimensions, including attitudes toward race, gender, sexual orientation, social relations, and privacy.

Attitudes towards health and health care have evolved too. The all-knowing authoritarian physician whose pronouncements were accepted passively has been replaced by clinicians who understand that the principle of patient autonomy (the right of patients to control what happens to them) deserves at least as much deference as the principle of beneficence (the ethical imperative to do what is best for the patient). **While truly informed consent and fully shared decision-making are quite difficult to implement in practice,**[40,41] **as principles they enjoy widespread acceptance by bioethicists and the public alike**. There is an edge case, however. When patient autonomy veers toward full-on consumerism, patients run the show. In the extreme, one might:

> Imagine a world in which patients trust television advertisements more than they trust physicians and insist that their doctors have nothing to offer them except cheerful compliance with their requests. In such a world, patients would shuttle between their televisions, on which they would watch DTC ads, their physicians' offices, where they would present a shopping list of "needed" drugs, and their computers, on which they would order pharmaceuticals directly from the Internet. The very involvement of doctors in care might soon be rendered irrelevant.[42]

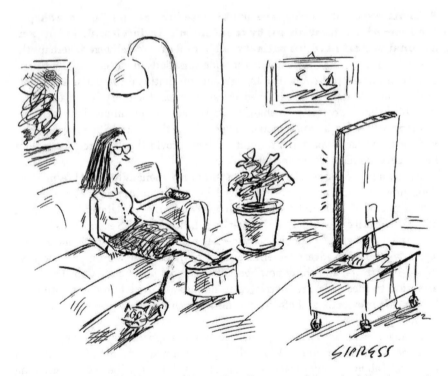

"Ask your doctor if taking a pill to solve all your problems is right for you."

Figure 2-2. Patient autonomy at the extreme. *Source:* ©David Sipress/The New Yorker Collection/The Cartoon Bank

This situation (illustrated comically in Figure 2-2) is probably not the kind of world most of us – health care providers and consumers alike – would want to inhabit. The trick for the thoughtful clinician is to respect patient autonomy while exercising the professional judgement that years of training and experience have produced. Getting better at this is really the whole point of this book.

As we have seen, patients' expectations are indeed shaped in part by broad societal forces. But they are also influenced by the specific organizational context in which care is delivered. For example, patients obtaining primary care in an isolated rural community may not expect to receive the same immediate access to an array of intensive diagnostic services and highly segmented sub specialty care as patients covered by indemnity insurance seeing their concierge care doctor on the Upper East Side in New York. Patients affiliated with an integrated health care services organization (such as Kaiser Permanente) can (and do) have different expectations than those getting care in smaller and more traditional fee-for-service practices.[43] There is some evidence that patients can adapt to their chosen practice settings and insurance plans over time – perhaps by finding a doctor they trust,[44] perhaps by "working the system" more effectively.[45] In any case, expectations, like politics, are local. Sometimes the best way to help a patient whose expectations are wildly at variance with what is possible is to explain to them how the system works.

SUMMARY POINTS:

- Expectations are what patients want, need, or think will happen; requests are what they ask for.
- Patients' expectations span both technical and interpersonal dimensions of care.
- Unmet expectations (including "perceptions of omitted care") are associated with worse patient experience.
- Sources of patients' expectations include somatic symptoms, perceived vulnerability to illness, previous experience, and acquired knowledge.
- Patients' expectations are shaped by broad societal forces as well as the specific organizational context.

QUESTIONS FOR DISCUSSION:

1. What are three reasons a healthy patient in her 20s with no personal or family history of significant illness might present to her new primary care physician requesting a battery of lab tests?

2. Dr. Smith operates a "cash-only" solo practice. Dr. Jones practices in a multi specialty group where most patients are covered by insurance plans that reimburse the practice "fee-for-service." Dr. Wesson is part of a large group-model health maintenance

organization which contributes capitated payments to providers as salary plus a bonus (which in turn depends on both efficiency and quality). What incentives does each physician have to practice in a cost-effective manner? Who would be most likely to accede to patients' requests for expensive services? Who would be least likely?

3. Despite the well-documented limitations of the physical exam, studies indicate that patients expect their primary care doctors to examine them, especially the heart and lungs. Why do patients harbor such expectations? How do you think these expectations will evolve as bedside ultrasound becomes more widely adopted in practice?

4. What is the importance of "mental representations" (mental models) of illness?

5. The text introduces somatic symptoms, perceived vulnerability, previous experience, and acquired knowledge as four separate categories or "sources" of patients' expectations for care. Yet these categories often overlap, as when a severe pain (somatic symptom) is reminiscent of a prior gallstone attack (previous experience). Give two additional examples of how two or more of these sources may intermingle.

6. A patient anxious about the COVID-19 pandemic contacts your office asking for hydroxychloroquine prophylaxis. You know that initial research provides no evidence of benefit and some possibility of harm. What factors may have motivated this patient's request? What might you, as the clinician, ask the patient to better understand his reasoning and inform the subsequent clinical negotiation?

References

1. Uhlmann RF, Inui TS, Carter WB. Patient requests and expectations. Definitions and clinical applications. *Med Care*. 1984;22(7):681-685.
2. Kravitz RL. Patients' expectations for medical care: an expanded formulation based on review of the literature. *Med Care Res Rev*. 1996;53(1):3-27.
3. Linder-Pelz S. Social psychological determinants of patient satisfaction: a test of five hypothesis. *Soc Sci Med*. 1982;16(5):583-589.
4. Brody DS, Miller SM, Lerman CE, Smith DG, Lazaro CG, Blum MJ. The relationship between patients' satisfaction with their physicians and perceptions about interventions they desired and received. *Med Care*. 1989;27(11):1027-1035.
5. Kravitz RL, Callahan EJ, Azari R, Antonius D, Lewis CE. Assessing patients' expectations in ambulatory medical practice. Does the measurement approach make a difference? *J Gen Intern Med*. 1997;12(1):67-72.
6. Thompson AGH, Sunol R. Expectations as determinants of patient satisfaction - concepts, theory and evidence. *Int J Qual Health C*. 1995;7(2):127-141.
7. Donabedian A. Evaluating the quality of medical care. 1966. *Milbank Q*. 2005;83(4):691-729.
8. Lazare A, Eisenthal S, Wasserman L, Harford TC. Patient requests in a walk-in clinic. *Compr Psychiatry*. 1975;16(5):467-477.
9. Hill JA. Therapist goals, patient aims and patient satisfaction in psychotherapy. *J Clin Psychol*. 1969;25(4):455-459.
10. Heymann J, Heymann M. *Equal partners: A physician's call for a new spirit of medicine*. University of Pennsylvania Press; 2000.

11. Kravitz RL, Cope DW, Bhrany V, Leake B. Internal medicine patients' expectations for care during office visits. *J Gen Intern Med*. 1994;9(2):75-81.
12. Cameron L, Leventhal EA, Leventhal H. Symptom representations and affect as determinants of care seeking in a community-dwelling, adult sample population. *Health Psychol*. 1993;12(3):171-179.
13. Kravitz RL, Callahan EJ, Paterniti D, Antonius D, Dunham M, Lewis CE. Prevalence and sources of patients' unmet expectations for care. *Ann Intern Med*. 1996;125(9):730-737.
14. van Tulder MW, Assendelft WJ, Koes BW, Bouter LM. Spinal radiographic findings and non-specific low back pain. A systematic review of observational studies. *Spine (Phila Pa 1976)*. 1997;22(4):427-434.
15. Kroenke K. A practical and evidence-based approach to common symptoms: a narrative review. *Ann Intern Med*. 2014;161(8):579-586.
16. Prohaska TR, Keller ML, Leventhal EA, Leventhal H. Impact of symptoms and aging attribution on emotions and coping. *Health Psychol*. 1987;6(6):495-514.
17. Grant LD. Effects of ageism on individual and health care providers' responses to healthy aging. *Health & Social Work*. 1996;21(1):9-15.
18. Klitzman R. "Am I my genes?": Questions of identity among individuals confronting genetic disease. *Genet Med*. 2009;11(12):880-889.
19. Becker SJ, Midoun MM. Effects of direct-to-consumer advertising on patient prescription requests and physician prescribing: a systematic review of psychiatry-relevant studies. *J Clin Psychiatry*. 2016;77(10):e1293-e1300.
20. Mackey TK, Cuomo RE, Liang BA. The rise of digital direct-to-consumer advertising?: Comparison of direct-to-consumer advertising expenditure trends from publicly available data sources and global policy implications. *BMC Health Serv Res*. 2015;15:236.
21. Kornfield R, Alexander GC, Qato DM, Kim Y, Hirsch JD, Emery SL. Trends in exposure to televised prescription drug advertising, 2003-2011. *Am J Prev Med*. 2015;48(5):575-579.
22. Niederdeppe J, Byrne S, Avery RJ, Cantor J. Direct-to-consumer television advertising exposure, diagnosis with high cholesterol, and statin use. *J Gen Intern Med*. 2013;28(7):886-893.
23. Frosch DL, Grande D, Tarn DM, Kravitz RL. A decade of controversy: balancing policy with evidence in the regulation of prescription drug advertising. *Am J Public Health*. 2010;100(1):24-32.
24. Donohue JM, Cevasco M, Rosenthal MB. A decade of direct-to-consumer advertising of prescription drugs. *N Engl J Med*. 2007;357(7):673-681.
25. Kravitz RL, Epstein RM, Feldman MD, et al. Influence of patients' requests for direct-to-consumer advertised antidepressants: a randomized controlled trial. *JAMA* 2005;293(16):1995–2002.
26. Korownyk C, Kolber MR, McCormack J, et al. Televised medical talk shows--what they recommend and the evidence to support their recommendations: a prospective observational study. *BMJ*. 2014;349:g7346.
27. Fox S, Duggan M. *Health Online 2013*. Washington, DC: Pew Research Center; 2013.
28. Moorhead SA, Hazlett DE, Harrison L, Carroll JK, Irwin A, Hoving C. A new dimension of health care: systematic review of the uses, benefits, and limitations of social media for health communication. *J Med Internet Res*. 2013;15(4):e85.
29. Kingod N, Cleal B, Wahlberg A, Husted GR. Online peer-to-peer communities in the daily lives of people with chronic illness: a qualitative systematic review. *Qual Health Res*. 2017;27(1):89-99.
30. Hoffman BL, Felter EM, Chu KH, et al. It's not all about autism: The emerging landscape of anti-vaccination sentiment on Facebook. *Vaccine*. 2019;37(16):2216-2223.
31. Mian A, Khan S. Coronavirus: the spread of misinformation. *BMC Med*. 2020;18(1):1-2.
32. Papanicolas I, Woskie LR, Jha AK. Health care spending in the united states and other high-income countrieshealth care spending in the united states and other high-income countrieshealth care spending in the united states and other high-income countries. *JAMA*. 2018;319(10):1024-1039.
33. Chassin MR, Kosecoff J, Park RE, et al. Does inappropriate use explain geographic variations in the use of health care services? A study of three procedures. *JAMA*. 1987;258(18):2533-2537.
34. Gawande A. The cost conundrum. New Yorker; 2009;June:36-44.

35. Enthoven AC. The history and principles of managed competition. *Health Aff (Millwood)*. 1993;12 Suppl:24-48.
36. Woolhandler S, Himmelstein DU. Medicare for all and its rivals: new offshoots of old health policy roots. *Ann Intern Med*. 2019.
37. Schwartz LM, Woloshin S. Medical marketing in the United States, 1997-2016. *JAMA*. 2019;321(1):80-96.
38. Gilbody S, Wilson P, Watt I. Benefits and harms of direct to consumer advertising: a systematic review. *Qual Saf Health Care*. 2005;14(4):246-250.
39. Wilkes MS, Bell RA, Kravitz RL. Direct-to-consumer prescription drug advertising: trends, impact, and implications. *Health Aff (Millwood)*. 2000;19(2):110-128.
40. Braddock CHIII, Edwards KA, Hasenberg NM, Laidley TL, Levinson W. Informed decision making in outpatient practice: time to get back to basics. *JAMA*. 1999;282(24):2313-2320.
41. Stiggelbout AM, Pieterse AH, De Haes JC. Shared decision making: concepts, evidence, and practice. *Patient Educ Couns*. 2015;98(10):1172-1179.
42. Kravitz RL, Halpern J. Direct-to-Consumer Drug Ads, Patient Autonomy, and the Responsible Exercise of Power. *Virtual Mentor*. 2006;8(6):407-411.
43. Lin CT, Albertson G, Price D, Swaney R, Anderson S, Anderson RJ. Patient desire and reasons for specialist referral in a gatekeeper-model managed care plan. *Am J Manag Care*. 2000;6(6):669-678.
44. Safran DG, Montgomery JE, Chang H, Murphy J, Rogers WH. Switching doctors: predictors of voluntary disenrollment from a primary physician's practice. *J Fam Pract*. 2001;50(2):130-136.
45. Cohn V. Working the HMO system. *Washington Post*. 1986.
46. Price DD, Finniss DG, Benedetti F. A comprehensive review of the placebo effect: recent advances and current thought. *Annu Rev Psychol*. 2008;59:565-590.
47. Tracey I. Getting the pain you expect: mechanisms of placebo, nocebo and reappraisal effects in humans. *Nat Med*. 2010;16(11):1277-1283.
48. Quartana PJ, Campbell CM, Edwards RR. Pain catastrophizing: a critical review. *Expert Rev Neurother*. 2009;9(5):745-758.
49. Tavel ME. The placebo effect: the good, the bad, and the ugly. *Am J Med*. 2014;127(6):484-488.
50. Malani A, Houser D. Expectations mediate objective physiological placebo effects. *Adv Health Econ Health Serv Res*. 2008;20:311-327.
51. Street RLJr, Cox V, Kallen MA, Suarez-Almazor ME. Exploring communication pathways to better health: Clinician communication of expectations for acupuncture effectiveness. *Patient Educ Couns*. 2012;89(2):245-251.
52. Benedetti F, Lanotte M, Lopiano L, Colloca L. When words are painful: unraveling the mechanisms of the nocebo effect. *Neuroscience*. 2007;147(2):260-271.
53. Colloca L, Finniss D. Nocebo effects, patient-clinician communication, and therapeutic outcomes. *JAMA*. 2012;307(6):567-568.
54. Friesen P, Blease C. Placebo effects and racial and ethnic health disparities: an unjust and underexplored connection. *J Med Ethics*. 2018.
55. Bensing JM, Verheul W. The silent healer: the role of communication in placebo effects. *Patient Educ Couns*. 2010;80(3):293-299.
56. Beck AT, Rush AJ, Shaw BF, Emery G. *Cognitive Therapy of Depression*. NY: New York: Guilford; 1979.
57. Tsui P, Day M, Thorn B, Rubin N, Alexander C, Jones R. The communal coping model of catastrophizing: patient-health provider interactions. *Pain Med*. 2012;13(1):66-79.
58. Peck BM, Asch DA, Goold SD, et al. Measuring patient expectations - Does the instrument affect satisfaction or expectations? *Med Care*. 2001;39(1):100-108.
59. Collins TC, Clark JA, Petersen LA, Kressin NR. Racial differences in how patients perceive physician communication regarding cardiac testing. *Med Care*. 2002;40(1 Suppl):I27-I34.
60. Smith SK, Trevena L, Nutbeam D, Barratt A, McCaffery KJ. Information needs and preferences of low and high literacy consumers for decisions about colorectal cancer screening: utilizing a linguistic model. *Health Expect*. 2008;11(2):123-136.

61. Tortolero-Luna G, Byrd T, Groff JY, Linares AC, Mullen PD, Cantor SB. Relationship between English language use and preferences for involvement in medical care among Hispanic women. *J Womens Health (Larchmt)*. 2006;15(6):774-785.

62. Quick BL. The effects of viewing Grey's Anatomy on perceptions of doctors and patient satisfaction. *J Broadcast Electron Media*. 2009;53(1):38-55.

63. Amundsen A, Bergvik S, Butow P, Tattersall MHN, Sorlie T, Nordoy T. Supporting doctor-patient communication: Providing a question prompt list and audio recording of the consultation as communication aids to outpatients in a cancer clinic. *Patient Educ Couns*. 2018;101(9):1594-1600.

64. Street RLJr, Slee C, Kalauokalani DK, Dean DE, Tancredi DJ, Kravitz RL. Improving physician-patient communication about cancer pain with a tailored education-coaching intervention. *Patient Educ Couns*. 2010;80(1):42-47.

65. Robinson JD, Tate A, Heritage J. Agenda-setting revisited: When and how do primary-care physicians solicit patients' additional concerns? *Patient Educ Couns*. 2016;99(5):718-723.

66. Mintzes B. Direct to consumer advertising of prescription drugs. *BMJ*. 2008;337:a985.

67. Kravitz RL, Epstein RM, Feldman MD, et al. Influence of patients' requests for direct-to-consumer advertised antidepressants: a randomized controlled trial. *JAMA*. 2005;293(16):1995-2002.

68. Street RLJr, Elwyn G, Epstein RM. Patient preferences and healthcare outcomes: an ecological perspective. *Expert Rev Pharmacoecon Outcomes Res*. 2012;12(2):167-180.

69. Paterniti DA, Fancher TL, Cipri CS, Timmermans S, Heritage J, Kravitz RL. Getting to "no": strategies primary care physicians use to deny patient requests. *Arch Intern Med*. 2010;170(4):381-388.

PART II

Barriers and Strategies

CHAPTER **3**

Clinical Negotiation in the Context of Modern Practice

Clinical Take-Aways

- Health and well-being are influenced by clinical and social determinants.
- As a form of interpersonal communication, clinical negotiation takes place within a broader ethical, policy, and organizational context.
- Clinicians should:
  - Acknowledge the importance of shifting societal norms, evolving policies, practice structures, time constraints, and reimbursement priorities as influences on the clinical negotiation.
  - Not be too hard on themselves when external factors pose challenges to finding common ground with patients.
  - Be prepared to advocate for public, organizational, and clinical policies that support the patient-clinician relationship.

SECTION 3.1: INTRODUCTION

So far, we have shown how every clinical encounter, from the most banal to the most challenging, can be understood as a kind of negotiation. As we hope we have made clear, we are not talking about the type of negotiation where there are winners and losers, though if the negotiation is managed poorly, it can surely feel that way. The clinical encounter is not a business deal. Instead, it is a dialog in which the clinician and patient seek mutual understanding and agreement about how to move forward. In other words, a successful clinical negotiation helps the clinician and patient find common ground.

We have also shown how patients' expectations for care are influenced by their experience of symptoms, their perceptions of vulnerability, their personal histories, and their exposure to outside sources of information. Toward the end of Chapter 2, we discussed how patients' expectations are shaped by the economic, sociocultural, and organizational context. In this chapter, we continue our investigation of context, but from a different perspective. Here we are interested not so much in how context shapes expectations as in **how context sets the stage for clinical negotiation and influences outcomes.** The clinician facing structural and organizational barriers to care must act like a swimmer in a riptide. It is futile to swim directly against the current. Rather, one must angle obliquely past the undertow, making one's way slowly to shore.

Mrs. G is a 68-year-old widow and retired bookkeeper who lives in one of the semi-rural exurbs within the catchment area of a large academic medical center. Her medical problems include hypertension, type 2 diabetes, stage 3 chronic kidney disease, recurrent sinus infections, and chronic low back pain. She has received care in the Internal Medicine resident clinic for 15 years. By now, she is used to the turnover of residents every 3 years. She just saw her new intern, Dr. P, last week. The visit was scheduled for 10:30 am, but Dr. P was running late, and Mrs. G was not seen until 11:15. When Dr. P missed noon conference last week, the chief resident admonished her that "attendance at noon conferences is mandatory for all residents. You really need to be there."

The visit was rushed. The chart had not been fully updated, and Mrs. G was not clear about which medications she was taking. The blood pressure was 156/92, and the last recorded hemoglobin A1 (measured 9 months ago) was 9.5%. Dr. P understandably focused on the patient's blood pressure and diabetes, but the patient seemed to want to talk only about her back pain, rating it an "11" on a 0-10 scale. After discussing the case with an attending, Dr. P ordered some lab tests; refilled prescriptions for lisinopril, amlodipine, metformin, and pioglitazone; and agreed to prescribe a small quantity of acetaminophen/hydrocodone for pain. Because Dr. P was starting a busy Intensive Care Unit rotation, she scheduled Mrs. G for a follow-up visit at her next available appointment in 5 weeks.

The phone calls started about 2 days later. The first time it was a request for antibiotics for Mrs. G's recurrent "sinus." (The patient was advised to double up on her nasal corticosteroid for a week.) The second time, a question concerning some transient upper extremity numbness: "could it be a stroke?" (The symptoms occurred only during sleep and resolved quickly with a change in position.) Next, and many times thereafter, a plea for additional Vicodin. These requests took many forms: "I misplaced the bottle;" "It's the only thing that gives me any relief;" "Without the pills I just stay in the house all day."

During the day and when she was on call, Dr. P took the calls herself. Sometimes she couldn't get to the phone until after ICU rounds, and occasionally she forgot to call back, which led to accusations from Mrs. G that "no one around here seems to care about patients." Dr. P had back-up from Dr. H, her clinic "firm attending." (In Dr. P's hospital, a firm attending is a senior clinic physician assigned to assist residents with their ambulatory care responsibilities.) He tried to be helpful, but in the end there were only two people on the phone: Mrs. G and Dr. P.

The calls from Mrs. G continued over the next several weeks. Ultimately, Dr. P paged Dr. H. It was not an easy call to make. Dr. P certainly didn't want to be characterized as a "weak intern." However, she had enough positive experiences with Dr. H that she was willing to reach out. "I need help with Mrs. G," she began.

Dr. H suggested they meet for lunch in the hospital cafeteria. Over sandwiches, they discussed Mrs. G's medical problems and Dr. P's concerns. By the end of the hour, they had a plan for trying to address Mrs. G's medical needs while also providing her with the psychosocial support she seemed to need so desperately.

Dr. P found the lunch meeting helpful. At first, she was surprised that Dr. H spent so little time on Mrs. G's medical problems. He did briefly review his approach to managing poorly controlled hypertension and explained why nasal steroids and sinus rinses, not antibiotics, are the mainstay of therapy for chronic sinusitis. But most of the time, they talked about the context in which they worked and how it made caring for patients like Mrs. G more difficult than it should be.

"Look," he said. "In our system, Mrs. G gets a new doctor every 3 years. By the time she trusts someone, that person moves on. But it's not just that. You are in training. You have inpatient responsibilities. You're not in clinic every week, let alone every day. This is nothing to apologize for. But to Mrs. G, this can amplify her sense of needful desperation. 'If I don't make myself heard by calling my doctor constantly, are they going to forget about me?' And what else? Phone calls don't always get passed on by the triage desk. Lab tests needing attention don't get flagged. Missed follow-up visits don't get rescheduled. And between us, our pain clinic is frequently over booked and often over focused on procedures, so multidisciplinary pain care—the best alternative to opioids—isn't always available to our patients, especially if they have public insurance like Mrs. G."

"That makes a lot of sense. But how does that help me with Mrs. G?"

"Why don't you try talking with her about some of these things? Not by griping, though that would be tempting. Instead, show her you've tried to see the world through her eyes. Acknowledge that she's had a rough month. That it must be frustrating trying to get through the hospital message center. That it must be hard living with back pain every day. Even that it must be difficult switching doctors every 3 years. The main thing is to pause long enough to let Mrs. G respond and to be attentive to both verbal and non verbal cues. If she nods or smiles, maybe you've touched a chord. If she frowns or remains passive like a Sphinx, perhaps you're off base. The main thing is to be curious."

"I'll try it," said Dr. P, finishing her last bite of sandwich.

"I won't be in clinic Wednesday, but let me know how it goes."

Dr. P's struggle to provide effective care for Mrs. G raises several key questions (Table 3-1).

We begin this analysis by considering five major forces shaping the clinician-patient relationship and in particular the clinical negotiation: norms and values, policies and systems, organizational structures, time constraints, and reimbursement methods (Figure 3-1).

As we examine these different contextual elements, we do not mean to minimize differences in communication style among individuals. Individuals are not only shaped by context, they interact with it.

Table 3-1 Key Questions About the Effects of Context on the Clinical Negotiation, with Special Reference to the Case of Dr. P and Mrs. G

Key Questions	Some Facts Relevant to the Case of Dr. P and Mrs. G
What are the contextual factors that influence how quickly and easily clinicians and patients can negotiate successfully and find common ground?	• Government-sponsored insurance (relatively low reimbursement) constrains Mrs. G's care options in private practice, effectively shunting her to the local academic medical center • Behavioral health support (for Mrs. G's anxiety and chronic pain) is limited • Pre authorization requirements slow referrals
How have these "contextual determinants" changed over time?	• Ratcheting up of payer initiatives to reduce fraud and abuse (e.g., pre authorization for referrals to pain management; see above) have placed new administrative burdens on physician practices • While legal constraints limit resident work hours, intensity (e.g., inpatient turnover) has increased, putting pressure on Dr. P to do more in less time
How do they vary across practice settings?	• Within Dr. P's teaching clinic, involvement of multiple personnel with limited personal contact (phone room, medical assistants, residents, attendings) creates potential communication gaps
And what can clinicians do to meet the challenges that their own practice environment presents?	• As her mentor advises, Dr. P can proactively invest in the relationship with Mrs. G • At the same time, she can work with fellow residents to bring proposals for clinic workflow improvements to the clinic director

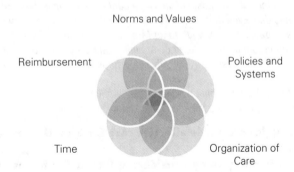

Figure 3-1. The contextual foundation of clinical negotiation.

SECTION 3.2: NORMS AND VALUES

Every clinical encounter is situated in a milieu defined by broad historical, political, and cultural forces. Many of the assumptions guiding modern practice in the United States would be foreign—and far from self-evident—to

Deeper Dive 3.1: Clinician and Patient Communication Styles

The embedded layers of influence on clinical negotiation depicted in Figure 3-1 parallel socio ecological models of contextual experiences affecting how people, including clinicians and patients, communicate with one another. At the core are one's personal experiences, which in turn are affected by relationships at the interpersonal level (family, co-workers), followed by involvement with organizations and institutions (workplace, religion, political affiliation, education), and community or identity (culture, race, ethnicity, geography, gender, and nationality).[85]

These different contexts of experience contribute to the formation of an individual's communication predispositions, or "styles." That is, each of us has a particular way of communicating across different situations.[86] For example, some people are generally talkative, others shy; some people try to control conversations, others are more passive; some people are expressive and animated, others are laid back. While we often attribute different communication styles to differences in personality, habitual ways of communicating with others have also been learned over a lifetime through experiences within these personal, relational, institutional, and cultural contexts.

Differences in individual communication styles can and do show up in clinical encounters. For example, some of the variation in clinician-patient communication is explained by differences across individual clinicians.[87,88] These findings comport with conventional wisdom among patients, who might be heard to say that "Dr. Kravitz is rather gruff," but not "Dr. Kravitz tends to be gruff when he is dealing with clinical conditions that puzzle him, especially when the patient is aggressive, the clinic is short-staffed, and it is near lunchtime." The same is likely true of patients in terms of how they communicate with different clinicians.

Differences in communication style may also be linked to social, educational, and cultural factors. For example, compared to men, women clinicians are more likely to talk with patients about feelings, family, and relationships.[89] Similarly, women patients tend to participate in more emotionally charged talk.[90] Both findings could be attributed to gender socialization.

Education and training matter as well. For example, family physicians report more interest in discussing patients' lifestyles and see themselves as more empathic than do specialists.[91] On the patient end, more educated and younger patients generally ask more questions, are more assertive, and have stronger preferences for involvement in decision-making.[92-94] Relatedly, patients with lower literacy tend to ask few questions and use less medical terminology than more literate patients.[95] Ethnic minority patients tend to be less verbally expressive and less assertive during the medical encounter than White patients.[96] These differences in communication style may reflect culturally embedded beliefs, social distance, or other factors yet to be elucidated. The differences, however, are not fixed: US-born Latinos exhibit "activation" behaviors that more closely resemble their White peers than foreign-born Latinos.[97]

While predispositions matter and communication "style" is likely real, the situation matters too. Our experiences *within* different communication contexts contribute to the development of communication styles we use *across* situations. Each of us has our own unique, routinely implemented repertoire of verbal and nonverbal behaviors, and these make up our typical communication style. These styles are comfortable, like an old suit. Sometimes, though, the situation demands a change of clothing. The ability to adapt requires deliberate practice.

practitioners of a different place and time. As introduced in Chapter 1, the dominant bioethical and legal principle of the current age is patient autonomy.[1] This was not always the case. Certainly, in the 1950s it was not uncommon for a diagnosis of metastatic cancer to be withheld from the patient, for surgeries to be performed without informed consent, and for physicians to play the pre-eminent, if not exclusive, agents of medical decision-making. These paternalistic behaviors were rooted in a sincere desire to benefit the patient. But to today's clinician or patient, rank paternalism as exhibited during the mid-20th century would be received as antiquated and unseemly, not to mention ethically and legally questionable.

Underlying the ascendency of autonomy is acknowledgement of the inherent worth of each individual, and by extension, the individual's right to shape his or her own destiny. The evolution of the concept goes back a long way, with early murmurings in Greek philosophy; further unfolding in the writings of Rousseau, Kant, Locke, and Mill; and codification in Nuremberg, Belmont, and modern bioethical discourse.[2] The right of patients to be the ultimate "deciders" was eventually codified in law and advanced by the information revolution.[3] In medical ethics, autonomy has traditionally been pitted against beneficence, the principle that physicians should do all they can to benefit the patient. **Conflict arises when the autonomous patient inclines toward decisions that, in the clinician's professional judgment, contradict the patient's best interests.**

The *solution* seems self-evident: provide the patient with the facts, explain the consequences of each option, and help the patient embrace their preferences.

This solution is simple, powerful, and wrong. To see why, consider three objections.

First, not all patients are autonomous at all times. Autonomy means deliberative self-direction. Deliberation implies both the inclination and capacity to ponder the possible consequences of an action and its reasonable alternatives. Self-direction means the ability to make choices and then to take action that meaningfully and consistently advances those choices. Deliberative self-direction is clearly absent in young children and in adults in stupor or coma. This is why we appoint proxies (parents or durable powers of attorney for health care) to help with decision-making in these cases. But autonomy in the fullest sense may also be beyond the reach of patients whose deliberative self-directing capacities are undermined by the urgency of the medical situation, anxiety, poor health literacy, distrust of the health care system, deep-rooted folk beliefs, or even repeated exposure to medical marketing campaigns. Furthermore, some cultures (in one study, Korean-Americans and Hispanics as opposed to Whites and African-Americans)[4] regard the family, not the individual, as the central decision-making agent.

Second, while patients have rights, so do health care professionals; these too should be respected. By virtue of training and experience, health care professionals have expertise that is not generally available to the public. They have earned the right to share this knowledge in the interest of the patient. Even in the edge case of rare diseases, where Internet-savvy patients may have acquired more factual knowledge about their specific condition than all but the most subspecialized physician, the clinician still brings value to the encounter by placing facts in context, correcting misconceptions, and identifying and reconciling contradictions. It would be in no one's interest to jettison useful knowledge and experience in pursuit of some idealized notion of autonomy.

Finally, there is the matter of **who defines what is beneficial for the patient.** The radical position would be that this is at the patient's sole discretion. After all, who but the patient is in a position to identify their own health-related goals and choose among alternative means for achieving them? The problem is one of identity: the patient today is not the same person as the patient 5 weeks, 5 months, or 5 years from now. Humans are uniquely bad at predicting how they will feel in the future.[5,6] Healthy persons, for example, consistently rate health states with disabilities worse than people actually living with those same disabilities.[7] Furthermore, fleeting changes in circumstances or mood can have an outsized impact on decision making (something decision scientists have called "projection bias").[8] This was seen in a study of Israeli criminal trial judges who issued harsher sentences just prior to lunchtime.[9] If being "hangry" can influence important judicial decisions, the role of emotional reactivity in medical decision-making is probably under appreciated.

These observations lead to an obvious question: might the patient wish to voluntarily constrain their own autonomy in the short term in order to derive greater benefit (as they themselves define it) in the long term? The answer would seem to be yes. This model of patient self-constraint is not a return to the medical paternalism of ages past. Rather, it is a means of acknowledging the centrality of patient's values while encouraging health care professionals to help patients develop more accurate beliefs about how medical decisions will affect their own future physical and emotional states.

As society continues to wrestle with these questions, clinicians need to meet patients where they are. Some patients in some clinical circumstances will veer towards radical consumerism ("I saw it on TV; please prescribe it."), while others will gladly relinquish decision-making to the treating physician ("What would you do if you were me?"). **The challenge is to identify where patients fall on the shared decision-making spectrum and to help them make decisions in the manner they prefer.** How to do this is part of the subject of Chapter 6.

SECTION 3.3: POLICIES AND SYSTEMS

Compared to most other developed countries, the US health care system provides patients on average with less access to essential care, more intensive use of technology, higher costs, and worse health outcomes.[10,11] Although the Affordable Care Act (ACA) of March 2010 dramatically increased the percentage of Americans with health insurance, coverage remains incomplete, particularly among certain populations (e.g., low- and middle-income adults, immigrants, Hispanics, and African-Americans).[12,13] Among those with health insurance, the main forms of coverage are employer-sponsored health insurance (55%), Medicare (18%), Medicaid (18%), and coverage through the military (including the privately managed TRICARE program) or the Department of Veterans Affairs (4%).[14] Each of these forms of coverage is further permuted through varying payment arrangements (e.g., indemnity insurance versus some form of capitation), the role of private intermediaries (e.g., Medicare Advantage plans), and contracting arrangements with hospitals and clinics.

Table 3-2 lists some characteristics of the US health care system that are particularly relevant for clinical negotiation from the perspective of clinicians (righthand column) and patients (lefthand column).

Table 3-2 Some Characteristics of the US Health Care System from the Perspective of Clinicians and Patients

Clinician Perspective	Patient Perspective
Multiple payers	Insecure access (including discontinuity of care)
Heavy administrative burdens	High out-of-pocket costs
Threat of litigation	Information asymmetry

Clinician Perspective

The existence of *multiple payers* means that clinicians (excepting those who practice in integrated health systems like Kaiser Permanente or Veterans Affairs) need to be familiar with different rulebooks for documenting clinical encounters, obtaining reimbursement for medical services, prescribing medicines with the lowest possible patient copayments, referring to specialists, and putting patients in the hospital. **Contending with multiple rulesets is not only annoying but potentially distracting from the fundamental task of attending to the patient's needs.**

Administrative burdens can make achieving clinical concordance challenging in other ways. Pre authorization requirements, in which physicians' orders require advance approval by insurance authorities, are particularly despised by both doctors and patients for several reasons: the implication that the physician's judgment may be in error; the implied endorsement of "cookie-cutter" medicine; the inherent delays in treatment; and the nagging suspicion that the underlying purpose is to raise the "hassle factor" enough so that clinicians and patients will just give up. In private practice, pre authorization imposes a per-physician cost of up to $3000 per year.[15] Other forms of utilization management, including pre admission certification, concurrent stay review, and retrospective review, are similarly two-edged swords that can at times avert unnecessary care but may also foment conflict between the patient (and the family) and the clinician—who they view as ultimately responsible. Even banal-seeming quality improvement interventions can have unintended consequences.

> Mr. J is a 72-year-old, generally healthy man who insists that "every time I take the flu vaccine I get the flu." Dr. J (a family physician) recommends the annual vaccine; Mr. J refuses. However, in December, Mr. J's health plan issues a list of "unvaccinated seniors" in the practice, and the practice manager asks one of the medical assistants to "call patients on the list and encourage them to come in and get vaccinated." Mr. J takes the call and becomes very angry. "I told Dr. M I'm not getting that damn vaccine. Why do you people keep haranguing me?"

In this example, the health plan's "vaccination algorithm" did not incorporate previously documented patient preferences.

Finally, US physicians perceive a uniquely hostile medical malpractice environment. Though *the threat of litigation* in any given year is low, most physicians can expect to be sued at least once in their career, suits can take many years to resolve, and physicians consistently list liability concerns as a principal cause of defensive medical practices (e.g., ordering more tests or hospitalizing patients more readily than necessary in order to reduce malpractice risk).[16,17]

Patient Perspective

From the patient's point of view, perhaps the most uniquely American influence on the clinical negotiation is *insecure access to care*. Unlike most other high-income countries, the United States provides no guarantee of health care access to its residents beyond emergency services. Large gains in insurance coverage followed passage of the ACA, but nearly 9% of US residents still lacked health insurance in 2017.[18] Some of the uninsured manage to get care through free clinics and other safety-net providers. However, short of dire emergencies, many still struggle. For this group (totaling close to 30 million people), the goal of successfully negotiating care with their practitioners is overshadowed by the challenge of obtaining care in the first place.

For those Americans *with* health insurance, *out-of-pocket health care costs* have been increasing.[19] These trends preceded Obamacare.[20,21] Holding patients responsible for a portion of their own health care costs has been applauded by those who believe that consumers should have "some skin in the game."[22] Indeed, from the decades-old RAND Health Insurance Experiment (HIE) we know that consumers enrolled in health plans with moderately high deductibles and copayments use 30% fewer medical services, with no apparent declines in health.[23] However, a lesser-known finding from the HIE is that, among vulnerable patients (particularly those who are both poor and sick), those saddled with copayments experience a 10% higher risk of death compared to those receiving free care.[24] For these individuals, having skin in the game could mean getting flayed.

Patients burdened by high medical expenses relative to income may forego recommended care, skip medications, or stint on other items (food, shelter, clothing, etc.) that may be equally important for preserving health. Consumers have adopted several strategies for contending with rising out-of-pocket costs: saving for future expenses, talking with providers about costs, comparing costs and quality across providers, and negotiating for prices.[25] However, not only do conversations about out-of-pocket costs take time, they also distract from other aspects of the clinical negotiation such as integrating patients' values and preferences with best practices and clinician experience.

Information asymmetry is a term that economists use to describe economic transactions where one party has more material knowledge than the other. With the possible exception of the VA and military health care systems, US health care is organized along quasi-capitalist lines, with private hospitals, medical groups, and pharmaceutical companies competing for business with health plans, employers, and individual patients. However, **whereas health care producers have reasonably good information about their own costs and some knowledge of their own quality, consumers know next to nothing about either.** In addition, patients are rarely in a position to evaluate the comparative costs and quality of different health care providers; they are sick and need care immediately. As a result, patients are at a structural disadvantage in the clinical negotiation.

SECTION 3.4: ORGANIZATIONS

Hospitals

Kerr White's depiction of the ecology of medical care in the United States (updated in 1997)[26] showed how only a small minority (<1%) of Americans are hospitalized in any given year. Yet **hospitalizations account for a plurality (40%) of US health care expenditures.**[27] US hospitals play above their weight in other ways. Hospitals are where many specialist and subspecialist physicians practice, where most complex procedures and surgical operations are performed, and where a sizeable fraction (currently around 20%)[28] of Americans die.

Unlike hospitals in many other countries, US hospitals are not readily classified into secondary care ("community hospitals") and tertiary/quaternary care (university hospitals and referral centers). Instead, hospitals compete with each other to offer specialized care, often emphasizing services (such as complex orthopedic procedures, heart surgery, and radiation therapy) that are most generously reimbursed by third-party payers. Depending on geography and insurance coverage, patients often have the choice of several hospitals for non emergency services. Even small hospitals are extremely complex organizations that, from the perspective of patients and families, can seem bewildering. The effects of these structural realities on the clinical negotiation are taken up in Chapter 9.

Physician Groups

Medical practices vary in how they are sized and organized. Three decades ago, most physicians in the United States practiced alone or in small groups. This form of organization allowed maximum clinical autonomy but required significant attention to the business of medicine. **By 2011, less than 20% of physicians practiced alone, another 25% in small groups of 2-10 physicians, and almost 30% in large groups (>100 physicians).**[29] The evolution has been most rapid for younger physicians and for those practicing primary care.

These changes have had mixed effects. On the one hand, larger practices can offer more diverse medical expertise and have budgets that can accommodate more specialized ancillary staff, more shared equipment, and more sophisticated electronic medical records systems. On the other hand, as practice size increases, contextual factors influencing the clinical negotiation are harder for individual clinicians to control. This may explain why some small group practices are able to deliver good outcomes[30] despite lack of sophisticated infrastructure.[31] Table 3-3 contrasts how the same problem might be addressed differently in solo or small group practices and in larger systems of care.

Of course, some of the potential disadvantages of large groups can be overcome with careful planning and artful execution, and there are also substantial opportunities resulting from scale. For example, a highly functional large group practice could route patient complaints about billing to a personalized "business concierge" empowered to solve such problems directly; arrange for after-hours patient transport to a radiology facility, with immediate reading of the imaging study by a radiologist; and, for patients not needing immediate in-person cardiology consultation, facilitate e-consults with less-than-24-hour turnaround. These are exactly the kinds of services delivered by many high-functioning

Table 3-3 **Differences in How Patient Care Problems Might Be Handled in Well-functioning Small Groups vs. Poorly-functioning Large Groups**

Patient Care Problem	Anticipated Response	
	Well-functioning Solo or Small Group	**Poorly-functioning Large Group or System**
Patient charged for clinical services not received	"Our business manager can zero that out for you."	"Call patient Financial Services between 9 and 12 or 1 and 4."
Delay in receiving durable medical equipment (DME) (e.g., nebulizer for delivery of inhaled bronchodilators)	Receptionist takes call from patient, contacts DME company, arranges for delivery. Problem solved within 24 hours.	Phone room takes patient message and delivers to physician's inbox; physician asks for more information; phone room responds next day; physician completes forms and places request in "DME Forms Box;" form faxed to DME company; company delivers machine next week. Problem solved in 8 days.
72 yo woman with COPD (last patient of day) has protracted productive cough and low-grade fever	Chest x-ray obtained in office shows left basilar streaking consistent with bronchopneumonia; patient started on azithromycin and improves rapidly. Clinician's reading confirmed by radiology the next day.	Patient referred to radiology department in next building; patient too dyspneic to walk and requests wheelchair; by the time patient arrives radiology has closed; x-ray and subsequent treatment delayed until next day.
83 yo man with atypical chest pain has nonspecific ST-T wave changes on office electrocardiogram	Primary physician places call to trusted cardiology colleague who reviews electrocardiogram and arranges for stress testing the next day.	Primary physician requests formal cardiology consult which is scheduled in 2 weeks.
29 yo woman concerned about sexually transmitted infection from casual partner	Nurse practitioner working with primary physician and medical assistant performs examination, testing, and empirical treatment according to protocol.	Physician temporarily assigned to examination room with inadequate physical setup for pelvic examination and staff unfamiliar with STI protocols. Empirical treatment not offered.

multi specialty groups and vertically integrated health care organizations such as the Mayo Clinic and Kaiser Permanente.

Another dimension of practice organization that matters for clinical negotiation is the mix of primary care and specialist physicians. In multispecialty groups that are "right sized" and well-organized, primary care clinicians have access to a broad range of specialists whom they can depend upon for both formal and informal consultation. Poorly integrated networks lack cohesion and trust. It makes a difference when the primary care practitioner can say, "I'm referring you to Dr. Edwards for that tremor. He is an excellent neurologist who will help us get to the bottom of this." The alternative (e.g., "Our neurology department will call you") is much less reassuring.

Primary Care

Primary care is widely acknowledged as the foundation of any well-functioning health care system.[32] Yet even as the clinical and administrative demands on primary care physicians, nurse practitioners, and physicians' assistants have increased, investment in primary care has not kept pace.[33] **The claim that primary care demands have increased even as investment has lagged is important, because if true, it suggests that reinvesting in primary care could improve outcomes at lower cost and create conditions for more successful clinical negotiation.** We'll briefly address each aspect of this claim.

- *Increased clinical demands*: Medical progress has resulted in the availability of many more effective treatments and preventive interventions compared to 20 or 30 years ago. As a result, the clinician's to-do list for prevention and chronic care has vastly increased,[34] and visit times have not kept pace.[35,36] One study showed that just complying with US Preventive Services Task Force guidelines would require 7.4 primary care clinician hours per day![37] At the same time, the number and variety of patient contacts outside of office visits (including communication via telephone, email, and patient portals) have exploded.[38]

- *Increased administrative demands*: Not all demands on primary care clinicians are clinical. Research has shown an increasing burden related to insurance paperwork, preauthorization requirements, documentation of quality metrics, and use of electronic health records.[38–40]

- *Insufficient investment*: Primary care is underfunded in the United States compared to the Organisation for Economic Co-operation and Development (OECD) average.[33] Doubling the percentage of health care resources expended on primary care (say from 5% to 10%) could facilitate longer office visits that might in turn decrease unnecessary testing and emergency room visits; promote better between-visit coordination; and support more effective teamwork.[41,42]

As it stands, primary care finds itself in a strange position. On the one hand, high-quality primary care is valued by patients, as reflected not only in surveys but in the popularity of concierge medicine and "direct primary care" among those who can access and afford these models.[43] While there is some evidence that younger generations ("millennials" and "generation Z") favor convenience over many of the defining features of primary care (e.g., continuity, comprehensiveness, and coordination), some may reconsider once they acquire chronic conditions.[19,44] On the other hand, within the profession of medicine, primary care is often viewed as underresourced, overburdened, and unworthy of consideration by the nation's most academically and clinically talented medical students.[45]

Where primary care is well-supported, clinicians can deliver high-quality technical and interpersonal care resulting in good outcomes and high patient satisfaction.[46] When primary care is not so well supported, physicians burn out and quality is degraded. Patients can often tell the difference.

SECTION 3.5: TIME AND THE PRACTICING CLINICIAN

Delivering health care takes time. The question is whether more time leads to better care and outcomes. Considering the importance of the question, the research landscape is remarkably sparse. Four empirical findings stand out:

- Time has always been a finite resource, and despite claims to the contrary, visit times in the United States at least through the 2000s were not shrinking.[47,48] Mechanic and colleagues examined national data on length of office visits between 1989 and 1998 and found that average visit duration had actually increased by 1-2 minutes over this decade.[35] In a more recent study, Chen et al. observed a 3-minute increase between 1997 and 2005.[49]

- With visit times at steady state, the *amount of work* physicians and patients must accomplish per unit time, particularly in primary care, has *increased*.[37] Abbo et al. found that between 1997 and 2005, average office visit duration increased from 18 to 21 minutes, while the number of clinical items to be addressed increased from 5.4 to 7.1. Thus the amount of time available *per clinical task* during the decade of observation shrunk by 14%—from 4.4 to 3.8 minutes. In addition, many nonclinical tasks (such as electronic health record documentation and phone calls with health plans) now occupy the physician's attention.[38]

- Evidence on the relationship between visit time and quality of care is unclear. Within certain broad limits (office visits between 15 and 30 minutes), there appears to be little effect of visit duration on technical quality.[50] This does not mean that visit times can be compressed indefinitely, however; in one British study, Roland and colleagues found that when visits were experimentally manipulated to last 10, 7.5, and 5 minutes, doctors spent progressively less time explaining the patient's problem and discussing prevention.[51]

- In primary care, patient satisfaction is related both to visit length measured by the clock[52] and to *concordance* between visit length expectations and experiences.[53] In other specialties, the relationship is fuzzier; for example, in one study, patients seeing hand surgeons were offended by long waiting room times but not by short visits.[54] Physician job satisfaction, in contrast, seems tightly bound to perceptions of having sufficient time with patients.[55]

Albert Einstein once joked that "The only reason for time is so that everything doesn't happen at once."[56] Innes and Skelton claim that there are three kinds of time: 1) clock time; 2) subjective time that is dependent on expectations for what might be typical and desirable; and 3) subjective time that varies according to corresponding emotional states such as anxiety, boredom, trust, security, and positive (or negative) mutual regard.[57]

From the physician's perspective, clock time matters (after all, there is a schedule to keep), but perceptions matter more. When rapport is well-established, good team support is available, needed equipment is at hand, and the clinical issues are challenging but not overwhelming, physicians can enter a "flow" state of peak experience where time slips into the background.

On the other hand, when the patient is distressed, clinical circumstances complex, and support thin, the visit can start to unravel. Repeated over the course of weeks or months, professional burnout is a definite hazard. In one national study, more than half of primary care physicians reported time pressure and 48% described their work pace as chaotic.[58] These perceptions are one likely explanation for the estimated 21% prevalence of physician burnout reported in a recent meta-analysis.[59]

Deeper Dive 3.2: Situational Influences on Clinician and Patient Communication

Previously, we discussed how over time individuals develop their own communication style that they tend to use across different situations (e.g., more or less talkative, more or less controlling, etc.). How can communication be both consistent (keeping with an individual's "type" or style) and adaptive (responsive to the situation)?

Consider this situation. Dr. Tang and Dr. Wilson have just finished a hectic 12-hour shift in the intensive care unit (ICU), where they jointly cared for several critically ill patients (including one who was successfully resuscitated). They agree to stop by a midtown bar/restaurant to unwind over a drink before heading home. Of course, we expect the content of the interaction at the bar to differ from the interaction in the ICU. But what about other features such as tone, pace, and nonverbal reactions? Psychologists have developed a heuristic pitting features of an individual that are relatively stable ("traits") against those that are highly responsive to the current environment or situation ("states").[98]

In this vein, we could ask to what extent any interactions between Drs. Tang and Wilson reflect their individual communication styles versus more immediate (situational) influences. For example, Dr. Tang immigrated from China with her parents, is a first-generation college graduate, is an only child who grew up in a small town where her parents worked at a meat processing plant, has a D.O. degree, and volunteers in her spare time at a homeless center. Dr. Wilson is a fourth-generation Harvard graduate (including medical school), the oldest of four children, grew up in Boston, is the of a divorced mother who is a highly successful personal injury lawyer, and is actively involved in the Harbor Sailing Club. Might these differences in experiences influence conversations both in the hospital and at the bar? They could. For example, Dr. Wilson talks a lot, is animated, and is direct in sharing his feelings and beliefs. Dr. Tang, on the other hand, is a good listener, polite, and less direct in communicating what she thinks and feels.

The same applies to clinician-patient encounters, and this has important implications for effective clinical negotiation. The ecological model of communication in medical encounters attempts to unravel the complexity of factors that could affect the way clinicians and patients communicate with one another.[99] The model describes three primary driving forces affecting clinician-patient communication during a specific visit. First, as noted, clinicians and patients have characteristic *communication styles* that they bring to the consultation.

Yet how each clinician communicates will depend on the situation. One source of situational variation is the *interactants' respective goals, feelings, and perceptions during the interaction*.[100] For example, a normally friendly, upbeat Dr. Wilson may assume a more serious, reflective demeanor if he perceives his patient to be confused or worried. Dr. Tang, who typically tries to spend time hearing the patient's story and uncovering the patient's agenda, may become more assertive and move the conversation along more quickly if behind schedule. Some research indicates that clinicians may engage in more patient-centered behavior (e.g., exploring the patient's concerns, partnership-building) with patients they like than with patients they dislike.[101] Similarly, patients who like their physician display more positive nonverbal behavior (e.g., approval, laughter).[102] Patients who have had a longer relationship with their physician may talk more than patients who have only known the doctor for a short time.[103] Another important situational factor is the emotional state of the parties. Low to moderate levels of worry, for example, can activate patients to be more engaged in health protective behavior. However, high levels of anxiety may inhibit patient participation in decision-making.[104]

Clinician and patient communication is also strongly affected by a second situational factor (the third of our "driving forces"): *mutual influence*. In other words, how the clinician communicates with a patient is affected by how the patient communicates with the clinician (and vice versa). For example, clinicians give more information to patients who ask more questions and express concerns.[105,106] Clinicians engage in more empathic and supportive talk when patients express concerns and worries.[107] Patients become more active communicators in consultations (e.g., asking questions, expressing concerns) when their clinicians encourage their involvement through partnership-building (asking for patient perspective, questions, or preferences) and offer supportive communication (reassurance, empathy).[103,108]

"Mutual influence" occurs because clinicians and patients are, in effect, creating one conversation. Thus, each has to work cooperatively to accomplish their agendas, coordinate their turn talking, and work toward shared understanding and agreement. In other words, most clinicians want to provide excellent care, address patients' needs and concerns, and provide information and support. Most patients also want to do their part by providing information and being explicit about what they need or want (although some patients may need to be encouraged to do so).

Given the multitude of processes that can influence how clinicians and patients communicate with one another during a specific encounter, how can we sort out the key drivers of the conversation? For our purposes, the rubber hits the road in the talk between clinician and patient. This is the place where clinical negotiation succeeds or fails. This does not mean that the broader contexts—social, cultural, institutional—don't matter. Rather, their influence will be manifest in the interactants' respective goals, perceptions, beliefs, communicative choices, and how they respond to the communication of the other.

In summary, clinicians and patients bring their communication "tool box" into the encounter, and some of these tools are used routinely (according to one's characteristic "style"). However, more often, the tools deployed depend on the situation: what one needs to do as a communicator to achieve effective clinical negotiation will depend on what clinician and patient perceive as need, what each hopes to accomplish, how each responds to the other, and how they work together to move the conversation toward mutual agreement.

Patients' perceptions of time are similarly subjective, affected by a range of behaviors that can make short visits seem long and long visits short. Some of these behaviors have been summarized by Lussier and Richard and are paraphrased in Table 3-4.[60] We will take up many of these in subsequent chapters, but suffice it to say that small changes in behavior by physicians or support staff can make a big difference in patient perceptions. For example, in a simple experiment conducted by John Heritage and colleagues, training doctors to ask patients if there was "something else" they wished to discuss reduced the

Table 3-4 Behavioral Interventions For Managing "Subjective Time" In Clinical Encounters

Category	Specific Behavior
Setting	Put patients in a quiet environment where confidentiality is preserved
	Keep the physical environment tidy
	Minimize interruptions
	Be familiar with the patient's medical history before entering the room
Nonverbal Behavior	Sit down if possible (try not to stand over the patient)
	Keep body turned towards and slightly inclined towards patient
	Adopt an open expression and avoid frowning, which can suggest annoyance
	Maintain eye contact when you or your patients are speaking
	Do one thing at a time, if possible
Verbal Behavior	Address patients by name (and, unless otherwise agreed, use an honorific such as Mr. or Ms. followed by last name)
	When eliciting the chief complaint and other items on patient's agenda, do not interrupt
	Show interest in patients as people
	Encourage patients to keep talking by using facilitators such as "what else," "mm hm," and "go on."
	Check your understanding of the patient's story by summarizing, then asking for verification
	When appropriate, express support, sympathy, or empathy

Source: Modified from Lussier MT and Richard C.[60]

prevalence of unmet concerns by 78%. In another study, just sitting down during hospital rounds was associated with significantly higher Press-Ganey physician satisfaction ratings.[61]

A major premise of this book is that successful clinical negotiation depends on mutual understanding nourished by trust. **Mutual understanding takes time to develop.** Within a single clinical encounter, the amount of time needed to foment such understanding depends on patient, physician, and organizational factors (Table 3-5). Patients who are biomedically or psychosocially complex (e.g., have or may have serious or life-threatening illness), or who lack trust in the current provider or in the health care system in general, will require more time. Physicians who know the patient well, who are familiar with the clinical presentation (and therefore able to invoke "pattern recognition"), and who speak the patient's language and are at least broadly familiar with the patient's cultural background will require less. Because all clinical encounters take place within an organizational setting, the degree to which support is available from medical

Table 3-5 Patient, Physician, And Organizational Factors Affecting Time Needed To Satisfactorily Complete A Single Clinical Encounter

Patient	Physician	Practice Organization
Biomedical complexity (symptoms, comorbidities, medications, etc.)	Prior knowledge of patient	Availability of front-line support (interpreters for patients with limited English proficiency; nurses and medical assistants practicing "at the top of their licenses")
Psychosocial complexity (mental health, substance use, family support, poverty, deprivation)	Experience with similar clinical presentations ("pattern recognition")	Availability of behind-the-scenes support (social work, case management, mental health liaison)
Prior experiences with (trust in) this and other health care providers	Cultural and linguistic competence (patient specific)	Functionality of physical space and equipment

assistants, nurses, social workers, mental health professionals, and others—as well as the functionality of the physical space itself—can meaningfully influence the amount of time needed to find common ground.

When patients feel pressured, they may fail to disclose important information, not discuss matters of concern, and ultimately feel unheard. Similarly, when doctors feel rushed, they are less able to listen attentively, demonstrate a sense of presence and compassion, and connect with patients in a way that fosters trust.

Harried conditions of practice—what some have called "hamster medicine"[62]—are not conducive to effective clinical negotiation. If the doctor is running behind, the patient will be seen late. If the doctor has managed to keep up but is not conscientious about maintaining a calm, unhurried stance, the patient will feel diminished.

Therefore, clinicians aiming to maximize patient satisfaction and engagement with care will need to be mindful of their own mental state,[63] how their demeanor can affect patients, and how they can interact effectively even when the context is unforgiving. Fortunately, evidence is accumulating that patients' perceptions of time can be influenced as much by the content of the visit as by its duration.[64-66] By applying some of the techniques described in Chapter 5 (Managing Emotions in Clinical Negotiation) and Chapter 6 (Strategies for Successful Clinical Negotiation), clinicians can make the most of the time they have.

Up until now, we have focused on the amount of time allocated for an individual patient encounter. However, encounter time is not the whole story. **In primary care especially, encounter time can be played off against longitudinal time**—what is commonly referred to as "continuity." When the clinician-patient relationship is durable (or at least expected to be so), not everything has to happen during a single visit. This is probably the reason that physicians in Japan (average visit length, 5-6 minutes)[67] or the United Kingdom (average visit length, 8-10 minutes)[68,69] can get away with encounter times that seem, to the American eye, almost shocking in their brevity. Continuity of care—seeing the same provider over time—has been associated with reduced health care utilization, costs, and complications and less overuse of low-value services. [70,71] Yet continuity may be an endangered species in the United States, threatened by many of the trends mentioned in this chapter (e.g., shiftwork, handoffs, poorly coordinated team care, the ascension of hospital medicine as a distinct branch of practice) but also by the willingness of Millennials and Gen-Z-ers to trade off continuity for convenience.

As seen in Figure 3-2, younger respondents to a survey of 4000 health care consumers in 2014 tended to value extended hours and free care over continuity (which remained importance to respondents over age 65).[72] At the same time, a small, largely affluent, and influential group of patients have endorsed continuity with their feet—and dollars—by signing up for concierge care or direct primary care. Both of these care models emphasize enhanced access, a focus on continuity, and a higher level of service in exchange for a monthly fee. In conclusion, though continuity can be a strong buffer against shorter visit times, the future of continuity is unclear and may depend on how the preferences of Millennial and Generation Z consumers evolve over time.

SECTION 3.6: REIMBURSEMENT

Payments to physicians account for about 20% of US health care costs, yet physicians (and other clinicians) strongly influence the other 80% by telling patients when to return to clinic, sending them to the emergency room, admitting them to the hospital, ordering tests, and prescribing medicines. There is no perfect way to pay doctors. At one extreme, the fee-for-service method (in which clinicians are paid for each medical service they render) encourages clinicians to provide more – and more costly—care.[73] At the other end, capitation (in which clinicians or their practice group are provided a fixed fee, sometimes risk-adjusted, for each patient assigned to their practice) can encourage stinting on needed care.

Other payment methods are hybrids of fee-for-service and capitation.[74] One common point of confusion is that the way funds flow from health insurers to provider organizations is not necessarily indicative of the way funds flow *within* a provider organization. For example, a large physician group might receive a monthly payment for providing comprehensive care to beneficiaries of a particular health plan, yet physicians practicing there might be paid a fixed salary; salary plus productivity and/or quality bonus; or fee-for-service (typically based on some accounting of work-based relative value units, a standard [albeit controversial] metric integrating the duration, intensity, and risk of providing a particular health care service, or some combination).[75] **The upshot is that the myriad ways that payment systems and structures are organized can influence the clinical negotiation.**

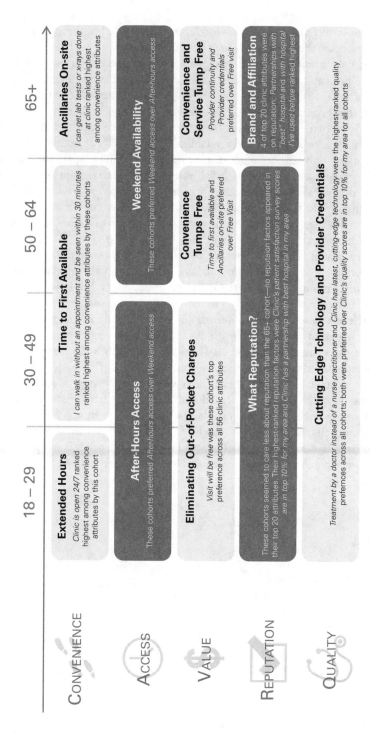

Figure 3-2. How primary care preferences vary by age. Source: Reproduced with Permission from Daugherty A. What Do Consumers Want from Primary Care? Advisory Board. June 25, 2014. https://www.advisory.com/research/market-innovation-center/expert-insights/2014/get-the-primary-care-consumer-choice-survey-results

How? When a physician is paid fee-for-service, there is a built-in incentive to do more. Sometimes the economics are powerful and the responses brazen. In one story of medical market economics gone wild, Atul Gawande describes McAllen, Texas, where per capita Medicare costs are twice as high as in neighboring El Paso.[76] The situation is typically more subtle. Nonetheless, much of medicine is practiced in the "gray zone," where "an intervention is neither clearly effective nor clearly ineffective—where benefits are unknown or uncertain and value may depend on patients' preferences and available alternatives."[77] For example, percutaneous coronary interventions such as stenting are lifesaving for patients having an acute ST-segment elevation myocardial infarction, but the benefits compared with standard medical therapy (statins, beta blockers, aspirin) are less clear in patients with chronic stable angina. Nevertheless, cardiologists have seen the procedure work in these patients, they know it is unlikely to cause harm, and in a fee-for-service system, they get paid handsomely for doing it.

Physician payment is only one part of the flow of funds through the health care system (Figure 3-3). Premiums from employers, taxes from citizens, and direct payments from patients all flow in the direction of providers. But how clinicians are paid, and for what, varies according to the specific arrangements of their work. **How patients react to these arrangements depends in part on their own insurance status.** Patients with generous insurance coverage who are shielded from most medical charges may be accepting of physicians' recommendations for more intensive (and expensive) care. They know that each additional specialty referral, test, and procedure will not cost them much; may do some good; and (with the exception of invasive procedures) carries little immediate risk. They are likely unaware of the so-called *cascade effect*, in which even noninvasive and seemingly innocuous diagnostic tests can lead to a heap of trouble.[78] We will take up this issue in Chapter 7 on negotiation about tests. On the other hand, patients whose insurance plans require large deductibles and copayments (features that

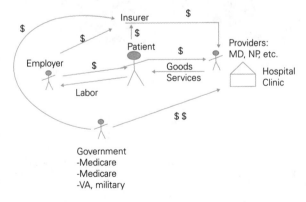

Figure 3-3. Flow of funds through the health system.

are increasingly part of most employer-sponsored plans as well as plans available through federal and state health exchanges) will be much more sensitive to costs.

Patients may not communicate about cost concerns with clinicians. A recent review suggests that patients and clinicians discuss costs of care in a minority of visits, ranging from 4% to 44% depending on the specialty, clinical population, and the definition of a cost discussion.[79] **In deciding whether and how to communicate about costs with patients, clinicians pursue multiple goals and use a common set of rhetorical strategies to manage these goals**[80] (Table 3-6). *Task goals* are related to accomplishing instrumental ends such as getting the patient to pick up the medicine at the pharmacy. *Identity goals* are related to preservation of some element of the clinician's self-image. *Relational goals* are about preserving the clinician-patient relationship. As Scott et al. emphasize, any of these goals may be advanced by direct discussion, derailed by false reassurance, or side-stepped by avoidance (Table 3-2).

The tendency to gloss over cost discussions is understandable, given short office visits and the competing demands of practice. The implications for clinical negotiation are twofold. First, patients may appear to accede to clinicians' recommendations but then balk at actually carrying them out due to high out-of-pocket costs. Second, to the extent that patients are aware of physicians' financial incentives (or believe they are aware of them), they may doubt that their doctor is acting fully in their interests. Ironically, the clinicians who have most fully mastered the art of cost conversations are those who provide "out of pocket services" such as cosmetic surgeons, cosmetic dermatologists, and concierge physicians. For most other practitioners, cost-of-care discussions are not part of the routine clinical dialog. However, the perils of avoidance are numerous.

Table 3-6 Communication Goals And Strategies For Talking About Costs Of Care

Communication Goals	Example	Common Rhetorical Strategies	Example
Task	Enhance adherence by identifying medication with lower out-of-pocket costs	Direct discussion	"I think this medicine is good for you, but I would like to make sure the price is ok."
Identity	Demonstrate commitment to patient (and identity as a "good doctor") by asking about affordability of care	Avoidance	"The most important thing is your health. Let's not focus on costs right now."
Relational	Avoid mentioning societal or health system costs as a reason not to obtain unnecessary imaging study	False reassurance	"Your insurance should cover most of these labs."

Source: Scott AM et al.[80]

Jules Benson, a 62-year-old UPS executive, has a new company insurance plan and schedules a "free" annual physical which has been advertised as a plan benefit. He makes an appointment with Dr. Jarvis, a family physician affiliated with the local medical school. The appointment goes well enough, but Dr. Jarvis determines that Mr. Benson's history of hypertension and mildly elevated cholesterol puts him at inter-mediate risk of coronary disease, so after discussion, he orders a coronary calcium scan along with a basic chemistry and lipid panel. The scan is consistent with mild atherosclerosis, and Mr. Benson is started on a statin. One month later, Mr. Benson receives a bill for $752 from the medical center, including $160 for a "new patient evaluation" and the balance for various tests. He is outraged, as he was led to believe his "physical" would be free. He makes a complaint to Patient Services at the medical center as well as to Human Resources at UPS, complaining that "this doctor is just out to make money." He never returns to see Dr. Jarvis.

When patients and doctors directly discuss out-of-pocket costs, they can often identify viable strategies for mitigating their effects. As revealed in a study of over 1700 doctor-patient encounters, these strategies may or may not involve changing the care plan.[81] Strategies not involving changes to the care plan include 1) changing logistics of care, 2) facilitating copay assistance, 3) providing free samples, and 4) changing/adding insurance plans. Strategies that involve such changes are 1) switching to lower-cost alternative therapy/diag-nostic, 2) switching from brand name to generic, 3) changing dosage/frequency, and 4) stopping/withholding interventions. In the absence of such discussions, however, misunderstandings can arise, and in extreme cases (as with Mr. Benson), these can disrupt the clinician-patient relationship.

When physicians are paid under a capitated or "prepaid" model, the incentive structure is reversed. Practices are rewarded financially for mini-mizing inappropriate care (which is relatively easy) and for moderating use of equivocally appropriate and unnecessary care (which is hard). Sometimes there are quality incentives designed to counteract the economic forces that would oth-erwise lead to stinting, but these are often insufficiently broad and financially robust to pack a meaningful punch.[82]

Aisha Collins is a 48-year-old, generally healthy, African-American middle manager at a state government agency. She has been followed by Dr. Jerilyn Chen, a gen-eral internist at Capital Associates, for 6 years. Capital Associates is a 100-physician multispecialty practice that has several full-risk capitated contracts. During a routine visit for gynecologic care, Ms. Collins mentions new-onset headaches. Dr. Chen notes a blood pressure of 146/85 but no neurological findings. She briefly considers ordering an MRI scan of the brain to rule out space-occupying lesions of the brain, but knowing that most headaches are benign, Dr. Chen suggests that Ms. Collins return to clinic the following week for a blood pressure check, and then a week after that for an office visit. By that time the headaches had vanished.

Was this stinting in the sense that necessary care was denied? Most likely not. Brain tumors and aneurysms are rare even among patients with new-onset headaches. Nevertheless, a case could be made for early brain imaging, and had Ms. Collins thought about it, she might have wondered whether one reason her doctor chose close observation over imaging was her form of insurance. Had Ms. Collins raised this concern explicitly, Dr. Chen might have artfully explained the clinical reality in a way that satisfied the patient's concerns and preserved trust. Or, she might have stumbled, unable to convincingly disentangle her own clinical reasoning from the financial incentive structure created by Capital Associates—of which both she and the patient were aware. Fortunately, the patient's headaches resolved spontaneously, her hypertension declared itself, and she was successfully treated with a low-dose diuretic.

SECTION 3.7: CLINICIANS AND PATIENTS IN A CHANGING MEDICAL LANDSCAPE

If a primary care physician fell asleep in 1970 and woke up in 2020, many aspects of medical practice would be familiar, but others would seem strange. Of course, our medical Rip van Winkle would gape slack-jawed on learning of new epidemics (AIDS, Ebola, COVID-19), new treatments (highly active antiretroviral therapy, coronary stenting), and new imaging modalities (magnetic resonance imaging, positron emission tomography). But Dr. van Winkle would also be surprised by changes in the rules and norms of practice: how physicians are expected to comport themselves, where their responsibilities begin and end, how they stand in relation to their colleagues, co-workers, and patients. In this final section we will address some of the ways that norms of practice have evolved in the last 50 years, focusing on changes with the greatest potential to affect clinical negotiation. Some of these changes are listed in Table 3-7.

From paternalism to shared decision-making. One of the main differences Dr. van Winkle would observe is the increased emphasis on patient involvement in care. With few exceptions (e.g., dire emergencies and when patients lack capacity for decision-making), rank paternalism has been replaced by other models of medical decision-making variably emphasizing information transfer, interpretation of medical facts, or mutual deliberation.[83] While truly informed decision-making is mostly honored in the breach,[84] this remains the modern ideal. **In short, the clinician's task is no longer to select the treatment that comports with**

Table 3-7 **Changing Practice Norms Over 50 Years**

Domain	Practice Norms in 1970	Practice Norms in 2020
Role of patient autonomy	Paternalism	Shared decision-making
Delivery of care	Visit-based	Multichannel
Locus of clinical responsibility	Individual physician	Team-based care
Longitudinal care	24/7 responsibility	Divided call and shift work

his or her own clinical experience. The task is rather to try to triangulate between best medical evidence, patient preferences and values, and clinical judgment.

From visit-based to multichannel care. Another difference that would no doubt surprise our medical time traveler is the **increased variety of communication channels in health care**. While in-person office visits remain the cornerstone of ambulatory care, new developments in home care, telephone care, telemedicine, emailing, texting, and secure electronic portals have pushed the boundaries of when and where care is provided. These developments, all of which have accelerated under pressure from the COVID-19 pandemic, have created new ways for clinicians to communicate, expanding the boundaries of care in time and space. A patient who wakes up at three in the morning fretting about something can send her doctor a secure message and expect to get an answer the next day. A primary care physician uncomfortable initiating treatment for hepatitis C might obtain the necessary support through an "e-consult" from an infectious disease specialist or hepatologist. An emergency medicine physician practicing in a small rural or suburban emergency department can get help managing a critically ill child via telemedicine from pediatric emergency medicine and intensive care specialists at the nearest children's hospital. On the other hand, telehealth makes some aspects of relationship-building more difficult.

From individual responsibility to team care. **In many practice settings, patient care involves teams.** Team members may include many individuals with familiar job titles (nurse, medical assistant, social worker) and some with new ones (health coach, community health worker). Smart use of teams has many advantages: access is enhanced, patients benefit from the differential expertise of team members, and sharing of clinical work can create both economic efficiencies and greater job satisfaction. However, despite recent hoopla around patient-centered medical homes, interdisciplinary teams, and interprofessional education, studies have yet to document definite and substantial clinical benefits or cost savings. One reason is that clinical environments are complex, and we have not yet created systems that efficiently coordinate the efforts of multiple team members.

From 24/7 responsibility to shift work. In the 1950s and early 1960s, residents in teaching hospitals were literally that, residing in the hospital nearly continuously. In subsequent decades, this tradition faded, to the disappointment of certain program directors, who lamented that their trainees on every-*other*-night schedules were "missing half the cases." Habits born of training carried into practice; graduates were imbued with the attitude that the physician—and the physician alone—is ultimately responsible for the patent's welfare and should be available when needed.

For medical postgraduate training programs, 1984 was a watershed year. In early March, Libby Zion, a freshman at Bennington College, died at New York Hospital from what was later thought to be a drug interaction between phenelzine (a monoamine oxidase inhibitor that she had been taking for chronic depression) and meperidine (an opioid analgesic administered by house staff physicians on duty that night).

Ordinarily the case might have been settled quietly, but because the deceased woman's father was a powerful journalist, a series of legal actions ultimately led to regulations limiting resident work hours in the state of New York. Similar limitations soon spread across the country, ultimately achieving the force of regulation. Residents were less bleary-eyed than in previous eras but often just as stressed, as they rushed to complete their work before the metaphorical buzzer. As in prior eras, attitudes developed in training were quickly adopted in practice; newly graduating physicians neither wanted nor expected to take up the mantel of 24/7 medical responsibility that would have been accepted by previous generations. No less interested in safe, high-quality care, this new generation has worked hard to create safe systems involving both collaboration and handoffs. But the resulting interruptions of continuity make the clinical negotiation more challenging.

Taken together, these trends (greater patient autonomy, more care delivery channels, more team care, and more handoffs) have placed greater demands on the clinician seeking to undertake successful clinical negotiation. At the same time, it is also true that no prior generation of physicians has had more options for connecting with patients, obtaining support from other health care professionals, and collaborating with colleagues.

SUMMARY POINTS:

- Contextual factors affecting the clinical negotiation include norms and values, policies and systems, organizational structures, time constraints, and reimbursement.
- Patients are and ought to be autonomous agents, but part of autonomy is choosing how much authority to cede to health care professionals. One of the fundamental tasks of clinical negotiation is to establish patients' preferences for decision-making.
- The complexity of the US health care system complicates the clinical negotiation. From the clinician perspective, relevant features include the multipayer system, heavy administrative costs and burdens, and the threat of medical liability. From the patient perspective, important aspects are insecure access to care, high out-of-pocket costs, and information asymmetry.
- At the margin, fee-for-service and capitated forms of payment have predictable effects on clinical care and utilization of resources (FFS encourages more care, capitated payment less), with downstream effects on patient trust and the clinical negotiation.
- Larger practices can provide greater support but tend to be more bureaucratic and less flexible than smaller ones, sometimes limiting the clinician's negotiating options.
- Time pressure is real, but time is also subjective; clinicians can invoke several strategies for making "short visits seem long."
- With change as the only constant, it is imperative to stay nimble and adopt flexible strategies for finding common ground.

QUESTIONS FOR DISCUSSION:

1. Name and briefly describe five sets of contextual factors affecting the clinical negotiation.

2. A decades-old study showed that patients were less confident in their physician's skills if the doctor consulted references (in this case, a textbook) within the exam room to address a clinical question than if the doctor provided the answer extemporaneously. Why do you think patients had this reaction? Do you think the same results would be obtained today?

3. Describe a time when you confronted a conflict between beneficence (doing good for the patient) and autonomy (respecting the patient's right to make their own decisions). How did you handle the situation?

4. In what ways do you think clinical negotiation is easier or harder in fee-for-service private practice compared to a group model health maintenance organization like Kaiser Permanente?

5. What are some ways in which clinicians can make a "short visit feel long"?

6. What are some ways in which "teams" can make patients feel well-cared for? What are some ways in which teams can fail?

7. Is continuity of care a fundamental building block of clinical quality or an outmoded concept? How does continuity make clinical negotiation easier? What strategies do you use in your practice to achieve rapport quickly (and advance the clinical negotiation) when covering for another clinician?

References

1. Schneider C, Schneider D. *The practice of autonomy: patients, doctors, and medical decisions*. Oxford University Press on Demand; 1998.
2. Saad TC. The history of autonomy in medicine from antiquity to principlism. *Med Health Care Philos*. 2018;21(1):125-137.
3. Rothman DJ. The origins and consequences of patient autonomy: A 25-year retrospective. *Health Care Anal*. 2001;9(3):255-264.
4. Blackhall LJ, Murphy ST, Frank G, Michel V, Azen S. Ethnicity and attitudes toward patient autonomy. *JAMA*. 1995;274(10):820-825.
5. Brickman P, Coates D, Janoff-Bulman R. Lottery winners and accident victims: Is happiness relative? *J Pers Soc Psychol*. 1978;36(8):917.
6. Halpern J, Arnold RM. Affective Forecasting: An unrecognized challenge in making serious health decisions. *J Gen Intern Med*. 2008;23(10):1708-1712.
7. Ubel PA, Loewenstein G, Schwarz N, Smith D. Misimagining the unimaginable: the disability paradox and health care decision making. *Health Psychol*. 2005;24(4s):S57-62.
8. Loewenstein G. Projection bias in medical decision making. *Med Decis Making*. 2005;25(1):96-105.
9. Danziger S, Levav J, Avnaim-Pesso L. Extraneous factors in judicial decisions. *Proc Natl Acad Sci U S A*. 2011;108(17):6889-6892.

10. Schneider EC, Sarnak DO, Squires D, Shah A, Doty MM. Mirror, Mirror 2017: nternationa Comparison Ref ects F aws and Opportunities for Better US Hea th Care. 2017.

11. Moseley GB III. The US health care non-system, 1908-2008. *AMA J Ethics*. 2008;10(5):324-331.

12. Moses H, Matheson DH, Dorsey ER, George BP, Sadoff D, Yoshimura S. The anatomy of health care in the United States. *JAMA*. 2013;310(18):1947-1964.

13. Garfield R, Majerol M, Damico A, Foutz J. The uninsured: a primer. *Key facts about health insurance and the uninsured in America Menlo Park, CA: The Henry James Kaiser Family Foundation.* 2016.

14. Berchick E, Barnett J, Upton R. Health insurance coverage in the United States: 2018 [Internet]. Washington (DC): Census Bureau; 2019 Nov [cited 2020 Jan 9].(Current Population Reports).

15. Morley CP, Badolato DJ, Hickner J, Epling JW. The impact of prior authorization requirements on primary care physicians' offices: report of two parallel network studies. *J Am Board Fam Med*. 2013;26(1):93-95.

16. Carrier ER, Reschovsky JD, Katz DA, Mello MM. High physician concern about malpractice risk predicts more aggressive diagnostic testing in office-based practice. *Health Affairs*. 2013;32(8):1383-1391.

17. Bishop TF, Federman AD, Keyhani S. Physicians' views on defensive medicine: a national survey. *Arch Intern Med*. 2010;170(12):1081-1083.

18. Berchick ER, Hood E, Barnett JC. *Health insurance coverage in the United States 2017.* US Census Bureau; September 12, 2018.

19. Ganguli I, Shi Z, Orav EJ, Rao A, Ray KN, Mehrotra A. Declining use of primary care among commercially insured adults in the United States, 2008–2016. *Ann Intern Med*. 2020;172(4):240.

20. Adrion ER, Ryan AM, Seltzer AC, Chen LM, Ayanian JZ, Nallamothu BK. Out-of-pocket spending for hospitalizations among nonelderly adults. *JAMA Intern Med*. 2016;176(9):1325-1332.

21. Cunningham PJ. The share of people with high medical costs increased prior to implementation of the Affordable Care Act. *Health Affairs*. 2015;34(1):117-124.

22. Herzlinger RE. *Consumer-driven health care: implications for providers, payers, and policy-makers.* John Wiley & Sons; 2004.

23. Manning WG, Newhouse JP, Duan N, Keeler EB, Leibowitz A. Health insurance and the demand for medical care: evidence from a randomized experiment. *Am Econ Rev*. 1987:251-277.

24. Brook RH, Ware JE Jr, Rogers WH, et al. Does free care improve adults' health? Results from a randomized controlled trial. *New Engl J Med*. 1983;309(23):1426-1434.

25. Kullgren JT, Cliff EQ, Krenz C, et al. Consumer behaviors among individuals enrolled in high-deductible health plans in the United States. *JAMA Intern Med*. 2018;178(3):424-426.

26. White KL. The ecology of medical care: origins and implications for population-based healthcare research. *Health Serv Res*. 1997;32(1):11.

27. National Center for Health S. Health, United States. In: *Health, United States, 2018.* Hyattsville (MD): National Center for Health Statistics (US); 2019.

28. Teno JM, Gozalo P, Trivedi AN, et al. Site of death, place of care, and health care transitions among US Medicare beneficiaries, 2000-2015. *JAMA*. 2018;320(3):264-271.

29. Welch WP, Cuellar AE, Stearns SC, Bindman AB. Proportion of physicians in large group practices continued to grow in 2009-11. *Health Aff (Millwood)*. 2013;32(9):1659-1666.

30. Casalino LP, Pesko MF, Ryan AM, et al. Small primary care physician practices have low rates of preventable hospital admissions. *Health Aff (Millwood)*. 2014;33(9):1680-1688.

31. Rittenhouse DR, Casalino LP, Shortell SM, et al. Small and medium-size physician practices use few patient-centered medical home processes. *Health Aff*. 2011;30(8):1575-1584.

32. Starfield B, Shi L, Macinko J. Contribution of primary care to health systems and health. *Milbank Q*. 2005;83(3):457-502.

33. Koller CF, Khullar D. Primary care spending rate—a lever for encouraging investment in primary care. *New Engl J Med*. 2017;377(18):1709-1711.

34. Abbo ED, Zhang Q, Zelder M, Huang ES. The increasing number of clinical items addressed during the time of adult primary care visits. *J Gen Intern Med*. 2008;23(12):2058.

35. Mechanic D, McAlpine DD, Rosenthal M. Are patients' office visits with physicians getting shorter? *New Engl J Med*. 2001;344(3):198-204.

36. Shaw MK, Davis SA, Fleischer AB, Feldman SR. The duration of office visits in the United States, 1993 to 2010. *Am J Manag Care*. 2014;20(10):820-826.

37. Yarnall KS, Pollak KI, Østbye T, Krause KM, Michener JL. Primary care: is there enough time for prevention? *Am J Public Health*. 2003;93(4):635-641.

38. Baron RJ. What's keeping us so busy in primary care? A snapshot from one practice. *N Engl J Med*. 2010;362(17):1632–6.

39. Doerr E, Galpin K, Jones-Taylor C, et al. Between-visit workload in primary care. *J Gen Intern Med*. 2010;25(12):1289-1292.

40. Tai-Seale M, McGuire TG, Zhang W. Time allocation in primary care office visits. *Health Serv Res*. 2007;42(5):1871-1894.

41. Goroll AH. Does primary care add sufficient value to deserve better funding? *JAMA Intern Med*. 2019;179(3):372-373.

42. Reid R, Damberg C, Friedberg MW. Primary Care Spending in the Fee-for-Service Medicare Population. *JAMA Intern Med*. 2019;179(7):977–80.

43. Adashi EY, Clodfelter RP, George P. Direct primary care: one step forward, two steps back. *JAMA*. 2018;320(7):637-638.

44. Glauser W. Primary care system outdated and inconvenient for many millennials. Can Med Assoc. 2018;190(48): E1430–E1431.

45. Kernan WN, Elnicki DM, Hauer KE. The selling of primary care 2015. *J Gen Intern Med*. 2015;30(9):1376-1380.

46. Sinsky CA, Willard-Grace R, Schutzbank AM, Sinsky TA, Margolius D, Bodenheimer T. In search of joy in practice: a report of 23 high-functioning primary care practices. *Ann Fam Med*. 2013;11(3):272-278.

47. Irving G, Neves AL, Dambha-Miller H, et al. International variations in primary care physician consultation time: a systematic review of 67 countries. *BMJ Open*. 2017;7(10):e017902.

48. Rao A, Shi Z, Ray KN, Mehrotra A, Ganguli I. National trends in primary care visit use and practice capabilities, 2008-2015. *Ann Fam Med*. 2019;17(6):538-544.

49. Chen LM, Farwell WR, Jha AK. Primary care visit duration and quality: does good care take longer? *Arch Intern Med*. 2009;169(20):1866-1872.

50. Dugdale DC, Epstein R, Pantilat SZ. Time and the patient-physician relationship. *J Gen Intern Med*. 1999;14(Suppl 1):S34-40.

51. Roland MO, Bartholomew J, Courtenay MJ, Morris RW, Morrell DC. The "five minute" consultation: effect of time constraint on verbal communication. *Br Med J (Clin Res Ed)*. 1986;292(6524):874-876.

52. Gross DA, Zyzanski SJ, Borawski EA, Cebul RD, Stange KC. Patient satisfaction with time spent with their physician. *J Fam Pract*. 1998;47(2):133-138.

53. Lin CT, Albertson GA, Schilling LM, et al. Is patients' perception of time spent with the physician a determinant of ambulatory patient satisfaction? *Arch Intern Med*. 2001;161(11):1437-1442.

54. Teunis T, Thornton ER, Jayakumar P, Ring D. Time seeing a hand surgeon is not associated with patient satisfaction. *Clin Orthop Relat Res*. 2015;473(7):2362-2368.

55. Konrad TR, Link CL, Shackelton RJ, et al. It's about time: physicians' perceptions of time constraints in primary care medical practice in three national healthcare systems. *Med Care*. 2010;48(2):95.

56. Arstila V, Lloyd D. *Subjective time: The philosophy, psychology, and neuroscience of temporality*. MIT Press Cambridge, MA; 2014.

57. Innes M, Skelton J. Different kinds of time. *Fam Pract*. 2005;22(4):470.

58. Linzer M, Manwell LB, Williams ES, et al. Working conditions in primary care: physician reactions and care quality. *Ann Intern Med*. 2009;151(1):28-36, w26-29.

59. Rotenstein LS, Torre M, Ramos MA, et al. Prevalence of burnout among physicians: a systematic review. *JAMA*. 2018;320(11):1131-1150.

60. Lussier MT, Richard C. Communication tips. Time flies: patients' perceptions of consultation length and actual duration. *Can Fam Physician*. 2007;53(1):46-47.

61. Tackett S, Tad-y D, Rios R, Kisuule F, Wright S. Appraising the practice of etiquette-based medicine in the inpatient setting. *J Gen Intern Med*. 2013;28(7):908-913.

62. Morrison I, Smith R. Hamster health care: time to stop running faster and redesign health care. In: British Medical Journal Publishing Group; 2000;321(7276): 1541–1542.

63. Epstein RM. Mindful practice. *JAMA*. 1999;282(9):833-839.

64. Lemon TI, Smith RH. Consultation content not consultation length improves patient satisfaction. *J Family Med Prim Care*. 2014;3(4):333.

65. Pollock K, Mechanic D, Grime J. Patients' perceptions of entitlement to time in general practice consultations for depression: qualitative study Commentary: Managing time appropriately in primary care. *BMJ*. 2002;325(7366):687.

66. Stevens R, Mountford A. On time. *Br J Gen Pract*. 2010;60(575):458-460.

67. Wooldridge AN, Arató N, Sen A, Amenomori M, Fetters MD. Truth or fallacy? Three hour wait for three minutes with the doctor: Findings from a private clinic in rural Japan. *Asia Pacific Fam Med*. 2010;9(1):11.

68. Jefferson L, Bloor K, Hewitt C. The effect of physician gender on length of patient consultations: observational findings from the UK hospital setting and synthesis with existing studies. *J R Soc Med*. 2015;108(4):136-141.

69. Orton PK, Pereira Gray D. Factors influencing consultation length in general/family practice. *Fam Pract*. 2016;33(5):529-534.

70. Kringos DS, Boerma WG, Hutchinson A, Van der Zee J, Groenewegen PP. The breadth of primary care: a systematic literature review of its core dimensions. *BMC Heath Serv Res*. 2010;10(1):65.

71. Romano MJ, Segal JB, Pollack CE. The association between continuity of care and the overuse of medical procedures. *JAMA Intern Med*. 2015;175(7):1148-1154.

72. Yakovenko A, Zuehlke E, Daugherty A, Reardon K. *Research Briefing: 2014 Primary Care Consumer Choice Survey*. Washington, DC: The Advisory Board Company; 2014.

73. Schroeder SA, Frist W, National Commission on Physician Payment R. Phasing out fee-for-service payment. *N Engl J Med*. 2013;368(21):2029-2032.

74. Quinn K. The 8 basic payment methods in health care. *Ann Intern Med*. 2015;163(4):300-306.

75. Stecker EC, Schroeder SA. Adding value to relative-value units. *N Engl J Med*. 2013;369(23): 2176-2179.

76. Gawande A. The cost conundrum. *The New Yorker*. Vol June 1, 2009. 2009:36-44.

77. Chandra A, Khullar D, Lee TH. Addressing the challenge of gray-zone medicine. *N Engl J Med*. 2015;372(3):203-205.

78. Mold JW, Stein HF. The cascade effect in the clinical care of patients. *N Engl J Med*. 1986;314(8):512-514.

79. Hunter WG, Hesson A, Davis JK, et al. Patient-physician discussions about costs: definitions and impact on cost conversation incidence estimates. *BMC Health Serv Res*. 2016;16(1):108.

80. Scott AM, Harrington NG, Spencer E. Primary care physicians' strategic pursuit of multiple goals in cost-of-care conversations with patients. *Health Commun*. 2020:1-13. doi: 10.1080/10410236.2020.1723051. Online ahead of print.

81. Hunter WG, Zhang CZ, Hesson A, et al. What strategies do physicians and patients discuss to reduce out-of-pocket costs? Analysis of cost-saving strategies in 1,755 outpatient clinic visits. *Med Decis Making*. 2016;36(7):900-910.

82. Newhouse JP. *Pricing the priceless: a health care conundrum*. MIT Press; 2004.

83. Emanuel EJ, Emanuel LL. Four models of the physician-patient relationship. *JAMA*. 1992;267(16):2221-2226.

84. Braddock CH III, Edwards KA, Hasenberg NM, Laidley TL, Levinson W. Informed decision making in outpatient practice: time to get back to basics. *JAMA*. 1999;282(24):2313-2320.

85. Pearce WB, Cronen V. Communication, action, and meaning: The creation of social realities. In. New York: Preager; 1980.

86. Norton R. *Communicator style: Theory, applications, and measures*. Vol 1: SAGE Publications, Incorporated; 1983.

87. Zandbelt LC, Smets EM, Oort FJ, Godfried MH, de Haes HC. Determinants of physicians' patient-centred behaviour in the medical specialist encounter. *Soc Sci Med*. 2006;63(4):899-910.

88. Street RL. Communicative styles and adaptations in physician-parent consultations. *Soc Sci Med*. 1992;34(10):1155-1163.

89. Roter DL, Hall JA. Physician gender and patient-centered communication: a critical review of empirical research. *Annu Rev Public Health*. 2004;25:497-519.

90. Hall JA, Roter DL. Patient gender and communication with physicians: results of a community-based study. *Womens Health*. 1995;1(1):77-95.

91. Barnsley J, Williams AP, Cockerill R, Tanner J. Physician characteristics and the physician-patient relationship. Impact of sex, year of graduation, and specialty. *Can Fam Physician*. 1999;45:935-942.

92. Street RL Jr, Voigt B, Geyer C Jr, Manning T, Swanson GP. Increasing patient involvement in choosing treatment for early breast cancer. *Cancer*. 1995;76(11):2275-2285.

93. Siminoff LA, Graham GC, Gordon NH. Cancer communication patterns and the influence of patient characteristics: Disparities in information-giving and affective behaviors. *Patient Educ Couns*. 2006;62(3):355-360.

94. Arora NK, McHorney CA. Patient preferences for medical decision making: who really wants to participate? *Med Care*. 2000;38(3):335-341.

95. Katz MG, Jacobson TA, Veledar E, Kripalani S. Patient literacy and question-asking behavior during the medical encounter: a mixed-methods analysis. *J Gen Intern Med*. 2007;22(6):782-786.

96. Schouten BC, Meeuwesen L. Cultural differences in medical communication: A review of the literature. *Patient Educ Couns*. 2006;64(1-3):21-34.

97. Alegria M, Sribney W, Perez D, Laderman M, Keefe K. The role of patient activation on patient-provider communication and quality of care for US and foreign born Latino patients. *J Gen Intern Med*. 2009;24(Suppl 3):534-541.

98. Fridhandler BM. Conceptual note on state, trait, and the state–trait distinction. *J Pers Soc Psychol*. 1986;50(1):169.

99. Street RL Jr. Communication in medical encounters: An ecological perspective. In: Thompson T, Dorsey A, Miller K, Parrot R, eds. *The handbook of health communication*. Mahwah, NJ: Erlbaum; 2003:63-89.

100. Greene JO. A cognitive approach to human communication: An action assembly theory. *Commun Monographs*. 1984;51(4):289–306.

101. Gulbrandsen P, Lindstrom JC, Finset A, Hall JA. Patient affect, physician liking for the patient, physician behavior, and patient reported outcomes: A modeling approach. *Patient Educ Couns*. 2020;103(6):1143-1149.

102. Cox ED, Smith MA, Brown RL, Fitzpatrick MA. Assessment of the physician-caregiver relationship scales (PCRS). *Patient Educ Couns*. 2008;70(1):69-78.

103. Zandbelt LC, Smets EM, Oort FJ, Godfried MH, de Haes HC. Patient participation in the medical specialist encounter: does physicians' patient-centred communication matter? *Patient Educ Couns*. 2007;65(3):396-406.

104. Sainio C, Lauri S, Eriksson E. Cancer patients' views and experiences of participation in care and decision making. *Nurs Ethics*. 2001;8(2):97-113.

105. Cegala DJ, Post DM. The impact of patients' participation on physicians' patient-centered communication. *Patient Educ Couns*. 2009;77(2):202-208.

106. Street RL Jr. Information-giving in medical consultations: the influence of patients' communicative styles and personal characteristics. *Soc Sci Med*. 1991;32(5):541-8.

107. Street RLJr, Krupat E, Bell RA, Kravitz RL, Haidet P. Beliefs about control in the physician-patient relationship: effect on communication in medical encounters. *Journal of General Internal Medicine*. 2003;18(8):609-616.

108. Street RL Jr, Gordon HS, Ward MM, Krupat E, Kravitz RL. Patient participation in medical consultations: why some patients are more involved than others. *Med Care*. 2005;43(10):960-969.

CHAPTER 4

How Communication Fails

Clinical Take-Aways

- The remarkable thing about clinician-patient communication is not how often it fails but how often it succeeds.
- Creating shared understanding is often complicated by differences in clinicians' and patients' life experiences and perspectives on health.
- Three types of communication failures are not understanding (the result of making unfounded assumptions), misunderstanding (saying it or hearing it wrong), and disagreeing (having different opinions).
- Clinicians should:
  - Cultivate curiosity, asking "what might it be like to be this patient?"
  - Cultivate humility, recognizing that it is easy to miscommunicate one's intentions or misunderstand patients' concerns.
  - Be alert to verbal, paraverbal, and nonverbal clues that the patient is confused about or skeptical of an explanation or suggestion.
  - Be aware of the potential for implicit bias related to race, ethnicity, gender, age, sexual orientation, and other nonclinical patient characteristics.

SECTION 4-1: INTRODUCTION

George Bernard Shaw famously observed, "The single biggest problem in communication is the illusion that it has taken place." While this may be true in nearly all literature and in much of life, the stakes in health care are such that illusory communication hardly suffices. We need the real thing. Miscommunication in health care has consequences—for medical decision-making, for patient satisfaction and morale, for professional self-regard and burnout. And not incidentally, for the clinical negotiation.

In her book *Of Two Minds*, which describes the way American psychiatrists are trained, anthropologist Tanya Luhrmann notes that "When young psychiatrists learn to diagnose and prescribe, they learn that a patient can hurt a doctor."[1] Later, "When young psychiatrists learn to do psychotherapy...they learn... that doctors can hurt patients." Luhrmann was talking about the power of words, and not just as wielded by psychiatrists. **Doctors' words can soothe, comfort, and empower—or frighten, disrupt, and undermine.** Furthermore, words are the raw material of negotiation, clinical or otherwise. In the struggle to find common ground with patients, clinicians must start with the right words. As even the most skilled clinical communicator will tell you, this is sometimes easy and sometimes exquisitely difficult. All of us can recall situations where communication simply went off the rails.

In this chapter our purpose is to promote a communication skillset that will facilitate the clinical negotiation. But to do so we work backwards. By looking at how communication fails, we see how it can succeed. By unpacking how things go wrong, we can see more clearly how to set them right.

Consider these patients.

> *Mr. Strahern, a 45-year-old man with alcohol-related liver disease, signs out of the hospital against medical advice when his medical team refuses his request for more opioid pain medication.*
>
> *Mrs. Ungerleider, an 86-year-old European immigrant who lives alone, calls the office repeatedly with minor concerns. She recently filed a complaint with the Patient Relations Department alleging that "Dr. Brown never calls me back."*
>
> *Ms. Coburn, a 20-year-old college student with lower abdominal pain is resentful when Dr. Melendez recommends a pregnancy test and screening for sexually transmitted infections.*

In each case, as the Captain in *Cool Hand Luke* famously lamented, "what we've got here is failure to communicate." Mr. Strahern believes his care team looks down on him because of his alcohol use and wants to punish him by denying pain medication. Mrs. Underleider has emotional needs that no mortal, medically trained or not, could possibly satisfy. And Ms. Coburn, perhaps the victim of past discrimination, medical mistreatment, or sexual harassment, carries her resentment into the examination room.

Yet to claim we need more or better "communication" between clinicians and patients underplays the complexity of the process. By joining in *interpersonal communication*, participants produce verbal and nonverbal behaviors to accomplish personal and mutual goals. **Communication is a process of action, interaction, and inference as the participants mutually construct a conversation by producing messages, responding to the behavior of the other, negotiating turn-taking, and making sense of what is being said and done.** Communication is behavior with a purpose—it is saddled with intent. And yet behaviors that aren't strictly intended to achieve any particular purpose can be interpreted as communicative. When Mr. Strahern's physician advises him to stop drinking, that's communication. But when the doctor rolls his eyes or cuts off the patient's rambling defense of how he "only drinks socially, and much less than in the past," that's communication too. In this sense, communication is identified by its consequences—it affects the way people think, feel, and act.

As described in Chapter 3, successful clinical negotiation depends not only on the primary parties to the dialog (e.g., clinician and patient) but also on any number of supporting actors (e.g., family members, medical office staff) and contextual factors (cultural, systemic, economic, organizational, and normative). When communication fails, the fault lies with all of these and more.

In this chapter, we first examine what makes clinical encounters such fertile ground for communication failures. We then take up the various ways that communication fails in clinical negotiation, the reasons for such failures, and how to preempt and remediate communication breakdowns. We organize our analysis around a taxonomy of communication failure that includes 1) not understanding; 2) misunderstanding; and 3) disagreement. We conclude by describing techniques for diminishing failures and optimizing success.

SECTION 4-2: THE CLINICAL ENCOUNTER: FERTILE GROUND FOR COMMUNICATION FAILURES

We began this book by acknowledging that most clinical encounters are routine, productive, and associated with positive health outcomes. However, this is also true of trips to the grocery store. Grocers and customers, however, are unlikely to disagree over where customers steer their pushcarts or when they plan to return for further shopping, let alone how the store stocks its shelves.[2] **Clinician-patient encounters, in contrast, are by their very nature ripe for communication failures. We advance three principal reasons.**

First, clinicians and patients approach the encounter from very different perspectives. Clinicians are in a familiar setting; patients find themselves in places (e.g., physicians' offices, emergency rooms, hospitals) that they visit only intermittently and may understand poorly. Clinicians are at work, such that clinical encounters are *part of* their daily routine; patients have taken time *away from* their routine. Clinicians see many patients during a given week; patients may see a doctor just once over many weeks. After some time in practice, clinical work does not generally stir up significant anxiety in the average clinician, whereas patients are often highly vulnerable to anxiety stemming from a health threat. The information environment within which clinicians create understanding consists of evidence from randomized clinical trials, clinical guidelines, expert opinion, and personal experience accumulated across encounters with multiple patients. The information environment within which patients create understanding includes patients' personal health experiences, social interactions with family and friends, mass media, social media, and the pronouncements of prior physicians (see Chapter 2). While clinician and patient may share the same goals, they come to the encounter differently prepared.

Second, patients differ in their capacity and preferences for participating in their own care; one communication style fits some but not all. Societal expectations for patient involvement in medical decision-making have evolved rapidly over the past 40 years. The 1990s were a particularly fertile time for the development of ideas around patient involvement in care. Emanuel and Emanuel proposed a four-part typology of the patient-physician relationship (paternalistic, informative, interpretive, and deliberative).[3] While acknowledging that each model had its place (e.g., paternalism is completely appropriate during life-threatening emergencies), they came down squarely in favor of the deliberative model, where physicians are enjoined not only to inform but also to (noncoercively) persuade patients to embrace care that advances health.

Several years later, Charles, Gafni, and Whelan distinguished between three types of clinician-patient relationships.[4]

- Paternalistic—the clinician is in charge, and the patient acquiesces;
- Shared—clinician and patient have relatively equal control over topics discussed and decisions made; and
- Informed—the patient has control over topics and decisions and views the clinician as a source of information.

Quill and Brody join many experts in what might be called the *normative model of shared decision-making*: that the ideal patient-physician relationship is one in which the doctor not only provides information but also seeks to understand the patient perspective; presents his or her own views; and joins the patient in wrestling actively with the question at hand.[5] Implicit in this view is the concept of emergent values—the idea that patients' inchoate preferences shift, take shape, and ultimately crystallize through active discussion with a caring, committed clinician.

What do patients think about all this? The literature seems to support the notion that most patients prefer to participate in medical decisions, while others choose to delegate. But participating and delegating are neither cleanly defined nor mutually exclusive. For example, some patients may wish to be highly involved in discussing their concerns and asking questions but defer to the physician on final decisions. Other patients may wish to participate in some decisions (or some *parts* of some decisions) and delegate others, depending on the health challenge they are facing. This may occur even during the same episode of illness. For example, a woman considering salvage chemotherapy for ovarian cancer might wish to have *full control* over the type of central venous port placed in her chest, to be *involved* in when to start and stop chemotherapy, and to *cede the decision* about choice of cytotoxic agents and antiemetics to her oncologist.[6,7,8]

Third, much of interpersonal communication is habitual and taken for granted. This is not all bad. During routine interactions with patients, clinicians often communicate in a subconscious or automatic fashion—selecting and pronouncing words, constructing syntax, making sense of what patients are saying, displaying nonverbal expressions, taking conversational turns, and maintaining connection (e.g., by smiling and being polite). Clinicians are simultaneously mindful of other pressing requirements such as discussing appropriate topics, staying on time, sharing essential medical information (e.g., test results), and making treatment recommendations. The *advantage* of being able to produce and interpret communication in a more "mindless" or automated manner with little cognitive effort is that clinicians can give more deliberate attention to monitoring the situation, making sense of what the patient is saying, and working with the patient to achieve the goals of the encounter. The *disadvantage* is that clinicians may be prone to cognitive laziness and take too much for granted. They may miss subtle clues to the patient's feelings (e.g., nonverbal reactions, verbal hesitancy, altered tone of voice), may be unaware of their own biases (e.g., towards obesity or substance use), or may be oblivious to skewed conversational patterns (e.g., clinician is doing most of the talking).

Deeper Dive 4.1: Meanings Are in People, Not Words

This oft-used quote highlights the point that words have no meaning in and of themselves. Rather, their meanings are generated (created) by the person making sense of the words. The reason we generally have few problems understanding one another is that in most conversations the interactants share the same meanings for most words. To English speakers, the meanings of words like "fever" or "nurse" are usually obvious, while "Qapla" or "Pah-tak" are obscure (unless they happen to have learned Klingon from long exposure to *Star Trek*).

In medical care, the fact that meanings are in people, not words, has important implications for achieving shared understanding. For example, a number of commonly used words may have one meaning for clinicians and another for patients: "positive," "undifferentiated," "sugar," "cancer," "high blood," and "lesion." In clinical negotiation, clinicians should as a matter of habit be alert for possible misinterpretations of words, their own as well as the patient's.

However, knowing what words *mean* requires us also to understand what words *do*. In his book, *How to Do Things With Words*,[53] philosopher John Austin argues that words are much more than a means to convey meaning, they "do things." Austin identifies three different levels of meaning— locutionary, illocutionary, and perlocutionary.

Suppose a clinician tells a patient: "Well, unfortunately your lab results indicate you have diabetes. However, I promise that, given a solid treatment plan, we can keep it under control and you can live a normal life."

Several different tasks are undertaken here. First, there is a report of lab test results coupled with a diagnosis. This represents the locutionary meaning, derived from the words alone. There also appears to be a "promise" being made. However, understanding whether this "counts" as a promise requires understanding the situation that goes beyond the words themselves. This represents the illocutionary level of meaning. For example, for the statement to be interpreted as a "promise" certain *felicity conditions* [54] need to be met: (a) the offer has to be perceived as having some value for the patient/recipient, (b) the clinician is sincere in making the promise, and (c) the clinician is capable of fulfilling the promise. If the patient harbors doubts that these conditions hold, then the clinician's statement will not be perceived as a legitimate promise.

Suppose the patient believes the clinician is sincere and capable of offering a plan that will benefit her well-being. The patient may experience hope and stay committed to the treatment recommendations (e.g., diet, exercise, medication). This represents the perlocutionary level of meaning—how the patient responds to the clinician's statement. Of course, if the patient has reason to doubt the clinician's sincerity (e.g., based on past promises made but not kept) or capability (e.g., based on skepticism that drug therapy will be free of unacceptable side effects), then the patient may not follow the treatment plan. Nonadherence would be the perlocutionary effect of the clinician's statement.

This deeper dive focuses on the pragmatics of language *in situ*. From a clinical negotiation perspective, it is important to recognize communicating through words requires more than two people knowing what the words mean in and of themselves. Words "do things" based on what we say and how we act, interpret, and respond. Effective clinical negotiation requires successful exchange of locutionary, illocutionary, and perlocutionary meaning. Or in plain English, do we understand what the words mean, are we communicating in good faith, and will we take steps to follow a plan?

If routine clinical care never wavered in its routineness, there would be nothing bad to say about automaticity. The problem, of course, is that routineness can never be counted upon.

Florence Chang is a 45-year-old Taiwanese immigrant who fell a few days ago and complained of vague lateral chest discomfort. Dr. Friedman tried to elicit further history about the circumstances, beginning with open-ended questions and then progressing, as he had been taught, to more specific questions about location, severity, radiation, time course, and aggravating and alleviating factors. The patient's responses were somewhat vague, but Dr. Friedman attributed this to cultural and language differences. He was reassured by the absence of symptoms suggesting syncope or vertigo; the fall must have been mechanical, and there didn't look to be any serious damage. On examination she was well dressed. Vital signs were normal. There was some tenderness over the lateral ribs, but the chest was clear when auscultated through the patient's blouse. At the last minute, Dr. Friedman asked if he could look at the patient's ribs by lifting her shirt. This revealed several large confluent ecchymoses. "Who did this to you?" Dr. Friedman asked. (Borrowed with modification from Feldman 1997)[9]

Dr. Friedman's encounter with Ms. Chang turned on a dime from a routine evaluation of a "fall" to suspected domestic violence. Communication rarely fails on the smooth terrain of the utterly routine. Communication failures are more common when the landscape abruptly shifts, where the seemingly routine turns out to be anything but. In subsequent sections, we discuss different types of communication failures and offer suggestions for ways to avoid them.

SECTIONS 4.3: TYPES OF COMMUNICATION FAILURES

As introduced in Section 1.2, clinical negotiation involves communication aimed at creating shared understanding and agreement between clinicians and patients. Communication failures encompass those situations where understanding and agreement are not achieved on an issue that matters.

As a form of information transfer, human language has some things in common with genetic material (DNA). Our language and our genome are both composed of symbols ("letters" of the alphabet and "bases" of DNA) assembled into complex strings that convey meaning. And both are subject to "failure": miscommunication in language, mutation in genetics. Scientists have described four types of genetic mutations: missense, nonsense, frameshift, and silent.[10] Without pressing the analogy too far, **breakdowns in clinical communication can be similarly divided into the following categories:**

- Not understanding
- Misunderstanding
- Disagreeing

Communication occurs through signs and symbols.[11] A sign is a consequence of a thought or feeling that is manifest to the observer. Stammering is a sign of anxiety, blushing a sign of embarrassment. A symbol is a signal that signifies something other than itself. The meaning of a symbol is defined by social convention and altered by context. Consider the three dialogs below:

Dialog 1

"Do you smoke?
"No, I quit."
"That's great. Not smoking is one of the most important things you can do for your health."

Dialog 2

"Those pills were just terrific, doc."
"Oh, I'm glad they helped."
"Yeah, who doesn't like non-stop diarrhea."

Dialog 3

"I'm worried about your drinking."
"Oh, don't worry, I've never had a problem."
"Still, I'm concerned that you might develop problems in the future."
"I'm fine. What are you going to do for my back pain?"

In the first dialog, the problem is not what has been said but what has been withheld. In reality, the patient quit smoking 3 days ago. Her risk for lung problems, cardiovascular disease and cancer remains high. This is *not understanding*, a problem of omission.

In the second dialog, the patient's meaning initially seems clear, and the doctor's positive response is appropriate. It is only in the context of the patient's vocal tone, facial expression, and subsequent statement that the physician recognizes the sarcasm that completely upends the message. This is *misunderstanding*, a problem of missed signs and crossed signals.

In the third dialog, the issues are clear, but the patient and physician disagree about problem prioritization and goals of care. This is disagreement, a problem of disputed facts or disparate values.

We now address these three types of communication failures in turn.

SECTION 4.4: NOT UNDERSTANDING.

The average American adult makes about three physician office visits per year. Assuming an average visit length of 18 minutes, that's 54 minutes with the doctor out of 525,600 minutes in a year. Acknowledging the long tail for patients with multiple chronic illnesses, it is still true that physicians witness only a very thin slice of patient's lives. Therefore, what physicians know of their patients depends on what physicians think to ask and what patients are willing to tell.

Mr. Kruger, a 45-year-old man with hypertension, has been taking 20 mg of lisinopril for the past 6 months. At this visit, the medical assistant records his blood pressure as 145/96. Dr. Aronow says the pressure is still high and advises Mr. Kruger to increase the dose of lisinopril. Mr. Kruger nods his head and says OK. Dr. Aronow writes a prescription for 40 mg and recommends follow-up in 2 months "to make sure we're on track." The visit is brief, Mr. Kruger doesn't have much to say, and Dr. Aronow silently congratulates himself for finishing early. Mr. Kruger, knowing that he has not been taking even the 20-mg dose regularly, leaves the office with no intention of filling the new prescription.

On the surface, this interaction appears routine and ends with a plausible plan for intensifying treatment of Mr. Kruger's hypertension. The conversation is pleasant. Care is conducted efficiently. Dr. Aronow knows that Mr. Kruger's blood pressure is higher than recommended by current guidelines and assumes the patient is amenable to an increase in medication.

However, this is a communication failure because of what the clinician has taken for granted. Dr. Aronow assumes his patient is taking 20 mg of lisinopril daily. In reality, Mr. Kruger has not been taking medication regularly at all. He suspects his blood pressure is artificially inflated at the clinic, particularly when he checks in with Martha, a medical assistant who has chastised him in the past for being late and whom he doesn't particularly like. Furthermore, blood pressure readings at home are averaging closer to 140/90. He considers himself in good health, exercises regularly, and feels well. When he starting taking lisinopril he had occasional bouts of lightheadedness that interfered with work. He is also afraid of what taking blood pressure medication means for his employment status, insurance eligibility, and self-image.[12] Rather than addressing these concerns with the doctor, he avoids the subject.

In this scenario, the communication failure is a *missed opportunity* for clinical negotiation. Assuming that the current lisinopril dose was ineffective, Dr. Aronow summarily increased the dose. In his haste to drive this "routine" visit to its conclusion, the physician missed important nonverbal cues (avoiding eye contact, neutral facial expression, verbal hesitancy). In turn, the patient failed to speak up about his concerns about medication side effects, did not ask about alternative treatment options, did not share his discomfort with being labeled as "sick," and did not ask about alternative treatments.

Communication is a two-way street. Both clinician and patient share responsibility for the outcome in this vignette. Mr. Kruger needed to more openly express his concerns about taking medication and enduring its side effects. Doctors know their patients better and can more accurately predict what patients are feeling and thinking when patients ask questions, state preferences, express opinions, and share concerns.[13-15] Mr. Kruger's silence was, in this case, poisonous. But Dr. Aronow's manner didn't help. **While the patient has the responsibility to speak up, the clinician needs to foster a communicative environment that promotes active patient participation.**[16] This requires a trusting patient-clinician relationship, one where both parties are comfortable talking openly and honestly with one another and where the patient is confident that the clinician is technically competent, interpersonally skilled, and invested in the patient's well-being.[17]

Trust is more readily established in existing patient-clinician relationships where there is already a history of positive interactions. For new patients, the onus on clinicians is greater: they need to communicate explicitly in a way that the patient interprets as, "I am here to help, I want to know what you think, and I am interested in what you have to say." This is accomplished through verbal statements (paraphrasing, asking "what else?"), paralinguistic utterances ("uh huh"), and nonverbal encouragement (friendly facial expressions, eye contact, listening without interruption, remaining silent).

In addition, clinicians can explicitly invite the patient to talk about their concerns, needs, and wants, drawing on techniques that are variously called partnership-building, soliciting the patient's agenda, and asking for the patient's story. Examples include statements such as "So how are things going with the..." "What concerns or questions do you have?" "Tell me more about that" and silence. Statements and questions that seek to elicit the patient's perspective are powerful communication strategies because they (a) explicitly communicate interest in what the patient has to say and (b) they invoke conversational norms for a response (i.e., something that counts as an "answer" is expected to follow a "question").[18,19] Importantly, these should occur early in the consultation so there is time to address issues important to the patient. If the solicitation of the patient's perspectives does not occur until the end of the consultation, patients are more likely to interpret this as the doctor signaling the consultation is over. Although some patients may need no encouragement to speak up, patients are more likely to ask questions, state preferences, make requests, and express concerns when clinicians explicitly solicit these issues.[20,21]

A somewhat more structured approach to agenda setting and negotiation is provided in Table 4-1. This approach, borrowing heavily from the work of Baker et al.,[22] emphasizes establishing the patient's agenda, assessing the patient's priorities, blending the patient's priorities with the clinician's, and dealing with items still pending or incompletely resolved. The purpose is to reduce the risk of "not understanding" by making the full spectrum of patient concerns as visible as possible.

Had Dr. Aronow applied these techniques, the visit with Mr. Kruger might have taken a different course.

> *Mr. Kruger, a 45-year-old man with hypertension, has been taking 20 mg of lisinopril for the past 6 months. At this visit, the medical assistant records his blood pressure as 145/96. Dr. Aronow asks how things are going with the medication. Kruger replies "fine, for the most part." Dr. Aronow asks him to talk more about that. Mr. Kruger elaborates on how side effects at work create some problems. The doctor listens and validates these concerns as side effects some patients experience and offers suggestions for how to manage them. Sensing the doctor has some empathy toward his situation, Mr. Kruger discloses he does not like to take medication and doesn't think he needs them because blood pressure at home is lower than at the clinic.*

The stage is now set for effective clinical negotiation.

SECTION 4.5: MISUNDERSTANDING

If *not understanding* is a kind of *information void*, *misunderstanding* is *information chaos*. Signals are being exchanged, but the fidelity of information

Table 4-1 **A Practical Approach to Agenda Setting**

Task	Strategy	Sample Language*
Establish patient's agenda	Begin with open-ended question Follow-up Gently redirect if necessary	*What brings you to see us today?* OR *What sorts of troubles are concerning you today?* AND *What else did you want to discuss today?* OR *Other than problems x, y, and z, what else did you want to be sure we begin to address today?* OR *What else did you need to have taken care of today?* PLUS *We can get into that in a moment, but first I'd like to hear about the rest of your concerns.*
Assess patient's priorities	Acknowledge length of agenda Ask for patient's top priorities Assure that lower priorities will not be neglected or forgotten	*There are a lot of issues for us to address. What were you most hoping we could accomplish today?* OR *What were you hoping I might be able to do about that today?* OR *What is the one thing you want to be sure happens before you leave here today?* OR *I see that you have several concerns today. Can you tell me what goes on the top of your list?* AND *We can make a plan for handling the rest later.*
Articulate clinician's priorities and forge consensus	Express clinician's priorities while reassuring patient that their concerns have been heard Suggest a combined agenda Solicit patient agreement	*As you know, I asked you back so I could [redo parts of the physical exam; see how the new medicine is working; etc.], and I heard you say that you were quite concerned about your _____. AND* *If it's OK with you, I think we can [check the things I need to see], and then take a look at your _____. AND* *Sound reasonable?*
Forge plan for handling incomplete agenda items	Acknowledge successes and failures (items covered and not covered) Suggest a follow-up plan Solicit patient buy-in	*I think we've done justice to the agenda we agreed upon at the outset, and I want to be able to give similar attention to the items we've left out. AND* *I suggest that we make a follow-up appointment and then we can reassess how you are doing and evaluate these other concerns at the same time. AND* *Sound reasonable?*

*Adapted with minor alterations from Baker et al.[22]

exchange is compromised. Finding common ground, achieving shared understanding, and reaching agreement mandate that clinicians and patients use a common language or "code" to create understanding. The most obvious way this process collapses is when the two speak entirely different languages (e.g., the clinician speaks only English, the patient only Spanish). But failure to establish a common communication code can occur easily enough even when clinician and patient both speak the language. In such instances, fault-finding is hazardous and ultimately unproductive. For example, if a patient is convinced that she need only take medicine for "high blood" when she is feeling "tense," the clinician might attribute such beliefs to poor health literacy and conclude that the patient does not have the requisite biomedical understanding for adequately managing her disease. However, one might just as easily argue the reverse, the doctor does not have sufficient "patient literacy" to understand the patient's perspective on health and wellness. **Two interlocking factors that contribute to limitations in communicative capacity are "not knowing the meaning of the words" and "not knowing what the words are meaning."**

The meaning of words

A prerequisite for effective clinician negotiation is that clinicians and patients use language each understands. This, of course, is a significant concern in settings where clinicians and patients speak different languages or cannot find a common language. Language discordance requires use of interpreters, which in turn adds another layer of complexity to clinical negotiation; now there are at least three parties who need to reach shared understanding.

In addition, the jargon of medicine is, in effect, a communication code with which many patients will have little or no familiarity. For example, if a patient appears confused when the doctor says, "the imaging shows a pulmonary nodule that could represent a malignant lesion," the patient may be confused about what "imaging," "pulmonary," "nodule," "malignant," or "lesion" even mean. Hence clinicians should steer clear of jargon-laden speech that patients may not understand. The jargon-tolerance threshold will depend largely on the patient's linguistic repertoire. For example, a laborer with a sixth-grade education, an accountant who frequently consults "Dr. Google," and an intensive care nurse will have variable familiarity with the technical language of medicine. **Thus, clinicians must have access to a mental dictionary of everyday language that is accessible to a spectrum of patients.**

Even experts struggle with this. Here is Medline Plus trying to explain diabetes in everyday language (https://medlineplus.gov/diabetestype2.html):

Diabetes means your blood glucose, or blood sugar levels are too high. With type 2 diabetes, the more common type, your body does not make or use insulin well. Insulin is a hormone that helps glucose get into your cells to give them energy. Without insulin, too much glucose stays in your blood. Over time, high blood glucose can lead to serious problems with your heart, eyes, kidneys, nerves, and gums and teeth.

The word processor on which this chapter was composed puts the Flesch-Kincaid reading level for this paragraph from Medline Plus at half way through sixth grade. And yet, can the average sixth-grader explain what sugar is doing in the blood; what a hormone is; why "cells" need energy; or—most importantly—why it is important to keep the blood sugar controlled throughout the day, day after day? Language comprehension may not translate into practical understanding.

What the words are saying

A more common problem is that patients and clinicians share a common language but have difficulty understanding each other because of different connotative and contextual framings of what individual words, phrases, and sentences mean. This occurs at several levels. **First, the same word can mean different things to the interactants.** For example, a clinician understands that a "positive" result for cancer is bad, whereas a patient may interpret positive as, well, "positive." In relating that "your LDL cholesterol of 137 mg/dl puts you at higher risk of a heart attack," the doctor means to convey that the patient's chance of a heart attack in the next 10 years is around 8%. This requires deliberate action but not panic; 92 of 100 patients like this one will *not* have a heart attack over the next decade. However, the patient may interpret "higher risk" to mean that a heart attack is inevitable.

Just as patients misconstrue doctors, doctors also misconstrue patients. The African-American patient complaining of "high blood" has hypertension, not polycythemia. The Cambodian patient with "wind" has fever and dizziness, not flatulence. The patient (of any ethnic background) who complains of "dizziness" might mean they are lightheaded, vertiginous, unsteady while walking, or emotionally overwhelmed.

Second, clinicians and patients may have difficulty finding words to adequately describe or explain something. This is different from not understanding what individual words mean, but rather what the words are referring to. For example, if a patient were to ask about what causes a fever and how common remedies work, only a clueless physician would respond:

"Fever is a complex physiologic response triggered by infectious or aseptic stimuli. Elevations in body temperature occur when concentrations of prostaglandin E(2) increase within certain areas of the brain. These elevations alter the firing rate of neurons that control thermoregulation in the hypothalamus. Although fever benefits the nonspecific immune response to invading microorganisms, it is also viewed as a source of discomfort and is commonly suppressed with antipyretic medication." [23]

The many technical terms aside (prostaglandin, aseptic, antipyretic, etc.), many patients (even among the most educated) will have difficulty mapping the words in this paragraph to their own internalized knowledge matrix in order to create meaning. The skilled clinical communicator will try to attach their explanation to some plausible version of the patient's experience. For example:

When your body fights something that's gotten into it, such as a germ or a bug bite, your internal thermostat (yes, you have one!) gets adjusted upwards. So instead of your internal thermostat getting set at 98.6, it gets set at 99.5 or 100.3. Drugs like aspirin and Tylenol reset the thermostat back towards normal.

Patients, too, may have difficulty finding language to unlock biographical memory or describe internal sensations. **When taking a medical history, clinicians operate as both interlocutors and interpreters.** Different patients may describe the same symptoms in any number of ways. Migraine headaches can be throbbing, pounding, twisting, sharp, or sickening. Patients with a feel for metaphor might say the headaches are like "a sharp stick poking in my eye, along with a profound urge to vomit." Those more divorced from their own subjective experience might describe them as simply "painful." Similarly, a patient with diabetes and coronary artery disease might say, "sometimes when I'm walking and it's hot outside, I start feeling woozy." The clinician can only wonder: is she describing vertigo, lightheadedness, disequilibrium, or panic, and do the sensations reflect hypoglycemia, heat exhaustion, a transient ischemic attack, or a cardiac arrhythmia?

Clinicians can help patients by encouraging them to elaborate upon their symptoms, nudging them to "go on in your own words" and to "tell as best you can what that experience was like for you." Some patients will be tempted to interpret, categorize, or self-diagnose, but they should be urged to resist: "I find it so helpful to hear in your own words what that felt like." Patients can help clinicians by encouraging them to slow down, eschew jargon, and tailor the depth of information provided to the patient's interests and need for cognition.[24] Other valuable communicative strategies include use of everyday language, repetition, examples, analogies, metaphors, illustrations, and educational materials.[25,26]

Deeper Dive 4.2: Mindful and Mindless Communication

Have you ever reflected on how people pull off conversations effortlessly and effectively? Consider everything people are doing while talking to one another—articulating words, forming nonverbal expressions, deciding what to say, making sense of what the other is saying and feeling, coordinating turn-taking, and working toward achieving the goals of the conversation. Communication is both mindful (deliberate) and mindless (subconscious or habitual). Given all the things we do as communicators, it is actually quite amazing that communication works so well so much of time.

John Greene's action assembly theory provides a useful framework for understanding how human thought "assembles" or produces communication behavior.[55] The model identifies four hierarchical levels of cognitive processing that connect what we want to talk about (the topic); how we talk about it (communication approach); and how we produce the words themselves (air flow; tongue, mouth, and lip movements). The model also provides insight into how communication succeeds and fails.

At the most abstract level of conversational cognition is the *interactional representation*. These are the cognitions representing the interaction-goal objectives for the interaction. These thoughts include what one wants to accomplish in the interaction, perceptions of the other interactant, and anticipated actions (communication) needed to accomplish the goals and purpose of the interaction. With clinical encounters, a clinician's objectives and strategies will vary when seeing a complex, difficult, and demanding patient compared with a well-known patient seeking preventive care. To tap a musical analogy, the interaction representation is the score (key, notes, tempo, etc.) for one song ("musical conversation") versus another.

Below the interactional representation is the *ideational level*. This represents the conversational moves, transitions, shifts, and adaptations designed to accomplish desired ends. In clinical negotiation, a clinician taking a tough, business-like stand with a patient requesting an unwarranted work release will change his or her approach and goal if that patient suddenly starts to weep. A clinician with a long-standing, friendly relationship with an HIV-infected patient will become more serious and stern if that patient discloses he is having unprotected sex with a new partner. In the context of music, ideational moves occur during improvisation as players takes turns performing riffs and runs in response to their bandmates.

The third level of communication production is the *utterance level*. This is where actual phonetic, syntactic, and lexical options are selected. Selection is followed by the actual set of motor commands producing sound and movement (words and behavior); this is the *sensorimotor level*. While one might imagine that thinking of what to say automatically produces the sounds of oral communication, the two processes can suffer interruptions, as when someone stutters, is heavily intoxicated, or when a person struggles with pronunciation when learning a new language.

These four levels of cognitive processing are hierarchically related, moving from the most abstract (interaction representation) to the most specific and physical (sensorimotor). People tend to be more mindful of the abstract cognitive processes and less aware of the more specific processing occurring at the utterance and sensorimotor levels. Much of the cognitive processing to produce behavior is top-down; that is, our understanding of the situation and what we hope to accomplish activates the communication approach and behavioral actualization of what we say and do in the encounter. For example, a clinician's communication approach during a follow-up visit with a patient with diabetes is different from his or her approach when seeing a patient likely to have the flu: different situations, different goals, different patients, different communication behaviors (e.g., what questions to ask, what information to provide), and different negotiation strategies.

Yet cognitive processing can also be bottom-up. For example, a clinician might have a hard time pronouncing Mr. Zbigniew's last name. This specific sensorimotor failure creates self-consciousness, leading to use of a different salutation: "Hello Mr. Z. Good to see you." Similarly, at the ideational level, a clinician might struggle to respond to a patient's question about how ACE inhibitors work. To develop a reasonable interactional representation, the doctor must simultaneously make sense of what the patient is saying while also inventorying her own repertoire of available explanations.

The mindful (deliberate, conscious) and mindless (automatic, subconscious) aspects of communication are the yin and yang of communication competence. Given the complexities of all that is going on behaviorally, cognitively, and emotionally as we communicate, it is to one's advantage to have much of the communication automated or scripted in a way that it can be efficiently and effectively deployed to move the conversation forward. More attention can then be given to situational awareness, monitoring the patient's reaction, thinking about how to explain things, and developing treatment recommendations that fit the patient's condition and preferences.

Communication, and thus negotiation, will "fail" if there are broken links between the different levels of communication behavior production. In the midst of stalled clinical negotiations, self-aware clinicians may find themselves bereft of 1) a reasonable *communication approach*, as might happen when confronting unexplained symptoms or a demanding patient (interaction representation); 2) a sense of how to *respond appropriately* to unexpected or emotive behavior such as a contraindicated request or crying (ideational level); or 3) the *actual words* needed to convey information or offer comfort, such as when explaining a serious diagnosis (utterance level).

To develop a versatile toolbox of communication practices that have interchangeable parts—leading to effortless, effective, and ongoing adaptation over the course of the encounter—requires *practice* and *experience*. Just as public speakers become better the more times they lecture before different audiences, so do clinicians become more effective communicators the more interactions they have with different patients. Yet there is a caveat to the practice makes perfect analogy: clinicians can trip up badly if the communicative "script" (interaction representation) overrides situational awareness of patient clues—subtle hints of emotional distress, lack of understanding, helplessness, or resistance—that would inform a need to adapt one's communication to further the overarching goals of the encounter.

Clues to misunderstanding

Despite the clinician's best efforts, misunderstandings can and do occur. The question is how to resolve them. The first step is to recognize that a misunderstanding exists. **Clues to misunderstandings can be placed on a continuum from the obvious and explicit to the more subtle and implicit (Figure 4-1).** At one end of the spectrum are explicit clues, such as when one party draws attention to a gap in clarity by saying "I'm not sure what you mean," "Can you clarify that?," "Can you give me an example?," or perhaps most directly, "I don't understand." The same message can be conveyed nearly as plainly through prominent nonverbal reactions (e.g., blank stares, raised eyebrows). In the middle are nonverbal signals manifest in facial expressions indicating confusion, inattention, or lack of interest. At the far end of the spectrum are situations where the only clue is no clue at all. Here the clinician and patient proceed as if absolutely nothing is untoward. And from their vantage point there isn't—until the consequences of the buried misunderstanding become manifest.

    Wherever they are located on the spectrum of explicitness, clues to misunderstanding (and "not understanding" as well) will be more accessible to clinicians who are situationally attentive, undistracted, open to experience, and curious—a mental stance some have described as constituting *mindfulness*. Though mindfulness may be as much a virtue as a skillset (perhaps akin to "equanimity"),[27] "[mindful practice] can be modeled by mentors and cultivated in learners."[28] Clinicians who are so inclined can find many helpful articles, books, and courses on the topic.[29]

    As is likely clear by now, it is almost always a mistake to take understanding for granted, for as often as not, understanding will be far shallower than thought. **All clinicians should routinely check for understanding, especially when it comes to information the clinician considers critical**. There are several proven communication strategies for checking in, including the "teach back" and "tell-ask-tell" techniques.[30,31] With both approaches, clinicians

	Explicit	⟹	Subtle	⟹	Buried
Verbal Indicator	"I don't understand"	"Could you repeat that?"	"I see." (expressed hesitantly)	"Hm."	None
Nonverbal Indicator	Prominent raised eyebrows, bilateral shoulder shrug	Intense concentration (or distraction), lip biting	Furrowed brow, delayed verbal response	Verbal-nonverbal asynchrony	None

Figure 4-1. Spectrum of clues to misunderstanding along continuum of explicitness.

ask patients to summarize or paraphrase the clinician's instructions. Nuances matter, though, because casual deployment of these techniques can come off as patronizing or condescending. If the doctor commands the patient to "Now, explain back what I just told you," or asks "Ok, what are you going to do after you leave the clinic," the patient may feel embarrassed, belittled, or simply put-off. Better phrasing might include: "So I have given you a lot of information. What did you find meaningful or important?" and "How does what I told you fit with what you are thinking?' "Do you have any questions about the next steps?" These questions allow patients the opportunity to talk about what they think and know, thereby providing clues as to where patients might need some reinforcing explanation or clarification.

Misunderstanding due to implicit bias

As we have seen, misunderstandings during the clinical negotiation commonly arise out of what we might call semantical gaps—failure to choose the right words or to attribute a common meaning to the same words. However, another important source of misunderstandings in clinical settings derives from one of three forms of bias:

- Prejudice, reflecting an overall evaluation of a group;
- Stereotyping, in which specific characteristics are attributed to a group; and
- Discrimination, which describes biased behavior towards a group and its members.[32]

In health care, bias is rarely explicit. Most clinicians would like to believe that they treat members of all groups with an equal measure of caring and respect. **Nonetheless, a large body of research indicates that all of us (clinicians and nonclinicians alike) are prone to *implicit bias*.** Implicit (unconscious) bias is manifest in assumptions people make towards others based on their size, color, gender, dress, dialect, sexual orientation, religion, or other group-level characteristic. Making assumptions about people based on their group membership can be a useful heuristic; they speed us towards a conclusion and are often enough correct. But they can also be wrong. The concern is that these assumptions (biases) can create inaccurate, simplistic, and unfairly negative (or positive) views of patients. These views can in turn degrade clinical care, especially for marginalized groups.[33,34]

For our purposes, we assume that clinicians and patients alike have implicit biases, the mutability of which varies across people. We also assume that the potential harmful effects of implicit biases can be attenuated by reflection (a cognitive strategy) and encouraging active patient engagement in the consultation (a communication strategy).

Consider this example:

Karen Smith, a 45-year-old African-American woman, is new in town and needs a primary care physician. She contacts Midtown Physician Associates, the only medical group taking new patients. They assign her to Dr. Fukuhara, a family physician 6 years out of residency. Prior to their initial encounter, Dr. Fukuhara reviews the patient's Personal History Form and sees that she has type 2 diabetes and hypertension. On examination she is obese, her clothing seems worn, and she emits a slightly unpleasant odor. The blood pressure is 145/92, and she has moderately severe onychomycosis of the toenails. Dr. Fukuhara assumes Mrs. Smith has little or no motivation to manage health, lacks health literacy, doesn't care about her weight, and is likely nonadherent to medical management.

In Scenario 1, Dr. Fukuhara begins the visit in a friendly way, asks how the patient is doing, and then starts the consultation by focusing on medical issues. He asks if she brought her medications so he can be sure she has the right ones. She did not bring her meds. He mentions the importance of lifestyle changes to manage weight. He states walking is a good way to exercise and that Mrs. Smith should try walking 2 miles a day. He takes out a piece of paper, draws a circle on it, and states that this is a plate, then then divides the plate into sections, pointing out which is the part for meat, which part for vegetables, and so forth. He orders a refill of the two medications and recommends she get a pillbox to help with adherence. He concludes the visit by asking Mrs. Smith if she any questions and hearing none, wishes her a good day.

The problem, unbeknownst to Dr. Fukuhara, is that Mrs. Smith is neither able nor willing to carry out his instructions.

How did this interaction go wrong? First, the physician's implicit biases related to race, appearance, weight, and comorbidities invoke a set of assumptions about Mrs. Smith's behavior, motivation, and intelligence. Based on this initial impression, Dr. Fukuhara conducts the consultation in a controlling, paternalistic manner. In turn, Mrs. Smith's passivity does nothing to redirect the course of the consultation.

In Scenario 2, Dr. Fukuhara begins the visit in a friendly way, asks how the patient is doing, and then starts the consultation by focusing on medical issues. However, Mrs. Jones interjects an answer to the question of how she is doing before he goes further. She states that she is doing pretty well, but is still battling side effects of diabetes management. She discloses a lifelong struggle with weight, something that runs in her family, which complicates management of diabetes and hypertension. However, she has enjoyed some recent successes, managing to lose 40 pounds over the past 8 months with the help of an online support group. However, periodic episodes of hypoglycemia have become more frequent. She says she has been taking metformin and glipizide, but believes the meds need to be adjusted to address the hypoglycemia. She makes suggestions for what she thinks the doses should be. Finally, she apologizes for being curt. She reveals that she is tired because she was up most of the night at the Emergency Department with a resident of the homeless shelter where she volunteers; the resident was having a psychotic episode. As a registered nurse at a local high school, she thought she would be the best person to be there with the resident.

In this scenario Dr. Fukuhara's initial impressions of Mrs. Smith are dramatically altered, and the consultation unfolds in a very different way.

Implicit bias can contribute to communication failures when biased attitudes lead to presumptive judgments that 1) influence the clinician's

conduct of the consultation and 2) go unchecked. Because most medical consultations, like most interpersonal interactions, are processes of mutual influence, the communicative actions of one participant (e.g., the patient's active communication style) will have an effect on what the other interactant thinks and does (e.g., a physician allowing greater involvement and control by an activated patient). Of course, if a clinician is so strongly bigoted that there is little the patient can do to alter a stereotypic impression, that is another problem (and beyond the scope of this book).

The theme of mutual influence—already mentioned in the context of social and cultural factors impacting the clinical negotiation—is critical here. To drill down on this idea, we focus briefly on the topic of race. Numerous studies have shown disparities in the quality of technical care (as measured objectively) and interpersonal care (as reported on surveys) when comparing African-American patients with White patients.[35,36] Patient-centered communication is associated with better adherence and health outcomes. Physicians are more patient-centered when patients shower them with positive affect and are more involved in their care. African-Americans are somewhat less likely to display positive affect and to engage actively in care. However, these effects are mitigated when African-American patients are matched with African-American physicians.[37–39] **The good clinician treats everyone the same. The *very* good clinician tries to create an atmosphere where patients feel comfortable asserting themselves, knowing that additional effort may be needed when the clinician and patient are not a racial, ethnic, cultural, and/or linguistic match.**

Misunderstanding due to social distance

During the COVID-19 (coronavirus) pandemic, many of us have become painfully familiar with the term "social distance." But using the term to describe "telecommuting" or "sheltering in place" is really a misnomer, since the distancing advocated by public health authorities during epidemics is *physical*, not social. **Social distance refers to the degree of intermixing—or remoteness—between social groups, defined by factors such as age, race, ethnicity, socioeconomic status, politics, or culture.** The term encompasses not only who spends time with whom but also the degree to which individuals engage as equals and share common beliefs. Social distance exists on a continuum within multi-dimensional space, so that two individuals might be very close with respect to socioeconomic status but very far apart in their politics, or perhaps share nearly congruous religious beliefs but hold different views on the value of immunization. Clinicians will of course have more in common with some patients than others on the basis of gender, education, race, ethnicity, or perhaps a mutual love of sports or music. Sometimes the match is perfect. Sometimes clinicians and patients may share little other than a common humanity.

This is often but not always enough. Over the long haul, patients who have a choice tend to sortthemselves into practices where there is a modicum of mutual compatibility. This is one reason why continuity of care has been associated with increased patient satisfaction.[40] In the shorter term, it is the physician's responsibility to seek out commonalities and build bridges where possible and to carry on in the patient's best interests when not.

In *The Spirit Catches You and You Fall Down*, author Anne Fadiman describes the decades-long odyssey of a Hmong child with seizures in a small Central California city. The child's doctors try to save her but fail, in part because of the vast cultural chasm separating Western medicine from Hmong folk beliefs. But cultural gaps like this are relatively infrequently encountered in daily practice. More common are patients whose views of health and illness are molded in the crucible of their own experience. For example, in a series of interviews, Sharf et al. asked lung cancer patients why they had refused recommended tests and treatments. Some representative responses:

- "It's an itty bitty spot and I'm a big man."
- "Doctors have a bad habit of wanting to experiment...to find out things. They don't really care about you."
- "Sometimes miracles happen. You have to have faith and believe. If you don't believe nothing will get better."
- "I have lung cancer and found out exercising is real good for lung cancer. I'm doing much better. Almost back to normal."

From the medical perspective these comments seem unfounded. But to the patients themselves they are serious and credible. As discussed in Chapter 1, beliefs like these are rooted in patients' mental representations of illness. A mental representation or model represents how someone organizes knowledge and experience to make sense of the world. It is composed of cognitions (what I know), affect (how I feel), motives (what I want), and causation/forecasting (why I think something happened; what I think will happen). A mental model of health invokes health-related content. These mental models represent a web of cognition and attitudes related to various aspects of health and health care and represent a person's health-related experiences, beliefs, feelings, preferences, and goals.

By working backwards from what these patients with lung cancer *say*, we can make inferences about their underlying mental models.

- The first patient sees cancer as a problem of current proportion (small lesion, big man) and not as a future threat;
- The second patient is dissuaded from undergoing treatment by global distrust of the medical profession;
- The third patient believes that valuing faith means discounting medical evidence and practice; and
- The fourth patient privileges information gained from outside sources above medical advice, and he washes down what he thinks he knows with a big swig of denial.

Most medical and nursing practitioners trained in the modern era would undoubtedly consider beliefs like these not just factually inaccurate but medically dangerous. Yet within the patient's own frame of reference, these beliefs make sense. Tiny spots are not a threat to a strong person, doctors don't always have the patient's best interests in mind, God performs miracles, and exercise keeps you healthy.

The notion that clinicians and patients differ in terms of their goals and preferences has been demonstrated in clinical areas as diverse as chronic pain,[41] diabetes,[42] cardiovascular disease, cancer, obstetrics-gynecology, and acute respiratory illness.[43,44] In one of our own studies, patients and physicians assessed various health beliefs centered on biomedical causation, fault, control, effectiveness of "natural" treatments, importance, and preferences for partnership. Patients and physicians differed significantly across all seven dimensions, with patients generally scoring higher (e.g., patients rated the impact/importance of their condition higher than physicians).[45] The only domain in which physicians scored higher than patients was the belief that the condition had a plausible biomedical explanation.

Yet while gaps exist, they are not unbridgeable. Models of causation can be discussed. Feelings of being at fault or out of control can be soothed. Complementary and alternative treatments can, when unlikely to be harmful, be endorsed. The personal significance of symptoms and conditions can be established through sympathetic questioning. And well-established partnership-building behaviors (e.g., soliciting the patient's opinion, providing reassurance and encouragement) can be deployed.[16]

SECTION 4.6: DISAGREEMENTS

As we have seen, many communication failures in clinical practice arise from what is *not* said or understood ("not understanding") and from what is *mis*-articulated or *mis*-interpreted ("misunderstanding"). **However, there are times when differences in attitudes, beliefs, goals, or preferences are crystal clear, yet patient and clinician disagree.** In these instances, communication fails because the two parties cannot resolve differences of opinion. Table 4-2 provides examples of clinical conflict across multiple domains, showing not only the opposing views of patients and clinicians but their corresponding rationales.

In these examples, clinicians may very well attribute the totality of the conflict to the patient's misconstrual of the facts, hidden motives, ignorance, or stubbornness. However, clinicians contribute to these clashes through their own beliefs and actions. Sometimes the clinician's missteps result from lack of relevant clinical experience or slippery grasp of the evidence. And sometimes they are born of arrogance or inflexibility. However, as self-help author Melodie Beattie says, "We cannot change others, but when we change ourselves, we may end up changing the world." So while both clinicians and patients are responsible for working cooperatively to reconcile differences of opinion, we focus on the provider side. **Regardless of what the patient brings to the table, what clinicians think and how they act can make the difference between successful negotiation and communicative disaster.**

Table 4-2 Examples of Patient-Clinician Disagreements

Topic	Patient's View (Rationale)	Clinician's View (Rationale)
Treatment of child's fever and putative ear infection	Wants antibiotics (thinks this will get child back into day care faster, so parent won't have to miss work)	Wants to treat symptomatically (believes antibiotics are unnecessary and possibly harmful for what is most likely a viral infection)
Treatment of chronic pain	Wants opioids (most powerful pain treatment)	Wants to deploy alternatives first (concerned about opioid side effects and addiction)
Cancer screening	"Forgets" to attend mammography appointment (waffles between thinking the test unnecessary and worrying about what the test might show)	Irked that patient is not doing her part (worried for patient's health as well as clinician's own HEDIS statistics)
Evaluation of headache	Wants MRI (concerned about brain tumor)	Prefers expectant management (feels clinical likelihood of tumor very low)
Work release	Wants work release for minor musculoskeletal injury (concerned about reinjury and also needs break from "toxic" boss)	Reluctant to issue release (can see no obvious medical justification)
Smoking cessation	In "pre-contemplative" stage (has never had a problem from smoking; grandmother smoked and lived to 94)	If legally permitted, would discharge patient from practice (disinterest in smoking cessation signals patient's neglect of his health)
Safer alcohol consumption	Enjoys 3-5 drinks per day, more on weekends (sees no evident harm, and drinking with friends is focal point of patient's social life)	Recommends enlisting in alcohol cessation program (notes early signs of liver disease)
Childhood vaccination	Parent wants to defer MMR booster (has read that too many vaccines in close succession can harm a child)	In absence of a valid medical reason, insists on vaccination according to standard schedule (concerned about resurgent pockets of measles elsewhere in state)

Here are some **common clinician errors**.

- **Assuming that the doctor is right.** This assumption is understandable, and not just because some clinicians have sizeable egos. Personality aside, clinicians often have the medical knowledge and experience to accurately assess patients' health and direct their health needs. Yet approaching a problem with this mindset undermines effective negotiation; it is instead likely to result in a "loss" for the clinician because it leads to a patient's resistance, silence, and nonadherence. Patients may very well be "right" in two respects. First, they have access to information (e.g., Internet, family) that offers a credible alternative interpretation (e.g., hypertension is a result of anxiety and not diet). Second, while patients may not know what constitutes "normal" within a population, they may be quite knowledgeable of what is normal for *them*. Medical science is slowly catching up to this idea. For example, the classic fever threshold of 100 degrees Fahrenheit fails to account for inter- and intraindividual variability, and there is a growing literature in support of adjusting the threshold based on the individual's average temperature and the time of day.[46] The patient who claims, "Doc, I have a fever" when the thermometer at 8:30 am registers 98.6 degrees may be right!

- **Labeling the patient in a negative light.** Good faith negotiation is difficult when the clinician questions the patient's honesty, motivation, cognitive capacity, or character. Of course, it is a fact of life that some patients (as human beings) are indeed difficult, resistant, and even "hateful." Even so, the clinician is better served by reflecting than reacting. For one thing, as Groves asserts:

Negative feelings about . . . patients constitute important clinical data about the patient's psychology. When the patient creates in the doctor feelings that are disowned or denied, errors in diagnosis and treatment are more likely to occur. Disavowal of hateful feelings requires less effort than bearing them. But such disavowal wastes clinical data that may be helpful in treating the "hateful patient."[47]

Reflection—especially when accompanied by genuine curiosity about what the patient is going through—can transform anger into empathy and defensiveness into openness. Jodi Halpern has argued that clinical empathy has two components: *cognitive* (which involves curiosity and perspective taking) and *communicative* (which involves affectively attuned empathic communication).[48] When clinical empathy is achieved, good things happen, including detectable alterations in brain function and improved patient-reported outcomes.[49,50]

When clinicians jump to conclusions about patients too quickly, they risk closing themselves off to new information, responding in a reactive fashion, and missing opportunities for empathic connection.

- **Skirting the patient's best interests.** Notwithstanding the ethereal pronouncements of medical ethicists and academicians, there is hardly ever a time when clinicians act *solely* in the patient's best interests. Medicine always involves a *balancing* of interests: of self and other, of individual and population, of this patient and the next patient. The doctor *fully* committed to an individual patient's welfare would never leave that patient's bedside except to eat and sleep (certainly not to see another patient), and would (if she could) marshal infinite resources on that patient's behalf. This is not how doctors operate in practice, and for good reason: the physician's responsibilities begin with the individual but do not end there.

Deeper Dive 4.3: Lying and Deception: Do Clinicians Know If Patients Are Not Telling the Truth?

Effective clinical negotiation requires that clinicians and patients communicate openly and honestly with one another. However, personally sensitive topics such as substance use, medication adherence, sexual function, and depression are subjects about which patients sometimes shade, mischaracterize, or suppress the facts. (Clinicians do not always tell patients the truth either, but that is a separate matter.) Cues to deception are not as explicit as in the story of Pinocchio. Hence, a question of importance in clinical negotiation is, "How do we know if a patient is not telling the truth or not telling us the whole story?"

There is a large academic literature on nonverbal cues to deception. This literature has proved popular with the broader culture. The Fox television show, *Lie to Me*, for example, was inspired by the classic work of psychologist Paul Ekman.[56] The show portrays the escapades of Dr. Cal Lightman, who almost magically detects lying and truth-telling by closely analyzing body language and microfacial expressions. For those seeking to emulate Dr. Lightman, YouTube has dozens of clips on how to recognize deception by deciphering nonverbal behaviors such as lip twitches, eye narrowing, fidgeting, gaze aversion, pouting, hesitant speech, nostril flares, and filled pauses ("uh," "umm").

Unfortunately, there is a fundamental problem with trying to map these nonverbal behaviors onto lying. As noted by Joe Navarro in his blog for *Psychology Today*,[57] these nonverbal behaviors may indicate deception—but just as often represent some degree of psychological distress or discomfort such as nervousness, fear, embarrassment, upset, or preoccupation. When people are generating a spontaneous lie, they may display these behaviors because they are experiencing two kinds of stress: 1) conjuring up a fabrication (because they do not have a real experience to describe) and 2) committing a socially unacceptable act. Conversely, people who have prepared lies, or have been using the same lies over a period of time, can pull off the falsehood without any hint of deception because they are familiar with the made-up story.

Because nonverbal "tells" are neither sensitive nor specific for lying, a more useful question is perhaps what leads clinicians to *think* a patient is not being honest or forthcoming. In the mid 2000s, Charles Bond and Bella DePaulo conducted two meta-analyses of research on factors affecting accuracy in detecting lies and individual differences in perceptions of lying versus truth-telling.[58] On average, people correctly identified lies just over 50% of the time, and their accuracy depended on the medium (communication channel). People hearing voice only (as in an audio-recording) were the most accurate, followed by those watching audiovisual presentations; least accurate were those watching someone without sound. A casual insouciance seemed to support successful deception: participants were least likely to believe people they perceived as *trying hardest* to be credible. In the companion paper, Bond and DePaulo[59] examined additional predictors of whether someone was *perceived* to be telling the truth. They concluded, as anyone who has played any serious poker knows, that some people are better liars than others. In addition, the strongest predictor of whether one person believes another is the judge's *a priori* assessment of the narrator's credibility. If you believe someone is an honest person, you interpret what they say as truthful.

What are the implications of deception research for effective clinical negotiation? First, clinicians should be aware that whether or not they think a patient is telling the truth is largely determined by what they think of the patient's character. A "responsible" patient will be believed more than a "frustrating" one. Second, some patients are very good liars, others not so much, and it is difficult to accurately assess truth-telling based on nonverbal leakage alone. Finally, even if non verbal behaviors are poor predictors of deception, these behaviors are worth noticing because they may indicate psychological distress or discomfort in need of subsequent probing and validation.

Nevertheless, commitment to the welfare of patients is at the heart of medical professionalism, and being *unduly* influenced by external factors is not only ethically suspect but will inevitably degrade the likelihood of successful clinical negotiation. For example, the doctor who "churns" patients to generate additional resource-based relative value units (RVUs) is sacrificing the chance to create more secure physician-patient relationships. The physician who cuts off a critical conversation (e.g., while revealing a life-changing diagnosis) in order to stay on schedule may be undercutting that patient's resilience just when he needs it most. The clinician who accedes to a patient's unjustified request for advanced imaging may not only be putting that patient at risk of unpredictable "cascade effects"[51] but might be inadvertently subjecting future clinicians to similarly strident demands, this time reinforced by the contention that "my other doctor did the PET scan once a year, why can't you?"

SECTION 4.6: CASE STUDIES IN "FAILED" COMMUNICATION: AVOIDING AND OVERCOMING ERRORS

Communication failure is as much a part of human discourse as communication success. Health care is no exception; it's just that the consequences of failure are often weightier than in ordinary life. **Using the case study method, we now explore three examples of communication failure, emphasizing how things went wrong and how they might have been made right.** As the examples illustrate, communication failures can be overt or subtle. Either way, they undermine effective clinical negotiation and so need to be identified, addressed, and prevented.

Case 1

Carrie Midland, a 27-year-old woman with cerebral palsy who uses a wheelchair, presents to urgent care with symptoms she ascribes to a UTI. Her medical record is not available. Dr. Kovar greets the patient and learns of her presenting complaint. Ms. Midland's speech is slurred and output is slow, but the content is coherent. On questioning, she relates that she has had three similar episodes over the past 2 years, each time treated successfully with Bactrim® (trimethoprim-sulfa). Dr. Kovar agrees that her symptoms are consistent with a UTI. He then adds, "But before we decide how to treat this, can you tell me about your neurologic condition?" Ms. Midland's demeanor immediately changes. She becomes angry and says, "That's not why I'm here." Dr. Kovar apologizes, orders a urinalysis and culture, and prescribes trimethoprim-sulfa. He then slinks out of the room feeling awful, and when the culture results come back confirming an E. coli urinary tract infection sensitive to trimethoprim-sulfa, he decides no further contact with the patient is necessary. Ms. Midland recovers but makes a note to avoid Dr. Kovar in the future.

The communication failure here is Dr. Kovar's insensitivity to the stigma Ms. Midland has experienced during her life with cerebral palsy. Although Dr. Kovar had good intentions to learn more about his patient's health from her perspective, he was not "mindful" of how his question might be perceived by a person living with this condition. In many ways, his line of inquiry resembles a doctor asking a patient, "Tell me more about your weight" or "Tell me more about how you got AIDS." The good news is that Dr. Kovar recognizes the offense, is embarrassed, and is less likely to make the same mistake in the future.

In fairness, however, Ms. Midland also shares some responsibility for this communication failure. Although her angry reaction was understandable given her long experience interacting with people who were uncomfortable being around her and who treated her as handicapped, the encounter with Dr. Kovar could have ended better had she made the point assertively, but without anger. The point is that communication failures occur because of the communication choices of all the participants. In this instance, Dr. Kovar started down the wrong path.

Case 2

Georgia Collins is a 57-year-old woman who works as a high-ranking appointed official in state government. Due to a change in health insurance, she recently switched her care to Neighborhood Health, a large multispecialty group with offices near her home, and she was assigned to Dr. Angela Trivedi, a recent graduate of the nearby academic medical center's internal medicine residency program. Ms. Collins has a history of hypertension, dyslipidemia, intermittent insomnia, and retinal detachment (repaired but with some unilateral loss of vision). Medications include atenolol, atorvastatin, and zolpidem as needed. Examination shows blood pressure 152/94 and diminished visual acuity (20/50 corrected) on the right, but is otherwise unremarkable. Dr. Trivedi asks, "Is everything going ok with your current medicines?"; Ms. Collins says, "Yes, fine." Dr. Trivedi explains that atenolol may not be the best medicine based on "lots of studies that show no mortality benefit in patients with high blood pressure." Dr. Trivedi states she'd like to start amlodipine instead, mentioning that the only common side effect is "some minor ankle swelling." Ms. Collins is somewhat nonplussed, as she has been on atenolol for many years without incident, and she wonders whether this young doctor knows what she is doing. Nevertheless, she agrees to try the new medicine and to return for follow-up in 1 month.

After a week on amlodipine, Ms. Collins notices her ankles and lower legs are swollen to the point where she cannot put on her dress shoes for work. She stops the medicine and restarts her remaining atenolol. She is angry that Dr. Trivedi switched her medicine and decides to seek another primary care physician.

On one level, Dr. Trivedi's conduct in this case was impeccable. She identifies an opportunity to improve the patient's blood pressure care, she explains her reasoning, and she obtains patient consent. She even warns the patient of ankle swelling. However, Ms. Collins experiences more swelling than expected (or more than she can tolerate), switches back to atenolol, and asks for another primary care physician.

The communication failure here is subtle but significant, and both parties are responsible. As mentioned earlier in this chapter, clinicians are not the only party that may have implicit (or explicit) biases—patients have biases as well. In this case, Ms. Collins, a middle-aged, highly educated, and prominent state government official, questions the competence of a newly minted, much younger doctor. Ms. Collins liked her prior physician and is disgruntled by the recent insurance-related disruption in continuity-of-care. Before the visit even begins, Ms. Collins eyes Dr. Trevedi with suspicion.

For her part, Dr. Trivedi makes several strategic communication missteps during the consultation. She should have been mindful of how patients from an older generation may perceive younger physicians. She should have been more aware that someone who has had to switch health plans may be disappointed, angry, and anxious, especially if that patient has significant health concerns or multiple comorbidities. Very importantly, Dr. Trivedi did not make an effort to get to know her patient and to provide an adequate opportunity for the patient to get to know her. Although she did ask Ms. Collins how she was doing with her medications and what she thought about changing them, Dr. Trivedi did not follow up on Ms. Collins' laconic response. Dr. Trivedi failed to consider Ms. Collins' perspective on her medications, which might be summarized as "why change things when what I'm taking is working just fine." Finally, Dr. Trevedi "lost" this clinical negotiation because she neither made an adequate case for switching medicines nor followed up sufficiently to understand and address Ms. Collins' reticence.

The unfortunate result is that Ms. Collins believes:

- That Dr. Trivedi changed her blood pressure medicine unnecessarily;
- That this change resulted in unacceptable side effects; and
- That Dr. Trivedi may simply be too inexperienced to be trusted.

Case 3, Part 1

Mr. Armstrong is a 62-year-old man who suffers from a number of chronic health problems, including COPD, congestive heart failure with preserved ejection fraction, coronary artery disease, chronic low back pain, and a history of methamphetamine use. Although currently living in a board and care facility, he is intermittently homeless. He frequently fails to attend scheduled appointments at the primary care center. Two years ago, Mr. Armstrong came under the care of Dr. Harris, a newly hired female internist. Prior to that time, he had been assigned to Dr. Abella, who showed little interest in working with nonadherent patients. Mr. Armstrong also misses appointments with Dr. Harris. However, after each missed appointment, Dr. Harris calls to check on his status. Each time, Mr. Armstrong assures the doctor that he "is hanging in there," asks for a refill of his chronic pain medications (tramadol and gabapentin), and explains that he missed the appointment because "I had to take care of some things— sometimes life just gets in the way." He promises to make another appointment. Mr. Armstrong and Dr. Harris are both African-American, and despite Mr. Armstrong's inconsistent adherence, Dr. Harris remains optimistic that Mr. Armstrong's chronic health problems can be brought under better control.

From an effective clinical negotiation perspective, this is a challenging case at multiple levels. A patient like Mr. Armstrong no doubt evokes a wide spectrum of reactions that will vary from physician to physician. Dr. Abella believed that Mr. Armstrong lacked motivation to take care of himself, engaged in drug-seeking behavior, and faced insurmountable social and economic barriers. Dr. Abella therefore wrote Mr. Armstrong off as a lost cause. Communication failed from the start because Dr. Abella became discouraged and gave up. While potentially understandable as a manifestation of statistically grounded pessimism, professional burnout, or even clinical depression, Dr. Abella's reaction precludes effective clinical negotiation. Finding common ground is simply not possible when the clinician attributes missed appointments and requests for pain medications as manifestations of poor character and questionable motives.

Dr. Harris, in contrast, is more hopeful. However, a positive attitude is, by itself, insufficient for effective clinical negotiation. Mr. Armstrong, for whatever reasons, is clearly not doing his part. Yet Dr. Harris finds an opening. She reaches Mr. Armstrong by phone and convinces him to attend his scheduled medical appointments. This "baby step" may have required a combination of persuasion ("I really want to see you in clinic—it's very important that I have a chance to check your blood pressure and listen to your lungs"), self-efficacy enhancement ("You have been able to keep some appointments in the past, so I know you can do it"), and practical assistance ("I'll ask our social worker about bus passes"). At his next appointment, Dr. Harris learns that Mr. Armstrong is struggling with a number of medical and life events. She asks him to elaborate about "having to take care of some things" and "life getting in the way." Whether because Dr. Harris communicates a genuine interest in his well-being, or because she also is African-American, or both, Mr. Armstrong opens up about his situation.

Armstrong discloses that he was laid off from his job as a dishwasher at a local restaurant when he missed work because of his back pain. He is depressed about the fact that his estranged son has refused to see him in over 2 years. He also confesses, "No offense doc, but it's hard to trust doctors. My wife died in the ER 5 years ago because they waited too long to get to her. And my last doctor didn't seem to like me or care about me." Dr. Harris acknowledges his feelings, reassures him she is there to take care of him, and engages in some limited self-disclosure—sharing that her dad had a very hard time when her mother passed away, but that gradually he reconnected with his community and felt better.[52] Dr. Harris then transitions to how addressing his health conditions can help him feel better. She discusses several options for pain management that may help his back pain and improve everyday functioning. Together they work out a reasonable pill-taking schedule, and they both agree on a pain management regimen that includes gradual tapering of tramadol.

In this example, Dr. Harris averts the communication failures experienced by Dr. Abella because Mr. Armstrong feels heard and understood. Clinician and patient worked collaboratively to devise a treatment plan that was consistent with the clinical evidence and practical given the patient's current circumstances and needs. Communication failure was avoided because Dr. Harris and Mr. Armstrong worked together in good faith to create shared understanding and agreement on a plan of action.

But then....

<u>**Case 3, Part 2**</u>

After 8 weeks following the visit with Dr. Harris, Mr. Armstrong notes worsening of his chronic lower extremity edema over the past week; last night he was somewhat short of breath. He calls the clinic for a same-day appointment. On arrival at the clinic, his heart rate is 104, blood pressure 120/74. When greeted by Dr. Huang (the urgent care doc of the day), he frowns and says, "No offense, but where is <u>my</u> doctor?" Dr. Huang explains that Dr. Harris is unavailable today so he will be handling Mr. Armstrong's care. Mr. Armstrong asks, "Well call her so I can talk with her first." Dr. Huang says, "I'm sorry but that is against clinic policy since Dr. Harris is not on call." Mr. Armstrong angrily exclaims, "This place is full of it. You have an excuse for everything. You don't really care. I'm not sure why I even bother." After this brief exchange, Mr. Armstrong storms out of the office without being examined. Two days later he is admitted through the emergency department for an exacerbation of congestive heart failure.

Communication failed in this situation because Mr. Armstrong refused to cooperate and Dr. Huang was unable to accommodate. One could blame Mr. Armstrong for his refusal to see Dr. Huang, although his reaction can be explained by his distrust of health care providers and his disappointment in not being able to see "his" doctor, someone who finally cared about his well-being. One could blame Dr. Huang for citing clinic "policy" for not accommodating a request to call Dr. Harris. Dr. Huang's actions can be explained by his being caught off guard, needing to preserve workflow, and suddenly finding himself in a situation with which he had little experience. The outcome was not good.

In this scenario, the real failure is the missed opportunity to remediate. The situation in the clinic unfolded quickly. Nevertheless, Dr. Huang could have attempted to call Dr. Harris to explain the situation and get advice or at the very least promised to call Dr. Harris at the end of the day to confirm the plan. Either of these actions may have been sufficient to placate Mr. Armstrong and prevent his clinical decompensation.

An important lesson from this case is that clinician-patient encounters do not occur in isolation. They are historically embedded, meaning that what a doctor and patient do, think, and feel during the present encounter are heavily influenced by past experiences with the health care system. **Again, clinicians who remain open, reserve judgement, and exercise clinical curiosity will have a better chance at achieving communication success.**

In these examples, clinicians and patients talk past each other, misapprehend what the other is trying to get across, or outright disagree. Such lapses should not be viewed as aberrant, nor as permanent stains on either party. As a human activity, clinician-patient communication will inevitably go awry from time to time.

The main challenge for the skilled and caring clinician is not so much to avoid communication failure as to detect it early and make an effort to recover.

SUMMARY POINTS:

- Clinician-patient communication often "fails" because of clinician, patient, or contextual factors.
- Clinician-patient encounters constitute fertile ground for communication failures because patients and clinicians have different perspectives; because patients' preferences for involvement in care cannot be taken for granted; and because clinical communication "routines" can foster efficiency but also cognitive laziness.
- One way to classify communication failures is to separately consider not understanding, misunderstanding, and disagreeing.
- *Not understanding* occurs when clinicians make unwarranted assumptions about what patients are saying, doing, or meaning.
- *Misunderstanding* occurs when words, their connotations, or their interpretations differ between clinician and patient. Verbal indicators of misunderstanding can run from explicit ("I don't get it") to buried (vaguely puzzled look).
- *Disagreeing* occurs when clinicians and patients cannot readily settle a difference of opinion.
- Many communication failures can be reversed through expressions of genuine interest, curiosity, and empathy. This sets the stage for effective clinical negotiation.

QUESTIONS FOR DISCUSSION:

1. After waiting over an hour for his appointment, Mr. Lazarus is miffed. When he asks the receptionist what's happening, she says, "The doctor will get to you just as soon as he can." Finally he is ushered into the examination room, where he waits another 15 minutes. When Dr. Savalas finally appears, the visit is conducted skillfully and in a patient-centered manner. Yet on a post-visit survey, Mr. Lazarus gives all aspects of the visit a mediocre rating (3 out of 5 stars). What is your analysis of this case? In what sense (if any) did communication fail?

2. How is it that even a routine health maintenance visit can trigger low-grade anxiety for some patients? How might this anxiety become apparent to the alert clinician?

3. Provide an example of not understanding, misunderstanding, and disagreeing from your own practice.

4. Dr. Tollinger, a resident physician, undertakes a review of systems with his new outpatient, Mr. Basich, a 26-year-old man. As part of his review of the genitourinary system, he asks, "Any sexual problems." The patient says, "Nah, everything works fine." Several months later Dr. Tollinger sees that the patient visited the emergency

department for urethritis, acquired during frequent unprotected sex with multiple partners (some women, some men). How did this episode of "not understanding" come about? How could it have been avoided?

5. Analyze the statement, "You are at high risk for a heart attack," in terms of the potential for misunderstanding. Consider both the meaning of the words and what the words are saying.

6. In keeping with the standards established in her practice, Dr. Bass suggests that Ms. Armenta return in 3 months for follow-up of well-controlled hypertension. Ms. Armenta says, "I'd rather not come back that soon." Speculate on what each party may be thinking. Is this a case of not understanding, misunderstanding, or disagreeing? How can the case be resolved?

7. The same Dr. Bass asks Ms. Armenta to "stop by the lab for some blood tests" right after the visit. Ms. Armenta says "ok," but the next day Dr. Bass notices that no blood has been drawn. What might have been the source of this clinical disconnect? How might it have been avoided?

8. What are some special issues faced by patients with disabilities during ambulatory medical encounters?

References:

1. Luhrmann TM. *Of two minds: An anthropologist looks at American psychiatry*. Vintage; 2011.
2. Pollan M. *The omnivore's dilemma: A natural history of four meals*. Penguin; 2006.
3. Emanuel EJ, Emanuel LL. Four models of the physician-patient relationship. *JAMA*. 1992;267(16):2221-2226.
4. Charles C, Gafni A, Whelan T. Shared decision-making in the medical encounter: what does it mean?(or it takes at least two to tango). *Soc Sci Med*. 1997;44(5):681-692.
5. Quill TE, Brody H. Physician recommendations and patient autonomy: finding a balance between physician power and patient choice. *Ann Intern Med*. 1996;125(9):763-769.
6. Deber RB, Kraetschmer N, Irvine J. What role do patients wish to play in treatment decision making? *Arch Intern Med*. 1996;156(13):1414-1420.
7. Degner LF, Kristjanson LJ, Bowman D, et al. Information needs and decisional preferences in women with breast cancer. *JAMA*. 1997;277(18):1485-1492.
8. Say R, Murtagh M, Thomson R. Patients' preference for involvement in medical decision making: a narrative review. *Patient Educ Couns*. 2006;60(2):102-114.
9. Feldman MD. Pandora's box. *West J Med*. 1997;166(2):157.
10. Rauch A, Wieczorek D, Graf E, et al. Range of genetic mutations associated with severe non-syndromic sporadic intellectual disability: an exome sequencing study. *Lancet*. 2012;380 (9854):1674-1682.
11. Krauss RM, Fussell SR. Social psychological models of interpersonal communication. *Social psychology: Handbook of basic principles*. New York, NY: Guilford Press. 1996:655-701.
12. Haynes RB, Sackett DL, Taylor DW, Gibson ES, Johnson AL. Increased absenteeism from work after detection and labeling of hypertensive patients. *N Engl J Med*. 1978;299(14):741-744.
13. Cegala DJ, Post DM. The impact of patients' participation on physicians' patient-centered communication. *Patient Educ Couns*. 2009;77(2):202-208.
14. Cegala DJ, Street RL Jr, Clinch CR. The impact of patient participation on physicians' information provision during a primary care medical interview. *Health Commun*. 2007;21(2):177-185.

15. Street RL, Haidet P. How well do doctors know their patients? Factors affecting physician understanding of patients' health beliefs. *J Gen Intern Med*. 2011;26(1):21-27.

16. Street RL Jr, Millay B. Analyzing patient participation in medical encounters. *Health Commun*. 2001;13(1):61-73.

17. Thom DH, Hall MA, Pawlson LG. Measuring patients' trust in physicians when assessing quality of care. *Health Aff*. 2004;23(4):124-132.

18. Robinson JD, Tate A, Heritage J. Agenda-setting revisited: When and how do primary-care physicians solicit patients' additional concerns? *Patient Educ Couns*. 2016;99(5):718-723.

19. Marvel MK, Epstein RM, Flowers K, Beckman HB. Soliciting the patient's agenda: have we improved? *JAMA*. 1999;281(3):283-287.

20. Street RL Jr, Gordon HS, Ward MM, Krupat E, Kravitz RL. Patient participation in medical consultations: why some patients are more involved than others. *Med Care*. 2005:960-969.

21. Zandbelt LC, Smets EM, Oort FJ, Godfried MH, de Haes HC. Patient participation in the medical specialist encounter: does physicians' patient-centred communication matter? *Patient Educ Couns*. 2007;65(3):396-406.

22. Baker LH, O'Connell D, Platt FW. "What else?" Setting the agenda for the clinical interview. *Ann Intern Med*. 2005;143(10):766-770.

23. Aronoff DM, Neilson EG. Antipyretics: mechanisms of action and clinical use in fever suppression. *Am J Med*. 2001;111(4):304-315.

24. Williams-Piehota P, Schneider TR, Pizarro J, Mowad L, Salovey P. Matching health messages to information-processing styles: Need for cognition and mammography utilization. *Health Commun*. 2003;15(4):375-392.

25. Gülich E. Conversational techniques used in transferring knowledge between medical experts and non-experts. *Discourse Stud*. 2003;5(2):235-263.

26. Ong LM, De Haes JC, Hoos AM, Lammes FB. Doctor-patient communication: a review of the literature. *Soc Sci Med*. 1995;40(7):903-918.

27. Osler W. *Aequanimitas*. Ravenio Books; 1930.

28. Epstein RM. Mindful practice. *JAMA*. 1999;282(9):833-839.

29. Santorelli S. *Heal thy self: Lessons on mindfulness in medicine*. Harmony; 2010.

30. Back AL, Arnold RM, Baile WF, Tulsky JA, Fryer-Edwards K. Approaching difficult communication tasks in oncology 1. *CA*. 2005;55(3):164-177.

31. Badaczewski A, Bauman LJ, Blank AE, et al. Relationship between teach-back and patient-centered communication in primary care pediatric encounters. *Patient Educ Couns*. 2017;100(7):1345-1352.

32. Dovidio JF, Hewstone M, Glick P, Esses VM. Prejudice, stereotyping and discrimination: Theoretical and empirical overview. *The SAGE handbook of prejudice, stereotyping and discrimination*. Los Angeles, CA: Sage. 2010;80:3-28.

33. Dovidio JF, Fiske ST. Under the radar: how unexamined biases in decision-making processes in clinical interactions can contribute to health care disparities. *Am J Public Health*. 2012;102(5):945-952.

34. Green AR, Carney DR, Pallin DJ, et al. Implicit bias among physicians and its prediction of thrombolysis decisions for black and white patients. *J Gen Intern Med*. 2007;22(9):1231-1238.

35. Cooper-Patrick L, Gallo JJ, Gonzales JJ, et al. Race, gender, and partnership in the patient-physician relationship. *JAMA*. 1999;282(6):583-589.

36. Schneider EC, Zaslavsky AM, Epstein AM. Racial disparities in the quality of care for enrollees in Medicare managed care. *JAMA*. 2002;287(10):1288-1294.

37. Cooper LA, Roter DL, Johnson RL, Ford DE, Steinwachs DM, Powe NR. Patient-centered communication, ratings of care, and concordance of patient and physician race. *Ann Intern Med*. 2003;139(11):907-915.

38. Johnson RL, Roter D, Powe NR, Cooper LA. Patient race/ethnicity and quality of patient—physician communication during medical visits. *Am J Public Health*. 2004;94(12):2084-2090.

39. Street RL Jr, Gordon H, Haidet P. Physicians' communication and perceptions of patients: is it how they look, how they talk, or is it just the doctor? *Soc Sci Med*. 2007;65(3):586-598.
40. Saultz JW, Albedaiwi W. Interpersonal continuity of care and patient satisfaction: a critical review. *Ann Fam Med*. 2004;2(5):445-451.
41. Henry SG, Bell RA, Fenton JJ, Kravitz RL. Goals of chronic pain management: do patients and primary care physicians agree and does it matter? *Clin J Pain*. 2017;33(11):955.
42. Heisler M, Vijan S, Anderson RM, Ubel PA, Bernstein SJ, Hofer TP. When do patients and their physicians agree on diabetes treatment goals and strategies, and what difference does it make? *J Gen Intern Med*. 2003;18(11):893-902.
43. Montgomery A, Fahey T. How do patients' treatment preferences compare with those of clinicians? *BMJ Qual Saf*. 2001;10(suppl 1):i39-i43.
44. Starfield B, Wray C, Hess K, Gross R, Birk PS, D'Lugoff BC. The influence of patient-practitioner agreement on outcome of care. *Am J Public Health*. 1981;71(2):127-131.
45. Haidet P, O'Malley KJ, Sharf BF, Gladney AP, Greisinger AJ, Street RL Jr. Characterizing explanatory models of illness in healthcare: development and validation of the CONNECT instrument. *Patient Educ Couns*. 2008;73(2):232-239.
46. Sund-Levander M, Grodzinsky E. Time for a change to assess and evaluate body temperature in clinical practice. *Int J Nurs Pract*. 2009;15(4):241-249.
47. Groves JE. Taking care of the hateful patient. *N Engl J Med*. 1978;298(16):883-887.
48. Halpern J. *From detached concern to empathy: humanizing medical practice*. Oxford University Press; 2001.
49. Benedetti F. How the doctor's words affect the patient's brain. *Eval Health Prof*. 2002;25(4):369-386.
50. Di Blasi Z, Harkness E, Ernst E, Georgiou A, Kleijnen J. Influence of context effects on health outcomes: a systematic review. *Lancet*. 2001;357(9258):757-762.
51. Mold JW, Stein HF. The cascade effect in the clinical care of patients. *N Engl J Med*. 1986;314(8):512-514.
52. Morse DS, McDaniel SH, Candib LM, Beach MC. "Enough about me, let's get back to you": physician self-disclosure during primary care encounters. *Ann Intern Med*. 2008;149(11):835-837.
53. Austin J. *How to do things with words*. 2nd ed. Cambridge, MA: Harvard University Press; 1975.
54. Searle JR. *Speech acts: An essay in the philosophy of language*. Cambridge, UK: Cambridge University Press; 1969.
55. Greene JO. A cognitive approach to human communication: An action assembly theory. In. *Communication Monographs*. 1984;51(4):289-306.
56. Ekman P, Friesen WV. Nonverbal leakage and clues to deception. *Psychiatry*. 1969;32(1):88-106.
57. Navarro J. The end of detecting deception. In. *Spycatcher*. Vol 2020: Psychology Today; 2018. Accessed March, 2021.
58. Bond CF Jr, DePaulo BM. Accuracy of deception judgments. *Pers Soc Psychol Rev*. 2006;10(3):214-234.
59. Bond CF, Depaulo BM. Individual differences in judging deception: accuracy and bias. *Psychol Bull*. 2008;134(4):477-492.

CHAPTER 5

Managing Emotions in the Clinical Negotiation

Clinical Take-Aways

- Negative emotions are a threat to effective clinical negotiation. When negative emotions arise in patients, they are best recognized, explored, validated, and acted upon rather than ignored.
- There is no test or imaging study to aid in the recognition of negative emotions. However, humans are excellent emotion detectors, and clinicians can cultivate this innate capacity through curiosity and active listening.
- Naming emotions can itself be helpful to the patient.
- Negative emotions in clinical care cannot always be consistently and effectively managed.
- Clinicians should:
  - Ask patients about emotions directly or by inquiring about impact, attributions, and triggers.
  - Validate emotions by naming the feeling, expressing empathy, and offering support.
  - Tailor their response to negative emotions depending on whether the emotions are a clue to a mental health condition, a manifestation of psychosocial distress, or an impediment to participation in care.

SECTION 5.1: INTRODUCTION

In *The Death of Ivan Ilyich*, Tolstoy depicts a man transported from a banal middle-class life in the Russian countryside to the killing fields of an unnamed, savagely progressive illness. In a more modern telling, Alice Trillin reflects upon the psychosocial landscape traversed by patients newly diagnosed with a serious disease like cancer, calling it "The Land of the Sick People."[1] The experience of being a patient is not always so dramatic—sometimes a backache really *is* just a muscle strain—but the experience is nonetheless associated with a range of strong emotions. These emotions are sometimes positive (e.g., a feeling of deep affinity with the provider) but can be negative (e.g., fear, anxiety, irritation, anger, sadness, or revulsion). **Patients' emotional responses to illness or the threat of illness are important not only because they represent important health outcomes in their own right but because emotional distress can disrupt other biomedical healing processes.** Helping patients manage emotions, especially intensely negative ones, is one of the six core functions of patient-centered communication.[2] Yet this is a tall order on many levels.

> Kay S., a 45-year-old divorced female, has been an active runner for the past 25 years. She has run several marathons and logs about 30 miles a week. However, over the past 3 months, she has been experiencing joint pain in her knees, hips, and wrists. In addition, she has been more fatigued when running, something she attributed to warmer weather. Feeling a little feverish, she wonders if she picked up a virus at work. At first these were minor inconveniences, but they have steadily gotten worse to the point she decided to see the doctor. After undergoing various examinations and tests, Kay was diagnosed with rheumatoid arthritis. She is in shock, and over the next several months experiences denial, anger, and depression.

Kay will live the rest of her life with rheumatoid arthritis. She will take a variety of disease-modifying medications. Her quality of life will be affected by medication side effects, flare-ups, and unpredictable problems with pain and functional limitations. She will experience a number of negative emotions. Although rheumatoid arthritis is a manageable chronic condition, the many emotions unleashed by the diagnosis will challenge not only Kay's capacity to cope but also her ability to engage in effective clinical negotiation.

Kay may try to hide or withhold her feelings, which including anger, anxiety, grief, and fear. Or, like many patients,[3] she may not see it as the clinician's job to help with emotions, believing that is the role of family, friends, clergy, and therapists. She may find it difficult to pay attention to what is being said during clinical encounters, reducing her capacity to understand or retain important information. Even though she normally has well-defined expectations and clear preferences for health care, she may find it difficult to gather and express her thoughts because of feelings of helplessness and vulnerability.

Further complicating this issue is that Kay's physician, like many clinicians,[4] may not be comfortable talking with emotionally distressed patients or feel prepared to help patients with difficult feelings. Physicians can become emotionally reactive in these situations, letting their own sadness, frustration, or helplessness knock the conversation off course.[5]

In this chapter, we examine how suppressed, unexamined, or unconstrained emotions can interfere with effective clinical negotiation. **We organize the chapter around three well-recognized stages of managing emotional distress in medical consultations: recognition, exploration and validation, and action.** Specifically, we first highlight difficulties clinicians have in *recognizing* patients' negative feelings. Second, we discuss challenges associated with *exploring and validating* patients' emotions. Third, we suggest approaches for therapeutic action that may help patients not only cope with emotional distress but become better partners for clinical negotiation. We conclude by examining *variability* in patients' emotional fluency and preferences and by exploring ways of attending to these variations. But first we look at the nature of emotions themselves.

SECTION 5.2: THE NATURE OF EMOTIONS IN CLINICAL PRACTICE

In everyday usage, the word "emotion" has multiple connotations. People are labeled too "emotional" if perceived as having insufficient control over their feelings. Others may be accused of being emotionally stolid if their behavior is perceived as uncaring, "cold," or unsympathetic. Emotions can refer to types of feelings (e.g., sadness, anger, boredom), affective orientation (liking, repulsion), and arousal (energy, activation, apathy). Emotions can reflect internal states experienced by the subject or attributions applied by others.

Emotions are at the core of health communication, clinical negotiation, and outcomes. Emotions can motivate behaviors (binge eating, avoiding colonoscopies); are a topic of clinician-patient communication ("Doc, I'm really worried"; "I'm feeling blue"); and may constitute health outcomes (e.g., anxiety, depression, mania, hyperactivity). Furthermore, patient and clinician emotions are important drivers of sense-making and communication in clinical decision-making.[6,7]

Acknowledging these complexities, it may be useful to consider Russell's two-dimensional model of emotions.[8,9] According to this model, emotions can be located along two dimensions—positive/negative and high arousal/low arousal (Figure 5-1). An emotion such as "excitement" would be highly arousing and positive, whereas "depression" would be negative with low arousal. Being "happy" is positive but in the midrange of the arousal continuum.

Most clinicians will easily recall situations where strong emotions played an important role in shaping the outcomes of care. Arousing emotions, whether positive (enthusiastic) or negative (angry), can be drivers of behavior. For example, feeling hopeful has been associated with patients' adherence to treatment.[10,11] Patients who express contentment with their health care are often more committed to treatment recommendations.[12,13] Worry could motivate patients to take preventive action (e.g., obtain a mammogram),[14] but fear may lead to impulsive action (e.g., requesting bilateral mastectomy) or avoidance (e.g., missing an appointment for fine needle aspiration after a suspicious mammogram).[15,16] An angry patient may choose to change doctors or sue for malpractice.

Within the consultation itself, emotional states can contribute both positively and negatively to clinical negotiation. For example, patients' decision-making capacity could be diminished if negative emotions are ignored or suppressed, are

Two Dimensions of Emotion

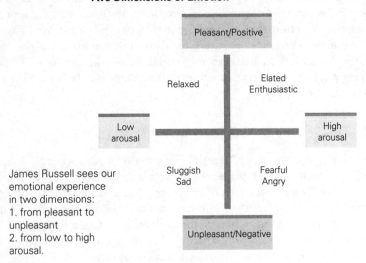

Figure 5-1. Russell's two-dimensional model of emotions.

unregulated, or lead to misinterpretation of information.[17] Positive emotions may, in contrast, foster attention, perceptual acuity, and awareness of the present moment (mindfulness), which in turn could facilitate discussions about diagnosis, prognosis, and treatment.[18] However, negative emotions can sometimes lead to positive outcomes (e.g., when a patient suffering from addiction "hits bottom" and resolves to change) and vice versa (e.g., when a patient with multiple cardiac risk factors is so elated about their "negative" exercise stress test that they stop their statin and ease up on dietary restrictions).

Conventional wisdom might suggest emotions interfere with "rational" decision-making, but growing evidence indicates that interplay between emotion, cognition, affect, and behavior is complex.[19] For example, wishful thinking may be deleterious to effective clinical negotiation, such as when a patient ignores evidence by substituting herbal remedies for chemotherapy to treat cancer. Yet optimism, a hopeful perspective that in the extreme can overlap with wishful thinking, can have substantial therapeutic benefits.[20,21]

When Kay starts to experience joint pain and fatigue, she attributes her symptoms to musculoskeletal strain and perhaps a viral infection. At first, she resists the possibility that she might have a serious condition. Wishful thinking leads to a delay in medical care-seeking. However, after symptoms persist and quality of life continues to decline, Kay seeks care and is diagnosed with rheumatoid arthritis. At first, she vacillates between anger and depression. Anger increases Kay's propensity for risk-taking (such as trying unproven therapies), erodes trust, and undermines shared decision-making. Depression results in emotional numbing and physical lassitude that make engagement in a therapeutic plan difficult.

During a follow-up consultation with her new rheumatologist, Kay remains angry about the disruptions her diagnosis has imposed and is sad about the turn her life has taken, but she seems invigorated, engaged by a fighting spirit and new willingness to work with her doctor to develop a viable treatment strategy. This collaborative approach is facilitated by her rheumatologist's warm manner and air of calm confidence. Kay begins to systematically process the evidence and share her preferences and goals as she and her doctor work through treatment benefits and risks and develop an action plan for treatment and follow-up.

Kay's evolution required acceptance of her new medical reality coupled with the knowledge that she has entered a true partnership that will adapt treatment strategies to her changing needs. The more success she has with treatment and maintaining her active lifestyle, the more likely an acceptance state can be sustained.

In summary, emotions are intricately tied to health behavior and decision-making and may function in both positive and negative ways. Hence, it is imperative that clinicians understand how to work with patients' emotions (and their own) when striving for shared understanding and agreement during clinical negotiation.

Deeper Dive 5.1: How Communication Heals

Figure 5-2 in this chapter presents what is known as a "pathway" model. Such models explicitly connect communication behavior to health outcomes. For many years, communication researchers were satisfied to examine the clinician-patient interaction itself as well as some interactional antecedents (e.g., differences in communication "style" between male and female physicians).

Over the past 15 years, however, researchers have demanded more of themselves. The critical question is no longer whether clinician-patient communication is meaningful to the participants but whether it helps patients achieve better health and well-being.

In work conducted in the 1980s, Greenfield and Kaplan analyzed recordings of physician-patient interactions and found that patients who talked more, were more assertive, expressed more negative feelings and concerns, and who saw physicians who were more liberal dispensers of information experienced better diabetes and hypertension control.[51,52] However, more information giving was also associated with *worse* self-reported functional status and well-being. Furthermore, the Greenfield/Kaplan findings have been inconsistently replicated.[53] Systematic reviews of the effects of clinician-patient communication (e.g., shared decision-making, patient communication skills, patient-centered communication) on health outcomes typically report few, if any, statistically significant associations.[54–58]

How then can one make sense of these conflicting and inconsistent findings? Much of the research examining relationships between clinician-patient communication and health outcomes suffers a "direct effects" fallacy—the idea that clinician-patient communication *directly* affects health outcomes. In reality, this is not typically the case.[59] Rather, communication may contribute to improved health outcomes *indirectly* by influencing more proximal outcomes of the consultation.[60] For example, better communication may lead to patients' achieving greater understanding of their conditions and treatments, a greater sense of being heard and understood, improved satisfaction with care, and health decisions more consistent with their own preferences and values. Such gains can lead in turn to intermediate outcomes such as better self-care skills, greater adherence to treatment, better access to needed health care services, and more robust patient engagement. These intermediate outcomes can then contribute to improved biomedical and psychosocial outcomes.

For example, in one of our own research collaborations, patients who talked more about pain-related concerns did not necessarily have better pain control following their consultation. However, these patients were more likely to have clinicians who adjusted their pain management regimen.[61] Those patients who underwent analgesic adjustments were more likely to have better pain control. Other studies also report indirect relationships between communication and outcomes. For example, a physician's participatory decision-making style (i.e., engaging patients in the decision-making process) has been linked to cancer survivors' mental well-being (through its effects on patients' self-efficacy with disease management)[62] and better metabolic control for patients with diabetes (through its effects on patient activation).[63] Among patients with inflammatory bowel disease, those more involved in the decision-making were more satisfied with their treatment, which in turn was associated with less anxiety about the treatment process.[64]

In this formulation, the causal chain linking communication to biological outcomes is long, with each factor acting as a kind of domino. The first domino is effective clinician-patient communication. The key to understanding how clinician-patient communication leads to better health outcomes is to first identify the pathway to better health and then engage in and facilitate the communication necessary to activate that pathway. For example, there could be two pathways to hypertension control, one involving greater commitment to lifestyle changes and the other involving better medication adherence. Clinician-patient communication about lifestyle changes (e.g., goal setting, overcoming behavioral barriers) is likely different from the conversation around medication (e.g., patient understanding of medication schedule, managing side effects, etc.).

This pathway model of how communication heals implicates two general mechanisms: direct and indirect. While not denying the possibility of a direct effect (with talk having therapeutic value in alleviating distress),[65] more sustained gains in well-being will likely depend on indirect effects involving motivation, self-efficacy, and ability to persist through challenges.

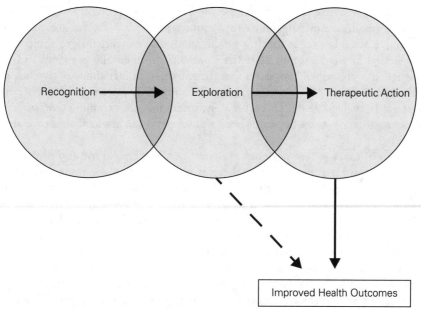

Figure 5-2. A three-stage model for dealing with patients' emotional distress. In adapting the model for this book, we include Validation as a task closely related to Exploration. *Source:* Reproduce with Permission from Dean M, Street RL, Jr. A 3-stage model of patient-centered communication for addressing cancer patients' emotional distress. *Patient Educ Couns.* 2014;94(2):143-148.

SECTION 5.3: RECOGNIZING CUES TO EMOTIONAL DISTRESS

In Dean and Street's three-stage model of patient-centered communication for dealing with emotional distress,[22] the first step in dealing with difficult emotions is recognizing them (Figure 5-2).

Why recognizing emotional distress is challenging

Recognizing patients' distress can be challenging for several reasons.
First, patients may try to hide their feelings, believing that expressing them
would be embarrassing, make them appear out of control, or create uncomfortable drama in the consultation.[3,23] In the early days following diagnosis, our
patient Kay may have openly expressed her dismay through verbal statements
("I'm scared that...," "I'm really frustrated with...") or explicit nonverbal cues (crying, head shaking, bowed head). Or, she may have tried to mask her feelings by
trying to appear calm, in control, and strong. This, of course, would make it more
difficult for the clinician to accurately assess her distress.

Second, a large body of research indicates that while clinicians are usually
responsive to explicit signs of distress, they are not good at recognizing more
subtle cues, especially those associated with confusion, fear, anxiety, worry,
and dislike.[24] Hence, when dealing with patients who are unable or reluctant to
express their emotions directly, physicians need to pick up on other indicators of
inner turmoil: stammering, limited eye contact, pursed lips, flat facial expression.
Failing to attend to these fleeting paralinguistic and nonverbal signs could leave
physicians falsely assuming that their patients are mentally prepared to fully
engage in a prescribed program of treatment when in fact they are psychologically immobilized. Unfortunately, physicians regularly miss signs of emotional
distress in their patients.[25,26] Fortunately, communication training (and perhaps
ardent self-study, as we hope this book will support) can markedly improve accurate detection.[27]

Even in cases where patients are emotionally transparent and physicians
sense that something is amiss, there is a third challenge: some physicians
"don't want to go there" because of their own discomfort.[28] Discomfort with
strong negative emotions is universal, and avoidance is natural.[29] In response,
clinicians may adopt "blocking behaviors" such as closed-ended questions,
multiple questions, leading questions, clarification with a physical focus, premature advice or reassurance, topic switching, and interruption.[30] Yet research
shows that acknowledging patient cues of emotional distress encourages further patient disclosure, whereas ignoring cues forces patients to amplify their
distress in an increasingly desperate effort to be heard or, alternatively, to
self-censor, sometimes feigning agreement with management plans where no
such agreement exists.

Specific techniques for recognizing emotional distress

**To more consistently recognize patients' negative feelings, clinicians can
draw on three tested communication strategies: situational awareness,
active listening, and emotional safety.**[22]

Situational awareness means taking in what is going on in both the *foreground* (moment to moment) and *background* (accounting for the totality of the patient's experience).

In the moment, as the encounter unfolds, situationally aware clinicians are attuned to subtle patient cues such as extended silences, verbal tics, fidgeting, sighing, changes in respiratory rate and depth, swallowing, blinking, blushing, and shifts in body position. At the same time, these clinicians contextualize the patient's current situation by reflecting upon similar situations arising in their own clinical or personal experience. For example, Kay's physician might wonder specifically about the implications of rheumatoid arthritis for an avid runner. A general tool for accomplishing this is to make a habit of asking oneself, *"What might it be like for a patient to experience that?"*

Developing awareness of patients' emotional experiences has an analogy in the way expert clinicians conduct the physical examination. Skilled physical diagnosticians pick up critical findings more often than average clinicians only in part because they are better at *eliciting* physical signs. Their main advantage is that, based on an informed differential diagnosis and a larger, richer catalog of illness scripts; *they know when to seek a finding.* A soft diastolic rumble is very easily missed—unless the physician, aware of the patient's history of rheumatic fever and the connection between chronic pulmonary congestion and mitral stenosis, tunes into it. In the same way, situationally aware clinicians have read about, observed, and reflected upon aspects of patients' lives that deserve further exploration. They pursue what they have trained themselves to consider.

Beyond awareness, clinicians need to be *active listeners*. Active listening is nonjudgmental attention directed to what the patient is saying, how they are saying it, and the patient's underlying perspective. In our running example, if Kay says, "I guess I'll just have to find a new form of exercise," the hurried, distracted, or detached clinician might respond, "Excellent—what a great idea." To a practitioner of active listening, however, this statement would trigger intense curiosity. After all, Kay has been an avid runner for years, and running is likely part of her identity. This active listener might ask, "What kinds of exercise are you thinking of?" and "How do you feel about switching over to walking and swimming, after so many years of running?" These kinds of questions will likely lead to a broader conversation that simultaneously clarifies the patient's concerns and helps her feel emotionally supported.

Finally, clinicians should work to create communication environments where patients can share their feelings, needs, and concerns, allowing unstated feelings to be expressed in an atmosphere of *emotional safety*. By not interrupting and by offering simple verbal responses such as "That must be hard" or "Can you tell me more about that," the clinician creates space for disclosure and sets the expectation that sharing is legitimate and welcome.

Through situational awareness, active listening, and creation of an emotional "safe space," clinicians may find that they have edged closer to what Zlatev et al.

(and later, Epstein and Peters)[31,32] call shared mind and what we will simply call shared understanding. These concepts are based on intersubjectivity, "the sharing of experiential content (e.g. feelings, perceptions, thoughts, and linguistic meanings)" among two (or more) people.[33] In health care, shared understanding is the collaboration patients and clinicians engage in when making treatment decisions, especially when patients' preferences are unstable or ill-defined. Turning again to our running example, Kay finds herself in a novel situation. She doesn't know what to do. Buffeted by unpleasant, highly arousing emotions (Figure 5-1), she may think mainly about short-term goals and immediate gratification at the expense of longer-term goals. Her doctor needs to walk a narrow line, avoiding paternalism (influencing Kay to think or act in a particular way), while not flatly accommodating Kay's possibly misconceived initial preferences. In short, clinician and patient must deliberate to jointly "create" mutual understanding about the evidence and the patient's goals. The endpoint is consensus achieved through attunement—the sense of being in synch or in stride with another person.[34] That such consensus is difficult to achieve (due in part to the many social and structural factors influencing both clinicians and patients) is a running theme of this book, but that hardly detracts from the importance of trying!

SECTION 5.4: EXPLORING AND VALIDATING EMOTIONS

Once a patient has revealed psychosocial challenges or displayed negative emotions, the clinician has two immediate tasks. The first, "exploring," is to tactfully encourage the patient to elaborate. The second, "validating," is to empathetically communicate understanding, respect, and support. While separating these two tasks has some heuristic value, there is obvious overlap. For example, naming the emotion ("You're smiling, but maybe you're feeling a little upset as well") may be intended to prompt further exchange of information (exploring), but it is also a way of signaling empathy. On the other hand, communicating respect ("You did the best you could under difficult circumstances") conveys empathy but also encourages additional disclosure.

Exploration

In their recommended approach to exploring patients' emotions, Fortin et al. advise four sequential steps beyond direct inquiry (e.g., "Can you tell me how you are feeling?"):

1. Inquiring about impact (e.g., "I imagine your pain must limit what you can do? Can you tell me about that?");
2. Eliciting beliefs/attributions (e.g., "How do you think the illness might have gotten started?");
3. Intuiting how the patient might be feeling (e.g., "Having a friend develop MS out of the blue could be very frightening"); and
4. Asking about triggers (e.g., "What else is going on in your life?").[35]

Deeper Dive 5.2: Empathy and Empathic Communication

Most advocates of effective clinician-patient communication highlight the value of clinician "empathy." But what does empathy really mean, and what does it look like?

A useful way of thinking about empathy is to distinguish between "inside" and "outside" empathy. "Inside empathy" is what the empathic person thinks and feels. The cognitive domain of empathy involves the ability to *understand* another person's perspective, whereas the affective domain involves the capacity to *experience* another's feelings.[66]

"Outside" empathy is what empathy looks like to an observer. As such, empathy is often communicated nonverbally. An important question, however, is how to know if someone actually feels empathy for another. To answer that question, it is important to distinguish between *representational* and *presentational* behaviors.[67] Emotions are feelings on the inside but they manifest as verbal and nonverbal expressions. This is how we know if someone is happy, sad, angry, surprised, or scared. These *representational cues* reveal what someone is feeling inside. *Presentational cues*, on the other hand, are controlled, internalized nonverbal expressions displayed to make another *think* we are feeling a certain way.

For example, when a clinician enters the examination room and smiles, has a friendly facial expression, makes eye contact, and says in an upbeat tone "How are you? Good to see you," she may certainly feel that way (in which case the behaviors are *representational*). Alternatively, she may merely be trying to get the patient to believe that that is how she feels (in which case the behaviors are *presentational*).

For the purpose of helping patients manage emotions during clinical negotiation, it is important for patients to *think* the clinician is having some form of an empathic reaction (e.g., compassion, support, sympathy) in response the patient's emotional state. Although we are not aware of any research on whether patients see through clinicians who fake their feelings, an interesting study suggests this may be the case.[68]

Yagil and Shnapper-Cohen surveyed 46 physicians along with 5 of their patients (230 patients total). The physician survey included a "surface acting" scale, a measure asking the doctors to report how often they fake their emotions at the clinic (e.g., "I put on a 'mask' to present the emotions I am required to display in my job"; "I fake a good mood"). Meanwhile, patients completed measures of perceived illness severity and satisfaction with the doctor following a consultation. The authors found a significant interaction between 1) physician regulation of displayed emotions and 2) patient perceptions of illness severity in predicting satisfaction. When patient perceptions of severity were high, patients were less satisfied with the physicians who self-reported higher faking of emotions. However, for those patients who were less concerned about severe illness, physicians who admitted to faking did just fine. The observation that patients in distress seem to want clinicians who are *actually* emotionally responsive to their suffering (whereas nondistressed patients don't register any disturbance as long as the doctor keeps up appearances) raises some important questions for further research. For example, are distressed patients more *sensitive* to their physicians' internal emotional states than nondistressed patients or do they simply *care* more?

Of course, feeling versus faking is not an either/or phenomenon; emotions are experienced in degrees. An optimal degree of empathic concern can contribute to better care for patients, as long as it does not lead to an excessive level of "compassion stress."[69] Although deep acting is preferred, physicians may rely on surface acting when immediate emotional and cognitive understanding of patients is impossible.[70] Importantly, patients who perceive their clinicians as having some empathic concern for their situation tend to be more satisfied with care[71] and derive therapeutic value from being heard and understood.[72]

Step-wise inquiry of this sort is a systematic and effective pathway to achieving what Matthews, Suchman, and Branch call *connexion*—a state of shared understanding that promotes healing.[36] This approach and others are worth practicing, and the interested reader is referred to Fortin's excellent book as well as other references.[37,38]

However, if you were to remember just one thing about exploring patients' emotions as part of the clinical negotiation, it's this: give patients the *opportunity* to talk about how they feel in a way that works for them. This can take persistence. Patients do not always recognize the emotions they are feeling. After all, the human emotional palate is broad: psychologists have identified at least eight families of facially evident emotion, including anger, fear, disgust, sadness, enjoyment, contempt, surprise, and interest,[39] not to mention the moral emotions such as shame, guilt, and self-consciousness.[40] It is sometimes hard to know what one is feeling. Even if patients recognize their emotions, they may have trouble naming or expressing them. And even if they can describe their inner experience, they may not see the relevance to the current problem—or to the current practitioner.

We found in our own research, for example, that patients with clinically significant depression do not necessarily see their primary care provider as interested, trained, or qualified to render treatment for what they think of as a "psychological problem."[41] Sometimes patients want to talk about their psychological state or the emotional impact of illness but believe it would be out of place to do so. Clinicians can help patients feel comfortable discussing such issues through gentle open-ended questioning ("What has it been like for you, getting to dialysis three times a week at the same time your granddaughter has been in and out of the hospital?") and sometimes explicit education ("Your mental health is just as important to me as your doctor as your high blood pressure and blood sugar.")

The use of open-ended questions and follow-up probes provides patients the freedom to talk about distressing situation on their own terms. For example, Kay might choose to share her feelings explicitly ("I am so depressed over this.") or might instead do so implicitly through think-aloud problem solving ("I could ride a bike, I guess").

Validation

Once emotions are on display, validation occurs through empathic statements (e.g., "I can see why that would be frustrating") and supportive responses (e.g., "We're here to help in whatever way we can"). In Kay's case, her physician could explicitly acknowledge the difficulty in changing exercise practices, express a commitment to work together to develop a treatment plan, and express confidence that they will together find a plan that works and is responsive to her needs and preferences.

As it turns out, this general approach matches up well with what experienced physicians do in practice. In one small but exquisitely detailed study, primary care clinicians revealed a uniform pattern during videotaped encounters with patients:

> The physician invited discussion through asking open-ended questions or by being generally open in approach; the physician followed up the patient's responses in different ways; and, finally, the physician showed empathy by asking about and acknowledging emotions as well as by emphasizing the element of cooperation with the patient.[42]

It is tempting to try to tamp down runaway emotions through reassurance. This is often a mistake. Reassurance is appropriate for actions or situations the clinician can control (e.g., promising that "I will be here to see you through this"; "We will get you to a rheumatologist by the end of this month"). However, there are many situations in which reassurance will be anything but reassuring. For example, if a patient worried about cancer feels that the clinician has not adequately assessed her complaints through careful questioning, physical examination, and diagnostic testing, she will view reassurance as lacking foundation and potentially dismissive—and she will still be worried about cancer. If a patient (like Kay) is concerned about the impact of a chronic condition on her ability to form relationships, start a family, continue to progress in her career, and live out a normal lifespan, easy reassurance ("Don't worry, you'll be fine") can feel fake and could lead to later disappointment. It can be tempting for clinicians to lend such glib reassurance in order to fend off what they perceive as potentially difficult conversations. But there will eventually be a price to pay. **On the other hand, *credible* reassurance—which is to say, reassurance supported by careful clinical investigation and material understanding of the patient's condition and concerns—can be powerfully healing.** Kay's physician offered this:

> *It's not easy to hear about a diagnosis like rheumatoid arthritis. But we caught the disease early, your x-rays show very little joint damage, and the treatments just keep getting better. So I am optimistic about getting you into remission and helping you develop an exercise program that works for you. Why don't we plan a follow-up visit after you've seen the rheumatologist?*

In four sentences, the doctor offers empathy, summarizes the clinical data, conveys hope, and commits to staying involved in the patient's care.

Managing difficult conversations

A persistent challenge in helping patients manage difficult emotions is knowing when—and when not—to press for details. Clearly, emotionally charged topics or subtopics will be off-limits for some patients all of the time and for most patients some of the time. At one end of the spectrum, patients with alexithymia lack "an ability to describe their feelings verbally, seem unable to fantasize, and report multiple somatic symptoms."[43] These patients need unhurried instruction; they should be taught that thoughts and feelings (like frustration) are linked to bodily sensations (like abdominal discomfort). However, other patients may simply prefer to avoid emotionally disturbing topics except under the most stringent conditions: in the presence of a clinician they trust, in a setting they find comfortable, at a time that seems right. For example, as discussed earlier, depressed outpatients may not believe that depression is an appropriate topic to discuss with a general physician. Along similar lines, gynecology outpatients (circa 1994) expected to discuss their general health, physical well-being, and vitality at an upcoming encounter but not their social functioning or role limitations (e.g., trouble fulfilling responsibilities at home and work) due to emotional problems.[44] An aversion to emotional topics is not the exclusive purview of the young and healthy. Resistance to such discussions is seen even in populations where the prevalence of social and emotional problems is very high, such as older adults with cancer.[45]

When the clinician detects negative emotions or significant psychological turmoil but the patient doesn't want to talk about it, the main thing to remember is that clinical care in general—and primary care in particular—is a *process*. **Just as one would not expect to achieve full and sustained control of type 2 diabetes or major depression after a single encounter (or even a year of encounters), it is not realistic to think that negative emotions can be instantaneously, consistently, and effectively managed.** Openness, equanimity, trust, and persistence will eventually win the day.

In summary, after recognizing that emotions are at play, the skilled clinical negotiator gently explores the contours of the patient's experience. One benefit of helping patients to elaborate on the emotions attached to their illness is that naming an emotion can itself be therapeutic. As Mr. Rogers (played by Tom Hanks) intoned near the end of *It's a Beautiful Day in the Neighborhood*, "Anything mentionable is manageable"—and, he might have added, "doctors can help" (Figure 5-3). **While few of us possess the reserves of emotional intelligence and warmth of Mr. Rogers, all clinicians can learn to lean in, make eye contact, exhibit curiosity, and listen intently.** Another benefit is that exploration opens the way to validation, whereby clinicians offer emotional resources (support, comfort, presence) that help patients stay resilient. These relational benefits aside, connecting to the emotional aspects of the patient's illness experience plays an important instrumental role, in that it prepares the clinician to take appropriate therapeutic action.

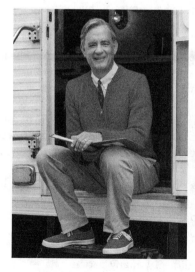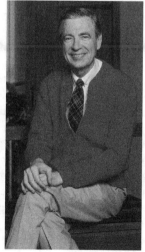

Figure 5-3. Tom Hanks and Fred Rogers.

SECTION 5.5: MANAGING EMOTIONS WITHIN THE CLINICAL NEGOTIATION

Sometimes naming, exploring and validating emotions are enough. But there are three situations where emotions must be explicitly *managed*. **The first situation is when emotions are a clue to an underlying mental health condition.** For example, sustained worry interfering with sleep, appetite, and social activities might signal generalized anxiety disorder; the frequent occurrence of sudden episodes of extreme dread, sweating, and palpitations might portend panic disorder. Similarly, sustained sadness, anhedonia, and diminished productivity at home and work would raise suspicion for clinical depression. These disorders require diagnosis (usually on clinical grounds) and specific treatment using evidence-based drug therapy, counseling by a mental health professional, or both. Whether due to stigma, fixed ideas about masculinity,[46,47] or fear of "addiction," resistance to drug treatment and psychotherapy is not uncommon among patients with mental health conditions. However, such resistance can often be overcome through skilled negotiation.

For example, imagine that Kay begins to ruminate incessantly on the disability her arthritis might impose and starts to experience early morning awakening, poor appetite, and social withdrawal. Her doctor recommends starting an antidepressant. Kay demurs. Through questioning, she reveals that she has heard "bad things" about antidepressants, "especially the sexual side effects," and she knows some people who "have been on them forever and can't get off." Knowing that Kay has a good health insurance plan and that several psychologists in the community offer cognitive-behavioral therapy (CBT, an evidence-based treatment usually lasting 10-12 sessions), the physician offers this as an alternative. Kay agrees enthusiastically. But suppose that access to CBT in Kay's community is limited (as is true in many places). Then her physician would need to draw on what he or she knows about Kay's reticence regarding antidepressants, acknowledging the sexual side effects but planting the idea that improved mood might actually help sexual function; urging Kay to think of starting antidepressants as a therapeutic trial that can be stopped at any time; and suggesting use of a longer-acting medicine to avoid withdrawal syndromes.

The second situation requiring explicit management of emotions is when psychological symptoms are distressing but do not rise to the level of a syndromic diagnosis. For example, patients may report problems with sleep, concentration, diminished motivation, impulse control, or anger management. Here the clinician's goal is to provide reassurance and supportive care, which may require time-limited treatment with a sedative-hypnotic or a recommendation to initiate a regular program of walking, yoga, mindfulness meditation, attendance at religious services, or other forms of social engagement. While behavioral treatments can be highly effective and are unlikely to do harm, clinicians should not underestimate the difficulty many patients have in accepting, initiating, and sustaining these behaviors.[48]

Two effective approaches for helping patients adopt healthful behaviors are motivational interviewing[49] and self-efficacy enhancing techniques.[50] However, motivational interviewing can be difficult to learn and requires in-depth training.

In contrast, self-efficacy enhancing techniques (Figure 5-4) are relatively simple and easy to apply in practice. For example, imagine that Kay was willing to try regular walks but without much enthusiasm. The clinician might begin by assessing her confidence for making a relatively small change: "How confident are you that you can begin by walking just 5000 steps a day, divided into two sessions?" He or she might then encourage Kay by referring to past successes ("remember when

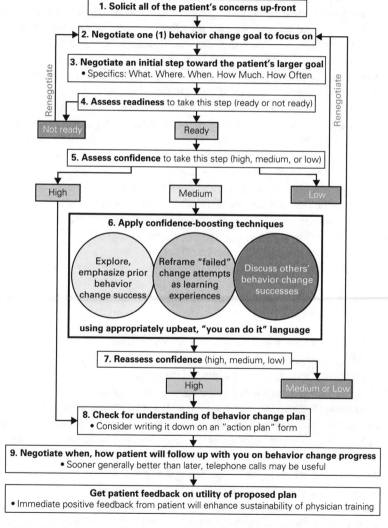

Figure 5-4. Self-efficacy-enhancing interviewing techniques. *Source:* Reproduced with permission from Jerant A, Kravitz RL, Tancredi D, et al. Training primary care physicians to employ self-efficacy-enhancing interviewing techniques: randomized controlled trial of a standardized patient intervention. Journal of general internal medicine. 2016;31(7):716–722.

you were determined to lose weight and you did it?"); reframing failures as steps on the path to success ("even if you don't make the full 5000 steps, every step you take is adding strength to your muscles and tendons, which will ultimately protect your joints"); and referring to others' success ("I've had several patients with inflammatory arthritis who converted to less intensive exercise but stayed in very good shape, and as a side effect, they are sleeping better too").

Finally, clinicians may need to take a patient's emotional state into account when making recommendations for management of acute or chronic medical conditions. For example, if Kay was feeling like she was "going to fight this," then the stage may be set for productive clinical negotiation. She and her clinician would engage in shared decision-making, discussing her preferences for treatment considering the trade-offs, e.g., restrictions she could live with versus those that might be unacceptable. Working together, they would establish realistic goals and agree to adapt the plan as needed. On the other hand, suppose Kay is disappointed and upset because treatment has not worked. Her physician doesn't seem to care. She is overtaken by anger, depression, and distrust. Obviously, effective clinical negotiation will be difficult here. Before the patient can be motivated, or self-efficacy enhanced, trust will need to be re-established. As described in Sections 5.3 and 5.4, the clinician's task is to identify, explore, and validate Kay's negative emotions ("It is distressing to me that our treatments haven't seemed to work very well so far; I imagine it must be that much more distressing for you.") Once this is accomplished, the clinician can start to encourage the patient to adopt small steps within a larger treatment plan (see Figure 5-4), hoping that even minor signs of progress will help to enhance self-efficacy, restore trust, and instill hope.

SUMMARY POINTS:

- Illness is almost always associated with a range of emotions.
- Russell's two-dimensional model classifies emotional states based on valence (negativity-positivity) and degree of arousal (high-low).
- Within the consultation, emotional states can contribute both positively and negatively to clinical negotiation. Negative emotions may heighten attention but can impair decision-making capacity. Positive emotions can foster mindfulness and perceptual acuity but if taken to extremes (e.g., unrealistic optimism) may derail rational decision-making.
- The three steps for dealing with emotions in the context of clinical negotiation are recognition, exploration combined with validation, and action.
- Recognizing patients' emotions can be difficult for reasons of deception, subtlety, or aversion, but clinicians can develop their "emotion detectors" by becoming more situationally aware, by listening actively, and by trying to create an emotional "safe space" for patients.

- One recommended approach for exploration of patients' emotions is to sequentially inquire about impact; elicit beliefs and attributions; intuit and comment upon the patient's feelings; and ask about triggers.
- Clinicians can validate patients' emotions by naming and normalizing the feeling, whether it is directly expressed or nonverbally implied.
- Negative emotions may be a clue to an underlying mental health condition (requiring specific treatment or mental health referral), they may be distressing in and of themselves (prompting brief supportive talk or symptom-directed therapy), and they may influence adherence to therapy and self-management of chronic illness (requiring team care and self-efficacy enhancement).
- Left to themselves, negative emotions are a continuing threat to effective clinical negotiation. They are best recognized, explored and validated, and acted on.

QUESTIONS FOR DISCUSSION:

1. A 24-year-old man has been having bloody diarrhea for 6 months. Colonoscopy with biopsies is consistent with ulcerative colitis. What emotions might he be experiencing? What strategies can his gastroenterologist deploy to help his adjustment?

2. The same patient is treated with 5-aminosalicylic acid and rectal corticosteroids for 6 months, with some improvement in symptoms. However, he continues to curtail work and social activities due to fear of "accidents." His physician advises treatment with infliximab, a tumor necrosis factor inhibitor, which is given by infusion every 8 weeks. The patient refuses, saying, "I'd rather have diarrhea than have something suppress my immune system, especially given what's happening with COVID-19." His physician believes the risks of opportunistic infection are low. What would you say to this patient?

3. How can patients' positive and negative emotions lead to behaviors that both foster and impede optimal health care?

4. A 54-year-old woman has an ovarian mass suspicious for cancer. To the physician, the way forward is obvious: surgical removal with the extent of the operation governed by operative findings. However, the patient refuses to sign the consent because it permits the surgeon to remove both ovaries, the uterus, and part of the bowel if cancer is found. "I don't want you taking half my organs. Just remove the mass and if it's cancer we can talk about it later." What can the physician do to better understand the source of the patient's resistance?

5. A 62-year-old woman with left shoulder pain for 6 weeks mentions that "my cousin had pain in the shoulder and ended up having cancer." Exam is consistent with rotator cuff tendinopathy. Before recommending physical therapy, what could you say to the patient to address her concerns?

6. What is an open-ended question? What is a follow-up probe? How can they both be used to explore patient's emotions?

7. What did Mr. Rogers mean when he said "anything mentionable is manageable"? How does this apply to dealing with patients' emotions? Are there circumstances where clinicians ought to "mention" (reveal) their own emotions to patients?

8. An 84-year-old woman has fallen twice in the past 6 months resulting in bruises but no fracture. Her nurse practitioner asks if she might consider Tai Chi, which has been shown to help with fall prevention. The patient is skeptical. How can her clinician apply self-efficacy enhancing techniques to encourage the patient's uptake of this fall prevention approach?

References:

1. Trillin AS. Of dragons and garden peas. In: *Coping with physical illness*. Springer; 1984:131-138.
2. Epstein RM, Street RL Jr. *Patient-centered communication in cancer care: promoting healing and reducing suffering*. Bethesda, MD 2007 2007. NIH Publication No. 07-6225.
3. Ryan H, Schofield P, Cockburn J, et al. How to recognize and manage psychological distress in cancer patients. *Eur J Cancer Care*. 2005;14(1):7-15.
4. Finset A. "I am worried, Doctor!" Emotions in the doctor-patient relationship. *Patient Educ Couns*. 2012;88(3):359-363.
5. Luff D, Martin EB Jr, Mills K, Mazzola NM, Bell SK, Meyer EC. Clinicians' strategies for managing their emotions during difficult healthcare conversations. *Patient Educ Couns*. 2016;99(9):1461-1466.
6. Martin EB Jr, Mazzola NM, Brandano J, Luff D, Zurakowski D, Meyer EC. Clinicians' recognition and management of emotions during difficult healthcare conversations. *Patient Educ Couns*. 2015;98(10):1248-1254.
7. Legare F, Thompson-Leduc P. Twelve myths about shared decision making. *Patient Educ Couns*. 2014;96(3):281-286.
8. Posner J, Russell JA, Peterson BS. The circumplex model of affect: an integrative approach to affective neuroscience, cognitive development, and psychopathology. *Dev Psychopathol*. 2005;17(3):715-734.
9. Russell JA. A circumplex model of affect. *J Pers Soc Psychol*. 1980;39(6):1161.
10. Legg AM, Andrews SE, Huynh H, Ghane A, Tabuenca A, Sweeny K. Patients' anxiety and hope: predictors and adherence intentions in an acute care context. *Health Expect*. 2015;18(6):3034-3043.
11. Lloyd SM, Cantell M, Pacaud D, Crawford S, Dewey D. Brief report: Hope, perceived maternal empathy, medical regimen adherence, and glycemic control in adolescents with type 1 diabetes. *J Pediatr Psychol*. 2009;34(9):1025-1029.
12. Fuertes JN, Anand P, Haggerty G, Kestenbaum M, Rosenblum GC. The physician-patient working alliance and patient psychological attachment, adherence, outcome expectations, and satisfaction in a sample of rheumatology patients. *Behav Med*. 2015;41(2):60-68.
13. Martin LR, Williams SL, Haskard KB, Dimatteo MR. The challenge of patient adherence. *Ther Clin Risk Manag*. 2005;1(3):189-199.
14. Hay JL, McCaul KD, Magnan RE. Does worry about breast cancer predict screening behaviors? A meta-analysis of the prospective evidence. *Prev Med*. 2006;42(6):401-408.
15. Glassey R, O'Connor M, Ives A, Saunders C, Hardcastle SJ, kConFab I. Influences on decision-making for young women undergoing bilateral prophylactic mastectomy. *Patient Educ Couns*. 2018;101(2):318-323.
16. Consedine NS, Magai C, Krivoshekova YS, Ryzewicz L, Neugut AI. Fear, anxiety, worry, and breast cancer screening behavior: a critical review. *Cancer Epidemiol Biomarkers Prev*. 2004;13(4):501-510.

17. Hermann H, Trachsel M, Elger BS, Biller-Andorno N. *Emotion and value in the evaluation of medical decision-making capacity: a narrative review of arguments. Front Psychol.* 2016;7:765.

18. Fredrickson BL. What good are positive emotions? *Rev Gen Psychol.* 1998;2(3):300-319.

19. Slovic P, Peters E, Finucane ML, Macgregor DG. Affect, risk, and decision making. *Health Psychol.* 2005;24(4S):S35-40.

20. Groopman J. *The anatomy of hope: How people prevail in the face of illness.* Random House Trade Paperbacks; 2005.

21. DeMartini J, Fenton JJ, Epstein R, et al. Patients' hopes for advanced cancer treatment. *J Pain Symptom Manage.* 2019;57(1):57-63.e52.

22. Dean M, Street RL Jr. A 3-stage model of patient-centered communication for addressing cancer patients' emotional distress. *Patient Educ Couns.* 2014;94(2):143-148.

23. Cape J, McCulloch Y. Patients' reasons for not presenting emotional problems in general practice consultations. *Br J Gen Pract.* 1999;49(448):875-879.

24. Mjaaland TA, Finset A, Jensen BF, Gulbrandsen P. Physicians' responses to patients' expressions of negative emotions in hospital consultations: a video-based observational study. *Patient Educ Couns.* 2011;84(3):332-337.

25. Levinson W, Gorawara-Bhat R, Lamb J. A study of patient clues and physician responses in primary care and surgical settings. *JAMA.* 2000;284(8):1021-1027.

26. Del Piccolo L, Saltini A, Zimmermann C, Dunn G. Differences in verbal behaviours of patients with and without emotional distress during primary care consultations. *Psychol Med.* 2000;30(3):629-643.

27. Roter DL, Hall JA, Kern DE, Barker LR, Cole KA, Roca RP. Improving physicians' interviewing skills and reducing patients' emotional distress: a randomized clinical trial. *Arch Intern Med.* 1995;155(17):1877-1884.

28. Maguire P, Faulkner A, Booth K, Elliott C, Hillier V. Helping cancer patients disclose their concerns. *Eur J Cancer.* 1996;32A(1):78-81.

29. Detmar SB, Aaronson NK, Wever LD, Muller M, Schornagel JH. How are you feeling? Who wants to know? Patients' and oncologists' preferences for discussing health-related quality-of-life issues. *J Clin Oncol.* 2000;18(18):3295-3301.

30. Soodalter JA, Siegle GJ, Klein-Fedyshin M, Arnold R, Schenker Y. Affective science and avoidant end-of-life communication: Can the science of emotion help physicians talk with their patients about the end of life? *Patient Educ Couns.* 2018;101(5):960-967.

31. Epstein RM, Peters E. Beyond information: exploring patients' preferences. *JAMA.* 2009;302(2):195-197.

32. Zlatev J, Racine TP, Sinha C, Itkonen E. *The shared mind: perspectives on intersubjectivity.* Vol 12: John Benjamins Publishing; 2008.

33. Atwood, GE, Stolorow, RD. *Structures of subjectivity: explorations in psychoanalytic phenomenology and contextualism.* 2nd ed. Routledge; 2014.

34. Epstein RM, Street RL. Shared mind: communication, decision making, and autonomy in serious illness. *Ann Fam Med.* 2011;9(5):454-461.

35. Fortin AH. Smith's patient-centered interviewing : an evidence-based method. In: Dwamena FC, Frankel RM, Lepisto BL, Smith RC, eds. *Patient-centered interviewing.* 4th ed. McGraw-Hill Education; 2018.

36. Matthews DA, Suchman AL, Branch WT. Making connexions: enhancing the therapeutic potential of patientclinician relationships. *Ann Intern Med.* 1993;118(12):973-977.

37. Henderson MR, Tierney LM, Smetana GW. *The patient history: an evidence-based approach to differential diagnosis,* Univerza v Ljubljani, Medicinska fakulteta; 2012.

38. Platt FW, Gordon GH. *Field guide to the difficult patient interview.* Vol. 719: Lippincott Williams & Wilkins; 2004.

39. Ekman P. Facial expression and emotion. *AM Psychol.* 1993;48(4):384.

40. Tangney JP, Stuewig J, Mashek DJ. Moral emotions and moral behavior. *Annu Rev Psychol.* 2007;58:345-372.

41. Kravitz RL, Paterniti DA, Epstein RM, et al. Relational barriers to depression help-seeking in primary care. *Patient Educ Couns*. 2011;82(2):207-213.

42. Arborelius E, Österberg E. How do GPs discuss subjects other than illness?: Formulating and evaluating a theoretical model to explain successful and less successful approaches to discussing psychosocial issues. *Patient Educ Couns*. 1995;25(3):257-268.

43. Lesser IM. Alexithymia. *N Engl J Med*. 1985;312(11):690-692.

44. Street RL Jr, Gold WR, McDowell T. Using health status surveys in medical consultations. *Med Care*. 1994:732-744.

45. Mazor KM, Street RL Jr, Sue VM, Williams AE, Rabin BA, Arora NK. Assessing patients' experiences with communication across the cancer care continuum. *Patient Educ Couns*. 2016;99(8):1343-1348.

46. Rochlen AB, Paterniti DA, Epstein RM, Duberstein P, Willeford L, Kravitz RL. Barriers in diagnosing and treating men with depression: a focus group report. *Am J Mens Health*. 2010;4(2):167-175.

47. Hinton L, Sciolla AF, Unutzer J, Elizarraras E, Kravitz RL, Apesoa-Varano EC. Family-centered depression treatment for older men in primary care: a qualitative study of stakeholder perspectives. *BMC Fam Pract*. 2017;18(1):88.

48. Organization WH. *Adherence to long-term therapies: evidence for action*. World Health Organization; 2003.

49. Britt E, Hudson SM, Blampied NM. Motivational interviewing in health settings: a review. *Patient Educ Couns*. 2004;53(2):147-155.

50. Jerant A, Kravitz RL, Tancredi D, et al. Training primary care physicians to employ self-efficacy-enhancing interviewing techniques: randomized controlled trial of a standardized patient intervention. *J Gen Intern Med*. 2016;31(7):716-722.

51. Kaplan SH, Greenfield S, Ware JE Jr. Assessing the effects of physician-patient interactions on the outcomes of chronic disease. *Med Care*. 1989;27(3 Suppl):S110-S127.

52. Greenfield S, Kaplan SH, Ware JE Jr, Yano EM, Frank H JL. Patients' participation in medical care: effects on blood sugar control and quality of life in diabetes. *J Gen Intern Med*. 1988;3(5):448-457.

53. Street RLJr, Piziak VK, Carpentier WS, et al. Provider-patient communication and metabolic control. *Diabetes Care*. 1993;16(5):714-721.

54. Saheb KM, McGill ET, Berger ZD. Shared decision-making and outcomes in type 2 diabetes: a systematic review and meta-analysis. *Patient Educ Couns*. 2017.

55. Schoenthaler A, Kalet A, Nicholson J, Lipkin M Jr. Does improving patient-practitioner communication improve clinical outcomes in patients with cardiovascular diseases? A systematic review of the evidence. *Patient Educ Couns*. 2014;96(1):3-12.

56. Rathert C, Wyrwich MD, Boren SA. Patient-centered care and outcomes: a systematic review of the literature. *Med Care Res Rev*. 2013;70(4):351-379.

57. Harrington J, Noble LM, Newman SP. Improving patients' communication with doctors: a systematic review of intervention studies. *Patient Educ Couns*. 2004;52(1):7-16.

58. Dwamena F, Holmes-Rovner M, Gaulden CM, et al. Interventions for providers to promote a patient-centred approach in clinical consultations. *Cochrane Database Syst Rev*. 2012;12:CD003267.

59. Street RL Jr. How clinician-patient communication contributes to health improvement: modeling pathways from talk to outcome. *Patient Educ Couns*. 2013;92(3):286-291.

60. Street RL Jr, Makoul G, Arora NK, Epstein RM. How does communication heal? Pathways linking clinician-patient communication to health outcomes. *Patient Educ Couns*. 2009;74(3):295-301.

61. Street RL Jr, Tancredi DJ, Slee C, et al. A pathway linking patient participation in cancer consultations to pain control. *Psychooncology*. 2014;23(10):1111-1117.

62. Arora NK, Weaver KE, Clayman ML, Oakley-Girvan I, Potosky AL. Physicians' decision-making style and psychosocial outcomes among cancer survivors. *Patient Educ Couns*. 2009;77(3):404-412.

63. Parchman ML, Zeber JE, Palmer RF. Participatory decision making, patient activation, medication adherence, and intermediate clinical outcomes in type 2 diabetes: a STARNet study. *Ann Fam Med*. 2010;8(5):410-417.

64. Veilleux S, Noiseux I, Lachapelle N, et al. Patients' perception of their involvement in shared treatment decision making: Key factors in the treatment of inflammatory bowel disease. *Patient Educ Couns.* 2018;101(2):331-339.

65. Fogarty LA, Curbow BA, Wingard JR, McDonnell K, Somerfield MR. Can 40 seconds of compassion reduce patient anxiety? *J Clin Oncol.* 1999;17(1):371-379.

66. Hojat M, Gonnella JS, Nasca TJ, Mangione S, Vergare M, Magee M. Physician empathy: definition, components, measurement, and relationship to gender and specialty. *Am J Psychiatry.* 2002;159(9):1563-1569.

67. Leathers DG, Eaves, M. *Sucessful nonverbal communication: Principles and applications.* 4th ed. Routledge; 2016.

68. Yagil D, Shnapper-Cohen M. When authenticity matters most: physicians' regulation of emotional display and patient satisfaction. *Patient Educ Couns.* 2016;99(10):1694-1698.

69. Zenasni F, Boujut E, Woerner A, Sultan S. Burnout and empathy in primary care: three hypotheses. *Br J Gen Pract.* 2012;62(600):346-347.

70. Larson EB, Yao X. Clinical empathy as emotional labor in the patient-physician relationship. *JAMA.* 2005;293(9):1100-1106.

71. Walsh S, O'Neill A, Hannigan A, Harmon D. Patient-rated physician empathy and patient satisfaction during pain clinic consultations. *Ir J Med Sci.* 2019;188(4):1379-1384.

72. Gramling R, Stanek S, Ladwig S, et al. Feeling heard and understood: a patient-reported quality measure for the inpatient palliative care setting. *J Pain Symptom Manage.* 2016;51(2):150-154.

Strategies for Successful Clinical Negotiation

Clinical Take-Aways

- Effective clinical negotiation rests on understanding the patient's concerns, developing realistic goals, and working collaboratively to achieve them. In this way, clinical negotiation overlaps with shared decision-making.
- The consumerist model of shared decision-making grants pre-eminence to patient preferences, while the clinical negotiation paradigm gives equal weight to professional expertise and experience.
- Clinicians should:
  - Take a few moments to mentally prepare for each encounter.
  - Allow the patient time to present their complete agenda.
  - Develop a chronological understanding of the current illness.
  - Conduct a focused physical examination, as the exam yields essential information, creates connection with the patient, and signals the clinician's unique expertise.
  - To better understand how the patient thinks about their illness, ask direct questions, show empathy, and pursue information uncovered in the history of present illness or suggested by the patient's own statements.
  - Generate a collaborative plan by *summarizing* what has been learned, *suggesting* a tentative course of action, *asking* for the patient's input, *integrating* the patient's feedback, and *proposing* a modified plan.
  - Confirm shared understanding.

SECTION 6.1: INTRODUCTION

When thinking of negotiation in ordinary life, most people probably imagine two parties with divergent interests facing off across a boardroom table. In clinical practice, however, negotiation mostly takes place between allies, is constrained by the guardrails of professionalism, and is often implicit. The clinician recommends something that is painful (like an injection or blood draw), inconvenient (like taking a medication daily for many years), expensive (like submitting to a treatment not covered by insurance), or risky (like surgery). In collaboration with the clinician, the patient decides whether the potential benefits are worth the costs—measured not just in dollars but also time, sequelae, and risks. Through a combination of words, gestures, and actions, the patient telegraphs their degree of enthusiasm for the recommended treatment. The patient who is not comfortable with a prescribed medication, for example, may not say so explicitly; rather he might simply miss pills, "forget" to obtain refills, or switch physicians. If the physician is attuned to subtle signs of the patient's unease, she might be able to produce an effective counter-offer: consolidating multiple blood draws, prescribing medicines that are easier to take and cheaper to purchase, suggesting a less-invasive surgical option. If not, the patient will find his own way.

However implicit or explicit the negotiation, it helps to have a strategy.

It is 10:15 am, and already family physician Dr. Charles Kramer has had quite a morning. His 8:20 appointment with Mrs. Lattimore ran over by 15 minutes because she is still grieving over her husband's death, and Dr. Kramer felt the patient needed extra time to unload. Fortunately, his 8:40 and 9:00 am appointments (an adolescent girl with well-controlled lupus and an older man with type 2 diabetes) went smoothly, and his 9:20 was a "no show," so now, at 9:40 am, he is caught up. Clicking on the next row of his electronic schedule brings up the chart of Sergei Gromyko, a 52-year-old man whom Dr. Kramer has seen twice before. Neither time went well. Mr. Gromyko immigrated from Belarus 20 years ago and speaks satisfactory if sometimes broken English. His medical problems include type 2 diabetes, hypertension, peripheral vascular disease, chronic low back pain on opioids, tobacco dependence, and possible depression. State disability payments are his major form of financial support. A quick review of the chart reinforces Dr. Kramer's recollection that Mr. Gromyko has many complaints, is poorly adherent to medical advice, and is easily provoked.

As Dr. Kramer walks toward the exam room, he bites his lower lip. What is on Mr. Gromyko's agenda? An early renewal of his opioid prescription? An MRI to "stop guessing and find out what's really going on with my back pain"? A new foot ulcer, undoubtedly exacerbated by poor diabetic control and continued smoking? Dr. Kramer breathes deeply and opens the exam room door.

As Texas oilman T. Boone Pickens once said, "a fool with a plan beats a genius with no plan."[1] Successful clinical negotiation doesn't just happen. You need a strategy. In this chapter, we present a process for understanding patients' needs, desires, and requests and negotiating towards solutions that satisfy patients while also maintaining the highest standards of medical practice.

A Seven-Step Strategy for Clinical Negotiation

Figure 6-1 lays out a seven-step strategy, born of our own experience, to which we have applied the mnemonic MASTerDOC. The acronym emphasizes both the

Mentally preparing
Setting the **A**genda
Constructing the **S**tory
Touching the patient
Seeking **D**yadic understanding
Outlining a plan
Confirming shared understanding

Figure 6-1. The MASTerDOC strategy for clinical negotiation.

challenges and gratification clinicians will find as they work towards *mastery* of these skills. In Step 1 (**M**entally preparing), the clinician prepares for the visit, attending both to the clinical issues that are likely to arise and to the clinician's own internal state. In Step 2 (**A**genda setting), the clinician elicits the patients' agenda and negotiates with patient as to what will be covered in this visit. In Step 3 (**S**tory building), the clinician joins with the patient to create a patient narrative that simultaneously builds rapport and supports problem formulation. Step 4 (**T**ouch) is a focused physical examination. In Step 5 (**D**yadic understanding), the clinician and patient work together to generate overlapping, if not necessarily congruent, mental representations ("models") of illness. Step 6 (**O**utlining a plan) is to develop, share, and iteratively negotiate a diagnostic and therapeutic plan. Step 7 (**C**onfirming shared understanding) closes the circle by checking in with the patient about the way forward.

Table 6-1 elaborates on the seven steps of the MASTerDOC strategy, highlighting the purposes of each step and the specific skills needed to carry out each step successfully.

SECTION 6.2: MENTALLY PREPARING

Abraham Lincoln claimed that if he had 6 hours to chop down a tree, he'd spend the first 4 hours sharpening the axe. Although most clinicians don't have that kind of time to prepare for a 15-minute office visit, Lincoln's attachment to the value of preparation is worth emulating. **Adequate preparation can make the visit run more efficiently, enhance clinical decision-making, and dampen the emotional toll of caring for patients who are grappling with serious physical illness, mental health conditions, or psychosocial stress.** In contrast, lack of preparation makes it more likely that the visit will suffer from interruptions (as the clinician seeks out missing data), mis-steps (as the clinician makes erroneous assumptions), and misalignment (as the clinician and patient pursue separate agendas).

Table 6-1 **Purposes of and Specific Skills Needed for Each Step of the MASTerDOC Strategy**

Step	Purposes	Specific Skills Needed
Mental preparation	Assume a mindset that facilitates a successful visit	Reflection; self-awareness; mindfulness
Agenda setting	Identify full spectrum of patient concerns; prioritize issues for discussion	Open-ended questioning; studied silence; repeated use of "What else?"
Story construction	Understand history of current illness in context of patient's life	Open-ended questioning, gentle redirection, and closed-ended questioning—all guided by an evolving set of diagnostic hypotheses
Touch	Obtain diagnostic information through physical examination; demonstrate caring and connection	Physical examination skills; interpretation of physical findings; sensitivity to patient's physical and emotional responses
Dyadic understanding	Elicit the patient's mental representation of illness and create shared understanding	Curiosity; cultural humility; empathic communication
Outlining a plan	Negotiating a mutually acceptable set of next steps	Clinical synthesis; eliciting feedback; art of compromise
Confirming shared understanding	Assure that clinician and patient are on same page; underscore patient's role as fully engaged partner in care	Summarizing key points of agreement; checking in

The Physical Environment

Being prepared for the visit starts with assuring that the physical layout of the office is optimized, clinical equipment and supplies are available, and needed clinical data are in hand. French chefs call this *mise-en-place*, which roughly translates to "having everything in its place before you start cooking."

Although clinicians increasingly have little direct control over the built environment in which they practice, a growing body of research indicates environmental features can have substantial impact on the quality, efficiency, and outcomes of care. Specifically, various design elements can facilitate or impede 1) access and wayfinding, 2) the waiting experience, 3) patient privacy, and 4) physician/staff-patient communication.[2] For example, clear signage can reduce stress and increase the likelihood that patients will find their way to the office on time; a clean waiting area enhances patients' confidence in their care; thick walls, solid doors, and soundproofing maintain patients' privacy; and arranging patient, clinician, and computer in a triangular configuration (so patients can follow what clinicians are doing on the computer) enhances patients' satisfaction and sense of connection.[2,3]

Having needed clinical equipment and supplies closely at hand not only improves visit efficiency but reduces the chance of "flails" that can undermine patient confidence. Patients cannot help but be unnerved when the otoscope doesn't function, clean examination gowns are missing from their usual place, or lighting is so poor that a rash cannot be adequately visualized. These problems are magnified for frail elderly patients or those with disabilities, for whom the simple act of moving from wheelchair to examining table may be difficult. **A comfortable, clean, well-organized examining room does not guarantee seamless clinical negotiation. But it is a minimal prerequisite.**

With that said, the physical environment in which many clinicians see patients (especially but not exclusively in under-resourced settings) falls well short of the ideal. Clinicians are good at "making do," but they can and should participate in administrative decision-making concerning their conditions of work.

The Information Environment

Beyond the physical environment, the way informational resources are organized can make a big difference in the clinical negotiation. Electronic medical records (EMRs) have revolutionized the capture and storage of medical data. Few physicians old enough to remember paper charts would want to return to a world where critical clinical information was buried deep within Volume VI of eight thick medical binders. But unfortunately, the EMR has failed to solve some important problems (e.g., integrating medical information from different health systems) and has introduced others (e.g., requiring multiple clicks to complete simple clinical tasks such as order entry; "alert fatigue"). EMRs are slowly adapting and improving; there is hope that innovations such as natural language processing and artificial intelligence will accelerate these improvements.

In the meantime, clinicians should learn to deploy the full capabilities of the EMR as best they can. They can also maximize the availability of clinical data needed for decision-making by doing some of tomorrow's work today.[4] For example, support staff can be charged with flagging key elements of clinical information (recent specialty consults, emergency department visits, hospital discharge summaries, abnormal imaging results) in advance of the visit. Patients can also be asked to obtain laboratory studies several days ahead of the visit. This allows the clinician and patient to make key decisions on the spot, without awaiting lab results that then require a follow-up phone call or clinical email.

Cognitive and emotional preparation

Having attended to the physical and information environment of the office, it is time to turn to two even more critical tasks. The first is *cognitive preparation*, in which the clinician familiarizes herself with key elements of the patient's medical and social history. For follow-up patients, this might be as simple as scanning the previous visit note, observing whether the patient is nearing (or just passed) a birthday, and refamiliarizing oneself with names of spouses or children. Such familiarity is reassuring to patients, foments trust, and is associated with visit satisfaction.[5] **While patients are generally forgiving, ignorance of important clinical data or key clinical events may leave the impression that the physician is careless or operating "on the fly."** For new patients (including those who ordinarily receive their care from a colleague or who are transferring their care from another practice), it is helpful to signal some familiarity with the clinical situation, either by alluding to some aspect of the case highlighted in the medical record ("I see that you saw Dr. Bederson for the same problem 2 weeks ago.") or—better yet—confirming that you have spoken or corresponded directly with the primary physician ("Dr. Bederson mentioned to me that your cough has not improved, and I'm glad you came in today to let us take another look.").

The second aspect of getting ready for the visit is emotional preparation. Clinical work can be physically and psychologically taxing, and some patients are more taxing than others. Several approaches to emotional preparation have been suggested in the literature. A 52-hour course in mindfulness meditation for physicians was associated with reduced burnout, greater empathy, and enhanced self-reported attentiveness to patient concerns.[6,7] However, few of us are likely to set aside the requisite 52 hours. Henry et al. have developed a simple approach to preparing for visits with patients experiencing chronic pain.[8,9] This method, which emphasizes monitoring one's own emotions (e.g., by articulating the biggest fears for an upcoming visit) and approaching the visit with an open, curious mind (e.g., by asking questions to discover the patient's perspective), may be generalizable to a broad range of primary care encounters.

A practical approach to incorporating these elements as part of visit preparation comes down to four steps:

- First, breathe. As you approach the examination suite or the patient's room, take a few slow deep breaths. This activates the parasympathetic nervous system and helps clear the head.
- Second, think. Anticipate any fears about the process or outcome of the upcoming visit (e.g., "I'm afraid this patient will resist when I suggest she needs to start tapering her opioids," or "I am worried about all the emotions this new diagnosis of hepatitis C will unleash.")
- Third, recognize negative emotions. As emphasized by internist Danille Ofri in *What Doctors Feel*, the practice of medicine is awash in both positive and negative emotions.[10] Among the negative emotions are anger, frustration, guilt, shame, sadness, and grief. In the few seconds a physician stands at the exam room threshold, there is little time for thorough self-analysis. But many clinicians will find that by silently and explicitly acknowledging "I'm really at a loss as to what's wrong here," "I'm feeling sad," or "This patient puts me on guard," they are better able to handle the encounter.
- Fourth, be curious. Delving into the patient's story enhances rapport, improves diagnostic accuracy, and acts as a counterweight to some of the negative emotions that have just been acknowledged. Equally important, curiosity fuels discovery that can sustain the immediate clinical encounter as well as an entire medical career.[11]

SECTION 6.3: SETTING THE AGENDA

Conducting the medical interview is a highly personal exercise. Highly skilled clinicians vary in their approach.[12-15] One element of consensus (embodied, no less, in the "Kalamazoo Consensus Statement"[16]) is the need to **elicit the patient's full range of concerns early in the visit.** Patients who are allowed to complete their opening statement without interruption or redirection generally do so within about 3 minutes, and they are less likely to bring up "surprise" topics at the end of the visit.[17]

> *"Hi Mr. Gromyko, what's going on?" Dr. Kramer asks as he walks into the exam room and sits down on the stool by the computer.*
>
> *"Pain, pain, and more pain," Mr. Gromyko replies in a thick Slavic accent, the sides of his mouth curling slightly upwards into a hint of a wry smile.*
>
> *Dr. Kramer knows that despite Mr. Gromyko's complex medical history and significant burden of illness, he maintains a sharp sense of humor. Though Dr. Kramer is often himself the victim of Mr. Gromyko's jibes (which sometimes veer towards the acerbic), he views humor as one of his patient's strengths.*
>
> *"Can you be a little more specific?"*
>
> *"My back still hurts. The physical therapy only made things worse. I had to stop after two visits. I picked up grandchild yesterday and knew right away I did something again to my back. I put grandchild down and called daughter."*
>
> *"Ok, so we need to talk about your back. Anything else?"*

By asking "anything else," Dr. Kramer indicates to the patient that he wishes to hear about his full array of concerns. Other clinicians may prefer "Something else?" or "What else?" Although we personally prefer the term "anything else" because it feels more natural, there is limited evidence from one randomized study that "Is there something else?" *may* be more effective in reducing the incidence of unmet concerns.[18] As seen in Table 6-2, asking "Something else" reduced the odds of postvisit residual concerns by 85% compared with control (p = 0.001), whereas "Anything else" reduced unmet concerns by a nonsignificant 79%.

In this study, there is substantial overlap in confidence intervals, so the main take-away is that eliciting the patient's list of concerns—*however it is done*—is better than the all-too-common approach of diving into the chief complaint and not hearing about the urethral discharge or squeezing chest pressure until the end of the visit. That is the conclusion of Dyche and Swiderski, who found that

Table 6-2   **Comparative Effectiveness of "Something Else" Versus "Anything Else" in Averting Unmet Concerns (*n* = 99)**

Phrasing*	Odds Ratio	95% Confidence Interval	P-Value
"Something else"	0.15	0.054-0.45	0.001
"Anything else"	0.21	0.30-1.5	0.122

*Adjusted for number of previsit concerns.
Source: Taken from Heritage et al.[17]

compared to allowing patients to spill their agenda uninterrupted, physician redi-rection (interruption) had little impact on subsequent concordance between the patient's (previsit) list of concerns and the physician's problem list (85% in the uninterrupted group vs. 82% in the interrupted group). However, *not soliciting an agenda at all* resulted in a significant drop in patient-doctor concordance (59%, p = 0.013).[19] This should be reassuring to those of us prone to interrupt but still committed to agenda setting.

When clinicians are told to elicit the patient's full set of concerns up-front, they typically respond in two ways. Some say, "I already do that." Others contend, "That would consume far too much time," or "If I elicit all these concerns, aren't I then obligated to deal with them?"

However, allowing patients to express all of their concerns appears to take very little additional time: patients allowed to complete their opening statement used only 6 seconds more than those who were redirected (i.e., asked to elaborate on a specific topic). Furthermore, patients allowed to complete their statement of concerns were less likely to bring up additional concerns at the end of the visit (15% vs. 35%).[20]

Furthermore, **while it is true that eliciting the patient's full set of con-cerns up-front will result in a longer list of potential topics, not every concern need be addressed immediately or comprehensively.** Visit agendas should not be established by physician fiat or patient demand. Like much else in clinical medicine, agendas themselves can and should be negotiated.

Gromyko: *The back is the main thing. But I also have headache and I think my blood sugars have been low sometimes.*

Knowing that Mr. Gromyko has complained on and off of chronic headaches for years, Dr. Kramer thinks this problem may be a lower priority for today. As he listens to the patient, he is also formulating a tentative proposal for today's visit agenda.

Doctor: *Ok, so you seem to have hurt your back in lifting up your granddaughter. We need to look into that. I would also like to see your blood sugar records, if you have them. And since your blood pressure was right on the border of what we're aiming for, I'd like to take the pressure again. Assuming your headaches are similar to what we talked about last time, we may not be able to address them today, but I do want you to continue to keep a headache diary, and if the headaches are still bothersome, we can discuss them next time.*

Gromyko: *That sounds ok. My headaches are about the same, no better, no worse.*

In this dialog, Dr. Kramer considers two sets of concerns: the patient's and his own. He then presents a tentative visit agenda to the patient. In this instance, the proposed agenda is accepted, and the visit is on its way. One can imagine other outcomes, however.

Gromyko: *Do you think the headaches are from high blood pressure? My sister had a stroke, remember?*

In this alternative scenario, Mr. Gromyko's question suggests worry that the headaches are a result of poorly controlled blood pressure. His concerns are amplified by a family history of stroke. On hearing these concerns, Dr. Kramer will need to do some mental reshuffling, balancing the need to rule out serious physical health conditions, address patient anxieties, and manage chronic conditions, all within the constraints of a time-delimited office visit.

> Doctor: *Well, let's recheck your blood pressure first thing, and also do a quick neurologic exam to make sure nothing's going on with your brain. Then I would suggest we spend some time looking into your back pain. Finally, I'd like to see your blood sugar records just to make sure your diabetes is on track. How does that sound?*

By recalibrating the agenda, Dr. Kramer nimbly addresses the patient's immediate concerns, while also leaving time to exclude significant pathology and do some chronic disease management. The skill and attention required to execute such recalibrations on the fly is significant (and unfortunately, not well-recognized by the Resource-Based Relative Value Scale [RBRVS]).[21]

The rationale for our approach to agenda setting is well summarized by Mauksch et al.[22]

> *Primary care physicians are generally presented with 3 to 6 concerns per visit and frequently more. It is not possible to address all concerns in detail in every visit. After initially checking in with the patient, the physician and patient can collaboratively create an agenda for the visit. Up-front, collaborative agenda setting is more thorough and efficient than the more common approach of addressing each issue as it surfaces. When physicians know [their] number, urgency, and importance...they will be more likely to address them, and they are also able to make rapid judgments about their time needs. Up-front agenda setting allows the physician and the patient to prioritize and explore the most important concerns and decrease the probability of "Oh, by the way" issues surfacing at the end of the visit.*

Avoiding surprises

Despite the clinician's best efforts, there will be occasions when the patient brings up important clinical material near the end of the visit. Such "oh by the way" or "hand on the doorknob" phenomena arise in about 20% of visits. The late-breaking revelation that a patient has been having significant chest pain or blood in the urine is not only jarring but can significantly disrupt the entire day's clinic schedule. Some evidence suggests that clinicians can reduce the incidence of such late-breaking surprises by incorporating three broad strategies.[23]

First, orient patients frequently during the visit. This may involve language such as "Let me save my note, examine you, and see if we can figure out what the problem is" or "Well, from talking and examining you, I think two things are going on.... Why don't you get dressed and we'll talk about next steps." By providing such ongoing cues, the physician helps the patient understand the structure of the visit and the relationship of its parts.

Second, in closing the visit, avoid asking patients whether there is something else they wish to disclose. Not only will such prompts often appear peremptory, they are much more appropriately utilized earlier in the visit.

Third, try to structure the visit so that the ending seems natural and unforced. As White et al. observed:

> ....only when both patient and doctor are ready to close the visit will they do so successfully. This is consistent with other work which suggests that asking patients about additional concerns early in the visit, allowing the patient to talk without interrupting, addressing psychosocial and emotional issues, and exploring patient beliefs may uncover hidden agendas before closure starts and decrease the number of new problems raised by patients late in the visit.[23]

SECTION 6.4: CONSTRUCTING THE STORY

A major premise of this book is that you can't negotiate what you don't understand. That is why obtaining a comprehensive and accurate medical history is so critical to the clinical negotiation. Taking a history affords the clinician the opportunity to characterize the patient's symptoms, develop a differential diagnosis, and uncover important information about the social and emotional context of the patient's illness. At the same time, skilled medical interviewing builds rapport—an essential prerequisite for obtaining necessary information and for healing itself.

There is both an art and science to medical history taking. As articulated by UC Davis master clinician Faith Fitzgerald, "Without a careful history, without knowing the patient's story of what happened to them and their unique circumstances...the practice of medicine becomes neither art nor science."[24] We refer to this process as *constructing* rather than *taking* a history to emphasize that the medical history is always a work in progress, built in layers through a combination of what Robert Smith, Auguste Fortin, and colleagues have called patient-centered and doctor-centered approaches.

Smith's approach is schematized in Figure 6-2.[25] As discussed already, the clinician begins by introducing herself and her role and negotiating an agenda. She then applies patient-centered interviewing skills to understand the evolution of the patient's chief complaint over time. Patient-centered interviewing emphasizes open-ended questions and judicious use of silence, neutral utterances ("uh huh," "go on"), and nonverbal encouragement (such as head nodding) to allow the patient to relay the history of the problem with minimal interruption. As the clinician listens, she remains alert to opportunities for relationship building. For example, if the patient says that her knee pain is starting to interfere with care of her grandson, the clinician can choose an appropriate moment to say: "You mentioned that at times your knees are so bad you can't keep up with your grandson. That must be difficult."

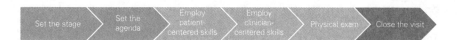

Figure 6-2. Smith's approach to patient interviewing. The interview is divided into beginning, middle, and end. The middle portion relies on both patient-centered and clinician-centered interviewing skills. *Source:* Reproduced with permission from Fortin AH. Smith's patient-centered interviewing : an evidence-based method. In: Dwamena FC, Frankel RM, Lepisto BL, Smith RC, eds. Patient-centered interviewing. Fourth edition. ed: New York: McGraw-Hill Education; 2018.

Sometimes this will be enough to prompt the patient to reflect on her situation, perhaps unfurling an important revelation: that her daughter has been away in rehab, that the patient is solely responsible for the child, and that she is seriously concerned about being healthy enough to fulfill her responsibilities. Other times the clinician may have to probe further.

Once the patient has had an opportunity to tell their story, the clinician adopts a more directive approach to flesh out the medical history. This might begin with a short synopsis of the clinician's understanding of the essential chronology of illness. Skeff and others have argued that explicitly detailing the chronological relationships among clinical events facilitates effective clinical reasoning.[26,27] These authors suggest that explicitly structuring the illness evolution in a chronological fashion enables the clinician to obtain key findings and clues that might otherwise be passed over as irrelevant. Chronological structuring thus provides the clinician with a more complete history, including symptoms or prior findings that may or may not be understood at the moment, yet can be pursued later through consultation or review of the pertinent clinical literature.

Summarizing the patient's story in a few short phrases or sentences is also an opportunity to check in with the patient and confirm that both parties agree with what happened. The clinician then asks additional questions (sometimes open ended, often much narrower) to characterize symptoms in terms of their seven fundamental dimensions (location/radiation, quality, severity, chronology, setting, modifying factors, and associated symptoms).[25] This is followed by questions aimed at filling in the remaining categories of the medical history: past medical history, medications, family history, personal history, and review of systems.

Broadly speaking, the purpose of the patient-centered portion of the interview is to understand the general chronology of the patient's current illness and to establish rapport, while the purpose of the clinician-centered portion is to amass evidence that supports or contradicts specific diagnostic hypotheses. Yet this dichotomy is an oversimplification. By letting the patient speak unimpeded, a skillfully conducted patient-centered interview is often sufficient to establish the diagnosis. On the other hand, skillful elicitation of pertinent positives and negatives, past history, family history (where relevant), and focused review of systems—aspects of the interview often considered more "clinician-centered"—signals the clinician's interest in understanding the patient's condition and doing his or her best to help.

SECTION 6.5: TOUCH (EXAMINE) THE PATIENT

This is a book about communication. The physical examination is not part of the clinical negotiation *per se*. So why do we elevate it to one of the seven steps of the negotiation process? The answer derives from the *instrumental* and *relational* value of the physical exam.

Instrumental value of the physical examination

While no one disputes the contribution of an accurate clinical *history* in establishing a diagnosis, the diagnostic value of the *physical examination* is more controversial—and probably more limited.[28] Among the specific physical examination maneuvers that have been rigorously studied, few have positive likelihood ratios above 5 or negative likelihood ratios below 0.2, suggesting that their pure diagnostic value is relatively weak. The truth is that many traditional physical findings, *considered in isolation*, are either too unreliable or insufficiently correlated with pathology to have much influence on the final diagnosis.

There are notable exceptions, of course.[29] Physical findings that contribute little in isolation can be useful in combination.[30] In an international survey, among a list of 58 maneuvers, the 5 most useful were listening for pulmonary wheezes and crackles; palpating the abdomen for tenderness; assessing muscular power and coordination; checking the pulse for heart rate; and evaluating gait.[31]

Beyond this small cache of high-yield physical maneuvers (some of which have been popularized as the "Stanford 25," touted as examinations "every clinician should know"),[32] new technologies are extending the diagnostic reach of the clinician's five senses. For example, point-of-care ultrasound (POCUS) allows nonradiologists to estimate cardiac ejection fraction, rapidly evaluate patients following major trauma, visualize intraabdominal organs, identify fluid collections, and more safely and reliably perform thoracentesis, paracentesis, and lumbar puncture.[33] Some medical futurists predict that pocket ultrasound machines, wirelessly connected to clinicians' personal smartphones, will become as ubiquitous as the stethoscope (and might well replace it).

However, a focus on special maneuvers, whether performed manually (splenic palpation; Lachman's test) or aided by instruments (ophthalmoscopy; cardiac auscultation; POCUS), ignores the two aspects of the physical examination which are most critical to clinical negotiation. **The first is the simple act of observation. A world of information is available by looking at the patient.** The patient seems older than their stated age? This observation by itself has prognostic value.[34] A man's belt appears to be engaged several notches past the prior, most-worn position? Consider recent weight gain, ascites, or mass. The belt has been taken in? Perhaps the weight loss is due to dieting, food insecurity, cancer, dementia, or chronic infection. The patient's movements and responses to questions seem slowed? Consider psychomotor retardation due to depression, organic brain syndromes, or substance abuse. The seasoned clinician takes in much of this information at a glance, contributing to those memorable moments when the master clinician, accompanied by students and residents, stands at the threshold of a patient's room and declares softly: "this patient has acute alcoholic hepatitis"—and is right.

In addition to observing the patient's clothing, appearance, and movements, careful attention to paralinguistic and nonverbal behaviors can provide information about the patient's understanding of their own condition, their emotional state, and their satisfaction with care. Does the young mother grimace when her child, in no obvious distress, is examined?[35] Is the patient's shrug of indifference when asked about her home situation accompanied by a noticeable cringe? When questioned about mood and anhedonia, is the patient's reticence accompanied by downcast, slightly glistening eyes? Does the patient nod in agreement with your instructions but appear confused or skeptical? The astute clinician registers these conflicting nonverbal inputs almost subconsciously. In the first instant, they trigger a sense of vague discomfort. On brief reflection, they trigger further questions, which if pursued can lead to a deeper understanding of the patient's illness and life context.

Relational value of the physical examination

Apart from all that the physical exam can do to inform medical diagnosis, a less obvious contribution is to enhance the clinician-patient relationship. As Constanzo and Verghese explain, **the physical exam is "an important ritual that benefits both patients and physicians; it helps to satisfy a patient's elemental need to be cared for, and a physician's need to make work meaningful."**[36] Bedell and Graboys expand on this theme with a focus on examination of the hands: "taking the hands conveys a sense of warmth and connectedness and is a means to communicate the physician's mindfulness."[37] Patients whose physicians fail to examine them sometimes react with strong emotion ("he didn't even touch me").[38] The focused physical examination is a tool that helps to locate the illness within the body (rather than in a laboratory result or on a radiograph), amplifies the placebo response, and can help clinicians find more joy in practice.[36]

Nevertheless, there are three caveats. First, if performed awkwardly or without adequate framing, patients may find the act of disrobing and subsequent examination invasive.[39] A reasonable introduction can be brief and matter-of-fact: "I'd like to do a physical examination now to see if we can zero in on the problem." It is increasingly expected that clinicians performing exams of sensitive areas (breasts, genital organs, rectum) will do so in the presence of a chaperone matched to the patient's sex. (This despite evidence that patients differ in their preference for a chaperone.)[40]

Second, in the era of COVID-19 (and any subsequent pandemics), physical examination (and for that matter, the entire interactional dynamic) may be changed by the need to use masks, gloves, or other personal protective equipment and/or to maintain physical distancing. In our experience, it is possible to establish a connection with patients by 1) referring directly to the elephant in the room ("I'm sorry about all this paraphernalia, but it's just part of the hospital [or clinic] routine these days.") and 2) performing necessary elements of the exam (beginning with a look at the hands) without haste and accompanied by a running explanation of the findings (especially if they are normal).

Third, certain cultural groups (Muslims, Orthodox Jews, and others) may be particularly sensitive to cross-gender interactions during the physical examination, and these should be respected and explored. Padela and del Pozo suggest the following language:

> *I know some people are very anxious about being examined or taken care of by someone who is not of their gender, do you have any concerns you want to share with me? This could be followed up by asking, Is there anything you want me to do differently or be cautious about during the physical exam?*

When the exam commences, it is recommended that the clinician diligently verbalize the purpose of each maneuver and uncover only those body parts that are integral to that portion of the exam.

SECTION 6.6: SEEKING DYADIC UNDERSTANDING—TOWARDS A SHARED REPRESENTATION OF ILLNESS

The experience of medical symptoms is as varied as humanity itself. Nevertheless, long before seeking medical care, **most patients with somatic symptoms are actively engaged in a struggle to understand them.** Returning to Tolstoy's *The Death of Ivan Ilyich*:

> *It could not be called ill health that Ivan Ilyich sometimes said he had a strange taste in his mouth and some discomfort on the left side of his stomach....But it so happened that this discomfort began to increase and turn, not into pain yet, but into the consciousness of a constant heaviness in his side and into ill humor.*

How exactly this struggle happens is a matter of contention among health psychologists. A useful framework is *Leventhal's common sense model of self-regulation*, which posits that cognitive and emotional representations of illness are related to coping behaviors aimed at managing illness threats and distress and to illness-related outcomes such as recovery or symptom management.[41,42] Consider again Dr. Kramer and his patient:

> *So what's going on with your back?*
> *Like I said, I picked up my granddaughter and knew right away something was wrong. I felt this sharp pain, here. (Points to low back just right of the midline.) For the last few days, I can barely walk.*
> *Pain down the leg? Numbness or tingling? Weakness? Difficulty urinating or losing urine?*
> *No.*
> *Well, let's examine you and see what we can learn.*
> *[Dr. Kramer's physical exam reveals some mild right-sided paraspinous muscle tenderness in the lumbar region with associated spasm, a halting gait, negative*

straight leg raise, and good strength, sensation, and reflexes. He begins to think Mr. Gromyko's problem is acute nonspecific low back pain, without alarm symptoms or other red flags.]

It seems like you overdid it a bit, but by taking it easy for a few days, then doing some gentle stretching and strengthening exercises, I think you'll be yourself again soon.

I was thinking I might need an MRI.

Different clinicians will hear Mr. Gromyko's declaration differently. Some might interpret the MRI request as indicating desire for a more definitive diagnosis, fear of cancer, pressure from worried relatives, or mistrust of the treating clinician.

However, Mr. Gromyko's request for an MRI is merely the surface manifestation of how he conceives of his illness. Given the opportunity to probe further, we might learn that the patient thinks he felt a slight "pop" as he set his granddaughter down. While his knowledge of spinal anatomy is rudimentary, he thinks he may have torn or broken something. Furthermore, he imagines that a mechanical defect, left unattended, will enlarge or worsen. Finally, he finds Dr. Kramer's suggestion to engage in graded physical activity as potentially dangerous, given that it was physical activity that caused the injury in the first place. This engineering perspective is logical, commonsensical, and probably wrong, given our current medical understanding of the typical course of acute uncomplicated low back pain.

Five dimensions of patients' representations of illness

In Leventhal's theory, which shares much in common with earlier work by Arthur Kleinman,[43] patients' mental representations of illness unfold along five dimensions: identity (the symptoms and an associated label); timeline (acuity and prognosis); putative causes; consequences (imagined and real); and control (degree to which the disease can be prevented, cured, or contained).[42]

As seen in Table 6-3, Mr. Gromyko experiences back pain and embraces a tentative label ("back injury"); believes the problem to be acute (although this could change were the pain to persist beyond a few weeks); ascribes this symptom to ripping or tearing of an important structure in the back; suspects that additional activity may cause further injury; and imagines that high-resolution imaging with MRI will show the site of injury and suggest a means of repair. Like most patients, Mr. Gromyko shares his mental representation of illness only haltingly and incompletely. Yet his perceptions are not completely inaccessible. Through gentle questioning, Dr. Kramer can learn enough about the patient's illness model to offer a reasonable and acceptable alternative.

It sounds like you are pretty worried about this pain. I get that—the pain is pretty bad and even your ability to walk is affected. What do you imagine might be going on?

With this question Dr. Kramer gives Mr. Gromyko license to advance some of his own views. Though some patients will respond by saying, "What are you

Table 6-3   Kleinman/Leventhal Model of Mental Representation of Illness as Enacted by Mr. Gromyko

Kleinman/Leventhal Construct	Mr. Gromyko's Enactment
Identity	Back injury
Timeline	Acute
Putative cause(s)	Lifting granddaughter
Consequences	Tearing/ripping of tissue; possible long-term disability
Control	MRI is key to identifying the injury and somehow creating conditions for repair

asking me for, you're the doctor!" most will appreciate the opportunity to share their concerns and diagnostic hypotheses. In one internal medicine clinic, 71% of patients thought it was necessary for the physician to discuss the patient's own ideas about managing their condition. They were also far less satisfied with the visit if this particular expectation went unfulfilled.[44]

It is possible for such questions to go astray. **Inquisitorial, rapid-fire questioning about the patient's own ideas can seem, to some patients, more like a trap than an opportunity.** The patient might view the question as a trick, with the doctor poised to demonstrate his or her superior expertise. Thus, Dr. Kramer starts the exploration of Mr. Gromyko's mental representation of illness with a brief demonstration of empathy. He acknowledges Mr. Gromyko's anxiety ("It sounds like you are pretty worried...") and registers understanding ("I get that—the pain is pretty bad..."). Observing the patient to visibly relax, Dr. Kramer can get to the heart of the matter—asking the patient for his own views on what is going on.

The gap between patients' and physicians' mental models or representations of illness can be wide, as in many of Kleinman's classic cross-cultural studies.[45] In one case, Kleinman et al. describe a 26-year-old Guatemalan immigrant admitted to a Boston hospital for total parenteral nutrition for Crohn's disease. She becomes withdrawn and uncooperative, believing her illness is the result of witchcraft by her fiancé's sister, and also that interruption of enteral nutrition means her doctors have given up on her. Once reassured by a psychiatric consultant that this is not the case, she reengages with care and begins to recover. But even a narrow gap can interrupt the delicate circuitry of the clinician-patient relationship. Mr. Gromyko suspects there has been a breach of vital tissue; if pressed, Dr. Kramer might guess that the patient has suffered some form of soft tissue injury resulting in low-grade strain or sprain, microhemorrhage, and possibly some degree of inflammation. But unlike Mr. Gromyko, Dr. Kramer is not particularly concerned about the precise pathophysiology of acute low back pain; he knows that most patients will recover within 4 to 6 weeks regardless of therapy.

The medical facts are certainly on Dr. Kramer's side. When hearing ideas that are medically inaccurate (and sometimes ludicrous), the practitioner's instinct is to correct the record by sharing her hard-earned, assiduously maintained medical knowledge. After all, the very word doctor is derived from the Latin word for "teach." But to think that education can bridge the gap between lay and medical models of illness is to underestimate how steadfastly patients cleave to their own deeply embedded, culturally molded illness representations. The wise clinician will first seek to understand, as thoroughly as possible, what ideas the patient harbors about the origins, nature, and consequences of his illness. Only then can the clinician bridge the "representations gap" and negotiate productively about management of the problem.

Getting at patients' mental representations

Table 6-4 outlines five ways of extracting information about patients' mental representations (a term we freely equate to "mental models") of illness. The simplest approach is to ask directly, starting with an open-ended question. If the patient is reticent, the clinician can try a series of closed-ended questions, guided by data on the prevalence of patient concerns in different clinical settings. One can also incorporate empathic encouragement, questions about illness representation as part of history-taking, and using the patient's own statements as a springboard for further inquiry as to how they think about their illness.

Lang et al. offer some additional specific recommendations for eliciting patients' perspectives (including diagnostic concerns). They tested their approach in a randomized trial of 46 patients videotaped while being seen in a family medicine residency clinic in East Tennessee.[46] The Lang algorithm, appealing for its directness and practicality, incorporates three questions:

- *What ideas or thoughts have you had about the possible cause of today's problem?*
  - *If patient balks, I know you may not know for sure the cause of your symptoms, but it would be helpful if you could share any ideas that crossed your mind.*
- *Besides that, did any other ideas occur to you of a serious or nonserious nature?*
- *Today people hear, see, and read a lot about health problems. I wonder if there is anything you have seen, read about, or heard someone mention that you connected with your symptoms.*

Although based on limited data, the Lang algorithm is appealing for its directness and practicality. Of 27 patients assigned to the intervention group (i.e., those who were asked the sequenced questions), 6 shared diagnostic concerns spontaneously, while the rest revealed additional concerns only upon sequential questioning. None of the 19 control patients made such disclosures. Among new patients, visit satisfaction was greater in the intervention group than the control

Table 6-4 Approaches for Eliciting Patients' Mental Representations of Illness

Approach	Suggested Language
Direct (open-ended) questioning	"Many patients have thoughts or worries about what's wrong. I was wondering if you could share any ideas you might have [about what's causing your illness]."
Direct (close-ended) questioning	"I was wondering if in light of [how bad the pain has been for you, your family history, what happened to your friend, etc.] you were worried this might be cancer?"
Empathic encouragement	"I can only imagine how you must have felt. That [loss of consciousness, episode of blurred vision, urethral discharge, etc.] must have been really frightening."
Illness representation as part of the history of present illness	"What did you think was going on the first time this happened? Did your thinking change over time?"
Using patients' own statements as a launching pad	"You mentioned earlier that this belly pain reminds you of the time you had appendicitis, only on the wrong side. In what ways is this time similar or different? What do you imagine might be wrong?"

group. Whether one adopts an algorithmic or more free-wheeling approach, it appears that asking about patients' concerns and diagnostic impressions is better than not asking.

Having encouraged the patient to disclose their previously unstated concerns, the clinician has options. She can address the concern directly, perhaps by suggesting a diagnostic plan or offering to make a specialty referral. She can place the concern in context by explaining how, even if the diagnosis in question is unlikely, "we will certainly keep that possibility in mind as we work together to figure this out." Or she can file the information away for use later in the visit or later in the illness course. Regardless, the effort isn't wasted. **Understanding how patients are thinking about their illness is a prerequisite for effective negotiation.**

SECTION 6.7: STEP 6: OUTLINING A PLAN

Up until now we have focused on gaining an understanding of the patient's perspective, particularly the visit agenda and mental representation of illness. If this exchange has been successful, the clinician will have a reasonable idea of the patient's starting point. Is this heavy smoker ready to quit? Is this patient who worries that their headache is due to a brain tumor prepared to accept that the diagnosis might be stress-related tension? Will this patient who asks to see a dermatologist for mild acne be open to a trial of empiric therapy instead? The answers to questions like these are tentative, with the clinician's initial hunch always subject to modification and dismissal based on accrual of evidence throughout the clinician-patient encounter.

Beyond understanding the patient's perspective, there is another obvious prerequisite to effective planning, and that is the clinician's own diagnostic formulations and thoughts about treatment, largely generated through "clinician-centered interviewing,"[25] an evidence-based physical examination,[28] and clinical reasoning skills acquired through training and experience. Although it is important to heed Osler's admonition to "listen to the patient; he is telling you the diagnosis," it is also important to recognize that what the patient is telling you may be wrong or misleading. Similarly, the patient's initial ideas about management may be dangerous, misguided, or misaligned with the patient's own goals. **In short, patients' thoughts on diagnosis and therapy should be taken seriously but not literally.** Patients' perspectives can provide important diagnostic clues and convey information about the kinds of management approaches that are most likely to stick. For this reason, the astute clinician enters the planning stage of the encounter with two mental rucksacks. The first is filled with educated guesses about the patient's understanding of their condition and preferences for management. The second is filled with medically informed diagnostic hypotheses and therapeutic recommendations. The task at hand is to organize the contents into a single package that constitutes both good practice (consistent with clinical evidence and professional standards) and good care (attuned to the patient's preferences, needs, and values).

This most critical part of the clinical negotiation—collaborative planning—is best approached in stages. Clinicians may have to cycle through the stages several times until agreement is reached. The stages of collaborative planning are:

- **Summarize** what has been learned during the encounter.
- **Suggest** a tentative assessment and plan.
- **Ask** for the patient's input.
- **Integrate** the patient's input with the initial plan.
- **Propose** a modified plan that melds clinical indications and patient preferences.
- **Repeat** until patient indicates agreement (verbally and nonverbally)

Let's examine how these stages might play out in the care of a specific patient.

Brenda Jackson is a 72-year-old woman with poorly controlled diabetes who comes to clinic with new-onset left-sided temporal headache and jaw claudication of 3 weeks duration which she thinks might be "sinus." There is minimal fatigue but no myalgias or arthralgias. She also has type 2 diabetes complicated by peripheral neuropathy that is suboptimally controlled (hemoglobin A1c, 8.4%) on glipizide and metformin, as well as hypertension treated with losartan. She has not had any significant hypoglycemic episodes. On examination, her blood pressure is well controlled. There is tenderness over the left temporalis muscle and over the left temporal artery. Laboratory studies obtained 6 months ago include an erythrocyte sedimentation rate of 84. Dr. Shreya Patel, a third-year resident, thinks the patient needs more aggressive diabetes control but she is also concerned about the possibility of giant cell (temporal) arteritis.

Dr. Patel: *Ok, so your exam is good, except for that tender spot over your temple. I wish your diabetes were under better control, but I think we need to focus on your headache.*

Mrs. Jackson: *Yes, I'm concerned. I've never had anything like this before.*

Dr. Patel: *I'm hopeful this is just a muscle thing, but I'm concerned as well, and I think we need to be sure this isn't something more serious. In particular, there's a condition in which the arteries in the head can become inflamed and cause headaches kind of like the one you're having—a condition called giant cell arteritis. The problem is that if not properly diagnosed and treated, this condition can sometimes lead to blindness in that eye.*

Mrs. Jackson: *Now you've got me scared.*

Dr. Patel: *I realize it can be frightening to hear this stuff. But I am glad you came in when you did, because if you do have giant cell arteritis, we can treat you to prevent that from happening.*

Mrs. Jackson: *So what do we do now?*

Dr. Patel: *Well, what I'd suggest is that we send you to the lab for another blood test. I'd also like to refer you to an eye doctor. In our medical center, they are the doctors who are best able to evaluate your condition. In the meantime, I'd like to start you on a medicine that will control the inflammation, maybe help your headache, and prevent any eye damage. It's called prednisone, and the dose is 60 mg every day.*

Mrs. Jackson: *Prednisone! My cousin was on that medicine and was bouncing off the walls.*

Dr. Patel: *Well, you're right, prednisone can have side effects. In the short run you might feel a little hyper, you could experience insomnia, and you might see your appetite increase. Your diabetes also might get worse, so it's important to keep checking your finger sticks, and we might have to temporarily put you on a nightly insulin shot. But it would be unusual to have the kind of reaction your cousin experienced. And if you take the medicine in the morning, and continue to regulate your diet and get some physical activity in every day, I think we can manage the side effects.*

Mrs. Jackson: *OK, if you really think it's necessary.*

Dr. Patel: *I do. One reason I'm sending you to the ophthalmologist is to see if they think you should have a biopsy—surgically removing a small piece of the artery in your temple to see if it's inflamed. That will help us decide whether you can stop the prednisone or need to stay on it a while.*

In this dialog, Dr. Patel does just about everything right. She summarizes her view of the situation, listens and responds to the patient's concerns, expresses empathy, and provides some reassurance in the context of a concrete plan for collaborative management. She is aided in this idealized conversation by a patient who is pliant, cooperative, and trusting. What if things had gone south?

> Dr. Patel: *I realize it can be frightening to hear this stuff. But I am glad you came in when you did, because we can try to prevent any of that from happening.*
> Mrs. Jackson: *I never heard of arthritis causing a headache. That doesn't make any sense to me. Are you sure it's not just sinus? I'm really congested.*

Here Mrs. Jackson is conveying misconceptions on several levels. She confuses arteritis with arthritis, and she continues to suspect that her chronic, bilateral allergic symptoms might be responsible for the unilateral headache. However, the most important message she's sending has nothing to do with the specifics of these inchoate diagnostic hypotheses.

Mrs. Jackson is saying that her *mental representation of illness* is a poor match with Dr. Patel's.

In this moment, Dr. Patel has several choices. She can correct some of Mrs. Jackson's misconceptions directly. ("Not arthritis, AR-TER-itis.") She can revisit the clinical evaluation for sinusitis ("Well, let's tap on your sinuses again and take another look in your nose.") Or she can explore and validate the patient's concerns while trying to edge towards a mutually satisfactory plan.

> Dr. Patel: *I'm glad you brought up these concerns. Can you share with me any other thoughts you might have about what's going on, either serious or nonserious?*
> Mrs. Jackson: *I guess it could be stress. And to be honest, I do sometimes think about cancer.*
> Dr. Patel: *That's very helpful. It can certainly be scary to experience headaches with no obvious cause. However, I don't think you have anything like a brain tumor, because the headache's only been going on for a few weeks, and your neurologic exam is completely normal. On the other hand, a sinus headache could certainly cause your symptoms, and we may need to look into that some more. In fact, it wouldn't hurt to restart the nasal steroid you were on and to increase your sinus rinses to twice a day.*
> Mrs. Jackson: *Ok, I can do that.*
> Dr. Patel: *In the meantime I'd really like you to start prednisone and see our eye specialist, just in case you have that serious but completely treatable condition called giant cell art-er-itis. It's a precaution, but an important one, because like I said we want to prevent complications. (Noticing patient's furrowed brow.) You look like you might still be worried about something.*
> Mrs. Jackson: *Yeah, what about my blood sugar? Did you say I have to go on insulin?*
> Dr. Patel: *Your blood sugar is definitely a concern. But I do think if you really pack on the vegetables, watch your intake of sugars and starches, and keep up with your daily walks, you'll probably be ok. You should also continue to write down your sugar levels in your log, and we should touch base by phone in 4 or 5 days.*
> Mrs. Jackson: *Well, ok. Where is that eye doctor's office?*

After making a supportive statement ("I'm glad you brought up these concerns."), Dr. Patel's next move is to ask, "Can you share with me other thoughts....?" She then follows the patient's lead. Mrs. Jackson mentions stress, but she also mentions fear of cancer. Judging this to be the more pressing concern, Dr. Patel addresses it directly. Even while talking, Dr. Patel is alert to the patient's nonverbal signals—something, we might add, that would be impossible were Dr. Patel more focused on *documentation* (in the electronic health record) than on *observation* of the patient. This leads to a discussion of diabetes control. Only then, her concerns fully addressed, does Mrs. Jackson indicate agreement with the plan.

Deeper Dive 6.1: The Role of Persuasion in Clinical Negotiation

Under the "deliberative model" of the clinician-patient relationship described in Section 1.6, persuasion is an accepted part of the clinician's role. But how does persuasion fit into clinical negotiation? To what extent should clinicians try to persuade patients to accept their assessment of the patient's condition and to implement the recommended treatment plan?

In the research on patient-centered communication and shared decision-making, the role of persuasion is like the "elephant in the room." Everyone knows it's there, but no one wants to talk about it. On the one hand, persuasion may lead to undue influence because of the clinician's position of power and expertise. On the other hand, clinicians have an ethical responsibility, based on the principle of beneficence, to advocate for a diagnostic and treatment plan based on scientific evidence and clinical judgment.

Dan O'Keefe[57] has defined persuasion as communicating with the *intention to influence* another's mental state (e.g., what to think, what to do) in a situation where the message recipient has the *choice* on whether to think and act in a manner advocated by the message sender. Using this definition, Sara Rubinelli[58] has identified three forms of persuasion that are applicable to clinical encounters. The "good" kind of persuasion is *rational persuasion*, which involves "making the case" for a particular belief or action based on evidence and reasoning. In clinical negotiation, this is where a clinician might argue against a parent's request for antibiotics by offering evidence that antibiotics are not effective for viral infections and raise the risk of antibiotic resistance. Rational persuasion complements the ideals of shared decision-making where quality decisions are those that are consistent with the patient's preferences and based on the best evidence.[59]

Other forms of clinician persuasion are more problematic. *Unintentional unreasonable persuasion* is where the clinician is ignorant of either the clinical facts or the pertinent scientific evidence. Imagine, for example, that the doctor caring for the patient requesting antibiotics had neglected to ask about fever or failed to note the patient's florid tonsillar exudate. In this instance, a bacterial strep infection becomes a real possibility, and persuading the patient to eschew antibiotics might be the wrong move.

Intentional unreasonable persuasion occurs when the clinician deliberately misleads or deceives a patient for either pro-social or self-serving purposes. In its most abusive form, a clinician advocates for a treatment or procedure because it is in the clinician's economic interest. The pro-social motive for intentional misrepresentation can be complicated. For example, effective clinical negotiation is not achieved if a clinician deliberately withholds information about different treatment options because he *assumes* the patient might not adhere to a thrice-daily pill and only offers one option (e.g., weekly injection at the clinic) without discussing the patient's perspective and preferences. On the other hand, in spirit of compassion, a clinician may disclose information about prognosis gingerly with a patient who has days or weeks to live.

This analysis focuses on the process of *persuading*. But persuading is not the same as being *persuasive*, which is the effectiveness of the efforts to persuade. While rational persuasion is appropriate during clinical negotiation, it doesn't always work. An older but still influential theory of persuasion, the Elaboration Likelihood Model,[60] explains why. In this model, the *central route* invokes rational elements like quality of evidence and reasoning. This route can lead to effective clinical negotiation unless thwarted by a patient's lack of capacity or motivation (e.g., apathy, strong opposition).

The alternate pathway involves peripheral processing where the patient is influenced less by what the clinician says and more by subjective considerations such as the clinician's credibility, interpersonal manner, and appearance. A focal point of the peripheral route is nonverbal behavior. For example, speakers are often more persuasive when they maintain eye contact, face the message recipient, gesture, display facial pleasantness, and vary speaking tempo.[61] In clinical settings, clinician affiliative nonverbal behaviors (e.g., smiling, eye contact, head nodding) are associated with greater patient satisfaction,[62] and presumably contribute to the clinician's persuasive effectiveness. As Cesario and Higgins[63] note, verbal messages packaged by nonverbal indicators of friendliness and competence create a sense of the message "feeling right." This in turn leads to a stronger persuasive effect.

Just like clinicians, patients too have considerable potential as persuasive communicators. By sharing their beliefs, opinions, concerns, and wants, patients can influence how a clinician thinks about a patient's health situation. For example, a clinician may think benzodiazepines could help a patient who occasionally suffers from acute anxiety. Yet the patient might push back against this recommendation, reminding the clinician that the main triggers are situations involving public performances. She may mention that a web search made her wonder whether beta-blockers might effectively treat symptoms with fewer side effects. This reasoning would likely "persuade" the clinician to prescribe propranolol.

In summary, clinical negotiation is a process by which clinicians and patients communicate to establish common ground. This requires both parties to collaborate, openly share relevant information, offer their respective opinions and preferences, resolve differences, and work toward agreement on a plan of action. Both parties are engaged in persuasion processes in that each are influencing what the other thinks, recommends, and accepts. As communication scientists David Smith and Lloyd Pettigrew[64] observed years ago, effective clinician-patient communication is most fundamentally a process of *mutual persuasion*.

SECTION 6.8: STEP 7: CONFIRMING SHARED UNDERSTANDING

The final step in the MASTerDOC approach to clinical negotiation is to check in with the patient, making sure that the plan suits the patient and that important concerns have not been overlooked. This check-in serves three basic purposes. First, it serves as a *reality check* on the plan. Does the patient understand and accept it? Will they follow it? Second, it provides an opportunity to *update the plan* based on new information. And third, it signals to the patient that they are an *essential partner* in care.

At this point in the visit, the clinician has already formulated the problem and a corresponding plan. But to what extent does the patient recall and understand the key components? **Many health communication texts and reviews recommend some version of the "teach-back" method.**[47] In this approach, the clinician asks the patient to summarize in their own words what they have heard the clinician say. In the context of the visit close, typical wording might be, "Just to make sure we're on the same page, would you mind summing up what we've agreed to do?" Limited evidence suggests that in certain contexts, the teach-back method enhances self-efficacy and may promote better patient outcomes, such as reduced hospital readmissions for congestive heart failure.[47]

However, it can be tricky to ask the patient to sum up without putting them on the spot. Some patients may be embarrassed by the request, fearing that they may be judged inattentive, ignorant, or otherwise unworthy. That's why it is important to direct the spotlight inward as much as possible. A reflective introduction can help. For instance, the clinician might say, "We've covered a lot of ground today. To make sure we're both thinking along the same lines, I was wondering if you'd be willing to sum up the plan as you understand it." If the patient's understanding diverges from the clinician's, any corrective should be gentle. "That's exactly right, except that it might be better to take your thyroid medication first thing in the morning, at least half an hour before break-fast." Once shared understanding is confirmed, the clinician can address shared commitment.

> "Does taking your thyroid medicine in the morning sound like something that would work for you?"
>
> "So you'll call me in 4 or 5 days to let me know how your blood sugar is doing while you're taking prednisone?"
>
> "While we're waiting for the physical therapy referral to get processed, do you think you could do some of the stretches on this handout?"

During more complex visits, some clinicians invoke a clinician-centered alternative to the teach-back. Here the clinician explicitly summarizes the formulation and the plan, following up with a question about the patient's commitment while carefully observing nonverbal expressions of discomfort, hesitancy, or resistance.

Deeper Dive 6.2: Metacommunication

Metacommunication refers to communication that is not *what* interactants are discussing but *how* they go about the discussion. In a clinical setting, the "what" of the conversation might be blood pressure control, but talk related to "how" would be reflected in comments like, "Well I've been doing most of the talking, what are some of your thoughts?" or "We're having difficulty agreeing on next steps." The term metacommunication has been used in the context of clinician-patient encounters to describe how the communication is or should unfold, such as when clinicians solicit patients' preferences for the way they want to hear about prognostic information (e.g., specific details vs. generalities),[65] what topics they want to talk about (e.g., agenda setting),[66] or how they prefer to be involved in making decisions about treatment.[67]

In this Deeper Dive we focus on a particular form of metacommunication called *reframing*, which is communication that seeks to redefine a communication situation. A classic example from politics would be the irreconcilable differences seen between pro-life and pro-choice activists. While the two would never agree on the legality of pregnancy termination, their conflict could be reframed as one that reflected not their differences regarding *abortion rights*, but rather their agreement on the need to *prevent unwanted pregnancies*.

Reframing is a strategy frequently used in bargaining and mediation in business and legal settings.[68] The approach has also been applied to couples and family therapy.[69] Imagine this dispute. A couple is arguing about uneven domestic workload and taking care of children. The disagreement could be framed as a conflict, with one partner concerned about the amount of effort the other was committing to family responsibilities, and the other feeling defensive. However, to get the couple to work together, the counselor could reframe (redefine) the disagreement as reflecting something the couple agreed upon. That is, both parties take the domestic needs of the family very seriously and are committed to a healthy and happy household. Having redefined the problem as how to best take care of the household, as opposed to who is at fault for not doing their share, the counselor could then suggest mutual starting points such as what chores each is willing to do, how to coordinate child care duties, and whether to hire outside help. By so doing, the counselor has shifted the situation from one of conflict to one of cooperation.

Although clinicians and patients rarely disagree openly over diagnosis or treatment, reframing may still be useful for clinical negotiation. For example, patients are sometimes resistant to guideline-recommended therapies. Consider this scenario: Mr. Gladstone's most recent lab work indicated a total cholesterol level of 240 mg/dL, which was slightly lower from 6 months before (260 mg/dL). The physician diagnoses Mr. Gladstone as having hyperlipidemia and recommends a statin. The patient disagrees with the diagnosis and says his health is very good. He also observes that his numbers "are getting better" because he recently changed his diet and started exercising more. Moreover, Mr. Gladstone worries about problematic side effects he has heard from others about statins, such as headaches, muscle cramps, and nausea. Doctor and patient are at an impasse. How could these differences be resolved?

Some researchers have argued that overcoming patient resistance requires clinicians to be better communicators to help patients understand their risks and the need for medication.[70,71] However, reframing might be more effective, particularly with highly resistant patients. For example, the apparent conflict revolves around taking statins and being labeled as sick. The clinician could reframe the situation by observing that, in spite of their apparent differences, clinician and patient both agree that high cholesterol can be a serious health risk and that Mr. Gladstone's cholesterol requires continued attention. Having established that common ground, clinician and patient can work together toward a plan and a goal. Working with the patient, the clinician could propose a plan that includes diet, exercise, and—if necessary—a trial of a low dose of medication, with careful follow-up to review both the benefits (in terms of cholesterol reduction) and harms (in terms of side effects).

SECTION 6.9: SPECIAL CASES

The MASTerDOC strategy for clinical negotiation is generalizable to a wide variety of patients and clinical situations. However, two circumstances deserve special consideration. First, clinicians in many countries, including the United States, are increasingly called upon to care for patients whose *linguistic and cultural background* are very different from their own. Second, every clinician will encounter patients they consider *"difficult."* **Whether clinicians come to regard these patients as a burden or a welcome challenge may depend in part on successful application of clinical negotiation strategies such as those described in this chapter.**

Fostering cultural humility

The United States is a diverse country, and it is getting more so. However, respecting racial, ethnic, linguistic, and cultural diversity in health care has been a challenge for the United States for many generations.[48]

Socioeconomic differences between health care professionals and patients are universal and inevitable. Even when clinicians and patients share similar ethnic or cultural backgrounds, medical professionals have their own specialized training, speak their own arcane vocabulary, and often occupy a higher rung of the socioeconomic ladder than their patients. These differences are magnified when patients are members of racial, ethnic, or linguistic minorities. Patients from these communities may be relatively distrustful of the health care system. Unfortunately, their fears are not entirely unfounded. Not only are there the numerous historical examples of overt moral collapse (Tuskegee Syphilis Study; Guatemala Sexually Transmitted Disease Inoculation Study),[49] there is ample contemporary evidence of health care disparities.

Differences in the quality of health care provided to different groups can be parsed into three sources: clinically appropriate differences, environmental factors, and discrimination (Figure 6-3). "Disparities" refer to differences in quality that cannot be explained by differences in clinical appropriateness and patient preferences.

This is not a book about the causes of health care disparities, nor about the societal-level interventions needed to address what the National Academy of Medicine has called "Unequal Treatment."[48] But we do feel compelled to acknowledge both the necessity of—and the challenges associated with—delivering the best possible care to all patients, regardless of racial, ethnic, cultural, or linguistic background.

Sometimes the solutions are straightforward, such as consistently using professional interpretive services (now available not only in person but often by video or telephone) to communicate with patients with limited English proficiency.[50] Just as often, the problems are deep-seated and the solutions murky, as in *The Spirit Catches You and You Fall Down,* introduced in Chapter 4. In this chronicle of

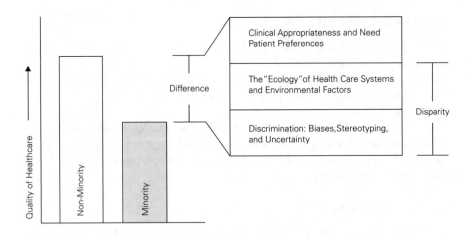

Figure 6-3. Differences and disparities in health care quality. *Source:* Gomes C, McGuire TG. (2001). Identifying the sources of racial and ethnic disparities in health care use. Unpublished manuscript.

cross-cultural medicine gone awry, Fadiman traces the story of Lia Lee's family who never fully accepts Western interpretations or prescriptions; the child ultimately suffers a massive seizure and dies. One sign of progress is that the medical education community has started to view "cultural competence" (which may be difficult, if not impossible, to achieve) through a more skeptical lens. "Cultural humility" may be a more realistic goal.

> *Cultural humility incorporates a lifelong commitment to self-evaluation and self-critique, to redressing the power imbalances in the patient-physician dynamic, and to developing mutually beneficial and non-paternalistic clinical and advocacy partnerships with communities on behalf of individuals and defined populations.* [51]

While the health care professions continue to strive for both competence and humility (it is unclear which goal is more distant), patients from diverse backgrounds will continue to need care. What to do in the meantime? "Matching" patients and clinicians according to race, ethnicity, and language has been shown to confer benefits [52] but seems unrealistic as a long-term strategy in a society as large, diverse, and geographically dispersed as the United States. Health care professionals have a moral and legal obligation to deliver the best possible care to their patients, regardless of social distance.

How to conduct effective clinical negotiation as social distance widens is an ongoing challenge. One approach is outlined by Teal and Street.[53] This approach incorporates four major elements: communication repertoire, situational awareness, adaptability, and knowledge about core cultural issues (Table 6-5). These elements are folded into three stages of the encounter: establishing the relationship, gathering information, and managing the problem.

Table 6-5 **Useful Behaviors for Bridging Social Distance and Potentially Reducing Disparities in Health Care**

Application to Functions of Clinical Encounter	Useful Behaviors
Establishing relationship	Ask "How do you prefer to be called?" and if necessary, "Can you help me pronounce your name?"
Gathering information	Assess patients' priorities for treatment ("What bothers you the most?") Ask about patients' acceptance of the plan ("How do you feel about this plan?") Assess self-efficacy for carrying out treatment ("Do you think you can follow the plan?" "What would help you to stick with the treatment?") Assess patients' concerns, expectations ("What worries you most about this diagnosis/treatment?" "Are you the kind of person who is most concerned about the risks and long term-complications of treatment, or are you more focused on doing whatever it takes?") Assess reluctance to make a choice ("You seem hesitant to decide one way or the other. Please tell me your concerns.") Include patient and family in determination of what information is sought and provided ("What else can you tell me that might be important for me to know?")
Managing the problem	Consider preferences
	Describe the clinician's treatment priorities and rationale
	Describe tests, procedures, and treatments in ways that are consistent with patients' education, medical knowledge and experience, health literacy, and explanatory model.
	Offer options and indicate that a choice needs to be made; share decisions when appropriate; affirm choices ("At this point, are you leaning towards treatment A or treatment B?" "You want to take medicine X and stop medicine Y? Assuming your insurance covers that, would you consider starting next month?")
	Work with family members
	Demonstrate willingness to work with alternative healers or treatments
	Supply information about community resources

Source: Teal CR, Street RL. Critical elements of culturally competent communication in the medical encounter: a review and model. *Soc Sci Med.* 2009;68(3):533–543.

The difficult patient

Every clinician who has worked in continuity settings knows that sinking feeling that comes with realizing that today's schedule includes a volatile, angry, uncommunicative, withdrawn, endlessly complaining, manipulative, or deceptive patient. Writing in the *New England Journal of Medicine* in the 1970s, John Groves described four classic stereotypes of the "hateful patient": dependent clingers, entitled demanders, manipulative help-rejecters, and self-destructive deniers.[54] **The lasting legacy of Groves' essay has been less the typology itself than the acknowledgement that physicians have feelings towards patients, that these feelings are sometimes negative, and that recognizing negative emotions can have real clinical value both in informing diagnosis and in shaping a therapeutic plan.**

It took nearly 20 years, but Groves's essay also stimulated a series of empirical studies concerning "the difficult patient." In a pioneering effort, Steven Hahn and colleagues developed a psychometric scale measuring "difficulty" from the physician's point of view; ultimately the full 30-item scale was reduced to a 10-item scale with little diminution in reliability. The 10 items shown in Table 6-6 measure both positive emotions (e.g., "enthusiasm") and negative emotions ("frustration").[55,56] Using a cutpoint of 30 out of 60, Hahn et al. concluded that about 15% of visits conducted in routine practice are experienced by physicians as "difficult."

We present these items in full not because we expect the scale to be used outside of research, but because it reminds practitioners of the range of emotions patients can trigger. By becoming more consciously aware of these emotions and their triggers, clinicians can more effectively support their patients while reducing the likelihood that they themselves will burn out.

Table 6-6   The Difficult Doctor-Patient Relationship Questionnaire (10-item Version) (*N* = 627)

Item
How much are you looking forward to this patient's next visit after seeing this patient today?
How frustrating do you find this patient?
How manipulative is this patient?
How difficult is it to communicate with this patient?
To what extent are you frustrated by this patient's vague complaints?
How self-destructive is this patient?
Do you find yourself secretly hoping this patient will not return?
How at ease did you feel when you were with this patient today?
How time-consuming is caring for this patient?
How enthusiastic do you feel about caring for this patient?

*A difficult patient had a score of >=30 out of a possible 60. (Each item scored from 1 [not at all] to 6 [a great deal].)
Source: Reproduced with permission from Hahn SR, Kroenke K, Spitzer RL, et al. The difficult patient. Journal of general internal medicine. 1996;11(1):1–8.

The approach to clinical negotiation with the "difficult patient" follows the same MASTerDOC strategy already described, but with a few twists. During the mental preparation phase preceding a potentially difficult encounter, it is particularly important to pause, mentally acknowledge the challenges ahead, and try to begin the visit in a calm and open frame of mind. Agenda elicitation and history taking ("constructing the story") can proceed as usual, except that patients with multiple somatic complaints may need to be gently reassured that the clinician is committed to addressing all of their problems, even though it might not be possible to talk about each one in detail today. Physical examination is particularly important here, as it signals nonverbally the clinician's interest in investigating the problem. As mentioned, it is striking how often patients complain, "he (or she) didn't even touch me."

Developing a shared mental representation or model of illness ("seeking dyadic understanding") with the difficult patient may be challenging for several reasons. First, both patient and physician may be in a high state of anxiety, one fearing rejection, the other worried about falling short of their own standards or the opinions of peers and supervisors. Unless managed deftly, high levels of atmospherics can impede the free disclosure of concerns that is necessary to forge a common mental representation of illness. Second, fearing rejection, some patients may unconsciously provoke the clinician in an effort to test the depth of their commitment. Even highly skilled clinicians can be distracted by these provocations, tending to strike back in subtle or not-so-subtle ways while ignoring the relationship-building task at hand. Third, their patience already exhausted early in the visit, clinicians may be tempted to rush this part of the process. **Giving short shrift to this critical step would, however, be a mistake.** We advise that instead, clinicians double down on empathic encouragement (Table 6-5). This allows the clinician to form an alliance with the patient while at the same time encouraging him or her to share critical information.

Patient: *Whenever I call the clinic, it rings forever, and when I do get through, no one ever calls back.*

Doctor (who has already called the patient back twice this week): *It must be very frustrating to be unable to get through to me or one of my colleagues when you have a concern.*

Patient: *You bet it is. I'm not blaming you, doctor. I'm just upset because I couldn't pick up my granddaughter from nursery school because my knee hurt so bad.*

Doctor: *I can only imagine! I know that girl means a lot to you, and you've been a special presence in her life.*

Patient: *That I have, that I have.*

Doctor: *Well, let's talk more about your knee.*

Patient: *It really felt like something was jammed up in there. One time I nearly fell over.*

This conversation, which could easily have gone off the rails, returns relatively quickly to a diagnostically useful offering: the patient describes a sensation consistent with a loose body or torn meniscus interrupting knee mechanics. While further investigation might be required, the doctor and patient are now in a position to come to terms about a plan.

In summary, as social distance (owing to language or culture) or psychological distance (owing to "difficulty") increases, the solution is—borrowing from Cheryl Sandberg—to "lean in" to the problem by adapting MASTerDOC to fit the circumstances specific to the patient and their illness. Doing so is hardly easy, but most clinicians will find it both meaningful and rewarding.

SUMMARY POINTS:

- Successful clinical negotiation requires a strategy.
- The MASTerDOC approach offers a useful roadmap.
  - Mentally prepare for the encounter.
  - Set the agenda.
  - Work with the patient to build a story.
  - Touch (examine) the patient.
  - Think dyadically. (Build a shared model of illness.)
  - Outline a plan.
  - Confirm shared understanding.
- Negotiating across cultures requires heightened sensitivity, resistance to stereotyping, and willingness to enlist available help (such as professional interpreters, trusted community members, etc.).
- Although clinicians rate only 15% of encounters as "difficult," these encounters can have outsized effects on clinician self-efficacy and burnout. Successful clinicians double-down on preparing mentally, showing that they take the patients' complaints seriously, and creating shared (dyadic) explanations for symptoms.

QUESTIONS FOR DISCUSSION:

1. Mr. Gromyko has been seeing Dr. Kramer for years, yet his health remains poor. Speculate on why Mr. Gromyko continues to seek care from a physician whose advice he often rejects?

2. Why is it often a mistake to begin a clinical encounter without at least a cursory survey of the medical record?

3. What are the tradeoffs involved in trying to elicit the patient's complete agenda at the beginning of an encounter?

4. It is sometimes said that the physical examination has both instrumental (diagnostic) and relational value. Drawing from your own practice, give examples of how the physical examination contributed to 1) making a diagnosis and 2) signaling interest in the patient's problem.

5. Two middle-aged men both experience significant central chest pressure lasting greater than 10 minutes. One seeks care in the emergency department, while the other decides to "ride it out at home." Suggest ways in which each patient might conceive of their problem. How do these opposing mental representations of illness lead to different courses of action?

6. What does it mean to assert that the patient's own ideas about their illness should be taken "seriously but not literally."

7. Why is the traditional "teach-back" method sometimes seen by patients as off-putting or condescending?

8. The sister of your patient confides that the patient has been seeing a traditional faith healer. Why would the patient do this? How would you approach the clinical negotiation in this case?

References:

1. Solomon D. In the air: interview with T. Boone Pickens. *New York Times Sunday Magazine.* 2008:MM11.
2. Gulwadi GB, Joseph A, Keller AB. Exploring the impact of the physical environment on patient outcomes in ambulatory care settings. *HERD.* 2009;2(2):21-41.
3. Frankel R, Altschuler A, George S, et al. Effects of exam-room computing on clinician-patient communication. *J Gen Intern Med.* 2005;20(8):677-682.
4. Sinsky CA., Sinsky TA., Rajcevich E. Putting pre-visit planning into practice. *Fam Pract Manag.* 2015;22(6):30-38.
5. Tallman K, Janisse T, Frankel RM, Sung SH, Krupat E, Hsu JT. Communication practices of physicians with high patient-satisfaction ratings. *Perm J.* 2007;11(1):19.
6. Beckman HB, Wendland M, Mooney C, et al. The impact of a program in mindful communication on primary care physicians. *Acad Med.* 2012;87(6):815-819.
7. Krasner MS, Epstein RM, Beckman H, et al. Association of an educational program in mindful communication with burnout, empathy, and attitudes among primary care physicians. *JAMA.* 2009;302(12):1284-1293.
8. Henry SG, Paterniti DA, Feng B, et al. Patients' experience with opioid tapering: A conceptual model with recommendations for clinicians. *J Pain.* 2019;20(2):181-191.
9. Henry SG. Opioids. In: *Behavioral medicine: a guide for clinical practice.* 5th ed. San Francisco: McGraw Hill; 2020:251-267.
10. Ofri D. *What doctors feel: how emotions affect the practice of medicine.* Beacon Press; 2013.
11. Fitzgerald FT. Curiosity. *Ann Intern Med.* 1999;130(1):70-72.
12. Stewart M. *Patient-centered medicine : transforming the clinical method.* 3rd ed. Radcliffe Publishing; 2014.
13. Novack DH, Dubé C, Goldstein MG. Teaching medical interviewing: a basic course on interviewing and the physician-patient relationship. *JAMA Intern Med.* 1992;152(9):1814-1820.
14. Kurtz SM. *Teaching and learning communication skills in medicine.* 2nd ed. Radcliffe Publishers; 2005.
15. Keller VF, Gregory Carroll J. A new model for physician-patient communication. *Patient Educ Couns.* 1994;23(2):131-140.
16. Makoul G. Essential Elements of communication in medical encounters: the kalamazoo consensus statement. *Acad Med.* 2001;76(4):390-393.
17. Marvel MK, Epstein RM, Flowers K, Beckman HB. Soliciting the patient's agenda: have we improved? *JAMA.* 1999;281(3):283-287.

18. Heritage J, Robinson JD, Elliott MN, Beckett M, Wilkes M. Reducing patients' unmet concerns in primary care: the difference one word can make. *J Gen Intern Med*. 2007;22(10):1429-1433.

19. Dyche L, Swiderski D. The effect of physician solicitation approaches on ability to identify patient concerns. *J Gen Intern Med*. 2005;20(3):267-270.

20. Marvel MK, Epstein RM, Flowers K, Beckman HB. Soliciting the patient's agenda: have we improved? *JAMA*. 1999;281(3):283-287.

21. Kumetz EA, Goodson JD. The undervaluation of evaluation and management professional services: the lasting impact of current procedural terminology code deficiencies on physician payment. *Chest*. 2013;144(3):740-745.

22. Mauksch LB, Dugdale DC, Dodson S, Epstein R. Relationship, communication, and efficiency in the medical encounter - Creating a clinical model from a literature review. *Arch Intern Med*. 2008;168(13):1387-1395.

23. White J, Levinson W, Roter D. Oh, by the way.... *J Gen Intern Med*. 1994;9(1):24-28.

24. Henderson MC, Tierney LM, Smetana GW. *The patient history : an evidence-based approach to differential diagnosis*. 2nd ed. McGraw-Hill Medical; 2012.

25. Fortin AH. Smith's patient-centered interviewing : an evidence-based method. In: Dwamena FC, Frankel RM, Lepisto BL, Smith RC, eds. *Patient-centered interviewing*. 4th ed. McGraw-Hill Education; 2018.

26. Mazer LM, Storage T, Bereknyei S, Chi J, Skeff K. A pilot study of the chronology of present illness: restructuring the HPI to improve physician cognition and communication. *J Gen Intern Med*. 2017;32(2):182-188.

27. Skeff KM. Reassessing the HPI: the chronology of present illness (CPI). *J Gen Intern Med*. 2014;29(1):13-15.

28. Simel DL, Rennie D. A Primer on the Precision and Accuracy of the Clinical Examination. In: *The Rational Clinical Examination: Evidence-Based Clinical Diagnosis*. McGraw-Hill Education; 2009.

29. Simel DL, Rennie D. Pretest Probabilities and Likelihood Ratios for Clinical Findings. In: *The Rational Clinical Examination: Evidence-Based Clinical Diagnosis*. McGraw-Hill Education; 2009.

30. Holleman DR, Simel DL. Quantitative assessments from the clinical examination: how should clinicians integrate the numerous results? *J Gen Intern Med*. 1997;12(3):165-171.

31. Elder AT, McManus IC, Patrick A, Nair K, Vaughan L, Dacre J. The value of the physical examination in clinical practice: an international survey. *Clin Med*. 2017;17(6):490.

32. Verghese A, Horwitz RI. In praise of the physical examination. In: British Medical Journal Publishing Group; 2009;339:b5448.

33. Andersen CA, Holden S, Vela J, Rathleff MS, Jensen MB. Point-of-care ultrasound in general practice: a systematic review. *Ann Fam Med*. 2019;17(1):61-69.

34. Christensen K, Thinggaard M, McGue M, et al. Perceived age as clinically useful biomarker of ageing: cohort study. *BMJ*. 2009;339:b5262.

35. Butler CC. The 'maternal grimace' sign. *Arch Fam Med*. 1995;4:273-275.

36. Costanzo C, Verghese A. The physical examination as ritual: social sciences and embodiment in the context of the physical examination. *Med Clin*. 2018;102(3):425-431.

37. Bedell SE, Graboys TB. Hand to hand. *J Gen Intern Med*. 2002;17(8):654-656.

38. Kravitz RL, Callahan EJ, Paterniti D, Antonius D, Dunham M, Lewis CE. Prevalence and sources of patients' unmet expectations for care. *Ann Intern Med*. 1996;125(9):730-737.

39. Iida J, Nishigori H. Physical examination and the physician-patient relationship: a literature review. *MedEdPublish*. 2016;5.

40. Baber JA, Davies SC, Dayan LS. An extra pair of eyes: do patients want a chaperone when having an anogenital examination? *Sex Health*. 2007;4(2):89-93.

41. Hagger MS, Koch S, Chatzisarantis NL, Orbell S. The common sense model of self-regulation: Meta-analysis and test of a process model. *Psychol Bull*. 2017;143(11):1117.

42. Leventhal H, Leventhal EA, Contrada RJ. Self-regulation, health, and behavior: A perceptual-cognitive approach. *Psychol Health*. 1998;13(4):717-733.

43. Kleinman A, Eisenberg L, Byron JL, Good. Culture, illness and care: clinical lessons from anthropological and cross-cultural research. *Ann Intern Med.* 1978;88(1).

44. Kravitz RL, Cope DW, Bhrany V, Leake B. Internal medicine patients' expectations for care during office visits. *J Gen Intern Med.* 1994;9(2):75-81.

45. Kleinman A, Eisenberg L, Good B. Culture, illness, and care: clinical lessons from anthropologic and cross-cultural research. *Ann Intern Med.* 1978;88(2):251-258.

46. Lang F, Floyd MR, Beine KL, Buck P. Sequenced questioning to elicit the patient's perspective on illness: effects on information disclosure, patient satisfaction, and time expenditure. *Fam Med.* 2002;34(5):325-330.

47. Dinh TTH, Bonner A, Clark R, Ramsbotham J, Hines S. The effectiveness of the teach-back method on adherence and self-management in health education for people with chronic disease: a systematic review. *JBI Database System Rev Implement Rep.* 2016;14(1):210-247.

48. Nelson A, Smedley BD, Stith AY. Unequal treatment: confronting racial and ethnic disparities in health care. *J Natl Med Assoc.* 2002;94(8):666-668.

49. Gamble VN. Under the shadow of Tuskegee: African Americans and health care. *Am J Public Health.* 1997;87(11):1773-1778.

50. Karliner LS, Jacobs EA, Chen AH, Mutha S. Do professional interpreters improve clinical care for patients with limited English proficiency? A systematic review of the literature. *Health Serv Res.* 2007;42(2):727-754.

51. Tervalon M, Murray-Garcia J. Cultural humility versus cultural competence: A critical distinction in defining physician training outcomes in multicultural education. *J Health Care Poor Underserved.* 1998;9(2):117-125.

52. Cooper LA, Powe NR. *Disparities in patient experiences, health care processes, and outcomes: the role of patient-provider racial, ethnic, and language concordance.* Commonwealth Fund; 2004.

53. Teal CR, Street RL. Critical elements of culturally competent communication in the medical encounter: a review and model. *Soc Sci Med.* 2009;68(3):533-543.

54. Groves JE. Taking care of the hateful patient. *N Engl J Med.* 1978;298(16):883-887.

55. Hahn SR, Kroenke K, Spitzer RL, et al. The difficult patient. *J Gen Intern Med.* 1996;11(1):1-8.

56. Hahn SR, Thompson KS, Wills TA, Stern V, Budner NS. The difficult doctor-patient relationship: somatization, personality and psychopathology. *J Clin Epidemol.* 1994;47(6):647-657.

57. O'Keefe DJ. *Persuasion: Theory and research.* 3rd ed. Thousand Oaks, CA: Sage; 2016.

58. Rubinelli S. Rational versus unreasonable persuasion in doctor-patient communication: a normative account. *Patient Educ Couns.* 2013;92(3):296-301.

59. Sepucha K, Ozanne EM. How to define and measure concordance between patients' preferences and medical treatments: a systematic review of approaches and recommendations for standardization. *Patient Educ Couns.* 2010;78(1):12-23.

60. Petty RE, Barden J, Wheeler SC. The Elaboration Likelihood Model of persuasion: developing health promotions for sustained behavioral change. In: DiClemente RJ, Crosby RA, Kegler MC, ed. *Emerging theories in health promotion practice and research.* Jossey-Bass; 2009:185-214.

61. Burgoon JK, Le Poire BA. Nonverbal cues and interpersonal judgments: participant and observer perceptions of intimacy, dominance, composure, and formality. *Commun Monogr.* 1999;66(2):105-24.

62. Mast MS. On the importance of nonverbal communication in the physician-patient interaction. *Patient Educ Couns.* 2007;67(3):315-318.

63. Cesario J, Higgins ET. Making message recipients "feel right": how nonverbal cues can increase persuasion. *Psychol Sci.* 2008;19(5):415-420.

64. Smith DH, Pettigrew LS. Mutual persuasion as a model for doctor-patient communication. *Theor Med Bioeth.* 1986;7:127-146.

65. Graugaard PK, Rogg L, Eide H, Uhlig T, Loge JH. Ways of providing the patient with a prognosis: a terminology of employed strategies based on qualitative data. *Patient Educ Couns.* 2011;83(1):80-86.

66. Meeuwesen L, Tromp F, Schouten BC, Harmsen JA. Cultural differences in managing information during medical interaction: how does the physician get a clue? *Patient Educ Couns.* 2007;67(1-2):183-190.

67. Chewning B, Bylund CL, Shah B, Arora NK, Gueguen JA, Makoul G. Patient preferences for shared decisions: a systematic review. *Patient Educ Couns.* 2012;86(1):9-18.

68. Putnam LL. Communication as changing the negotiation game. *J Appl Commun Res.* 2010;38(4):325-335.

69. Panichelli C. Humor, joining, and reframing in psychotherapy: Resolving the auto-double-bind. *AM J Fam THer.* 2013;41(5):437-451.

70. Djulbegovic B, Paul A. From efficacy to effectiveness in the face of uncertainty: indication creep and prevention creep. *JAMA.* 2011;305(19):2005-2006.

71. Faria C, Wenzel M, Lee KW, Coderre K, Nichols J, Belletti DA. A narrative review of clinical inertia: focus on hypertension. *J Am Soc Hypertens.* 2009;3(4):267-276.

PART III

Applications

CHAPTER 7

Negotiating Requests for Tests, Referrals, and Treatments

Clinical Take-Aways

- The clinical encounter affords patients and clinicians the opportunity to influence each other—patients by what they reveal and request, clinicians by what they ask and recommend.
- During a typical outpatient encounter, patients make requests for both information (e.g., about the significance of a symptom or lab result) and action (e.g., for medications, diagnostic tests, or referrals).
- Patients whose requests for services are denied tend to be less satisfied with their care, less likely to recommend the clinician to a friend, and (for acute conditions) less likely to report symptom resolution at follow-up.
- Clinicians are not obliged to accede to requests that are unreasonable, convey greater expected harms than benefits, or violate their own sense of professionalism. However, summarily rejecting a patient's request will reliably diminish the patient's care experience.
- Clinicians should:
  - Give the patient an opportunity to lay out their full agenda at the beginning of the visit.
  - Talk less and listen more—try to pick up on *why* the patient is requesting a potentially inappropriate service.
  - Focus less on *what* patients ask for and more on *why* they are asking.
  - Be alert to patient cues and respond to patients' emotions.
  - Be aware of their own emotional responses to patient requests.
  - When faced with a request for low-value care, consider *substituting* another service, stalling for time by offering a *contingency plan,* and providing clear instructions for *reconnecting* should the patient's clinical condition fail to improve.

SECTION 7.1: INTRODUCTION

The United States spends more on health care than any other developed nation. Yet the United States does poorly compared to other advanced economies in terms of life expectancy, maternal mortality, and hospitalizations for diabetes and hypertension, among other outcomes (OECD 2018 health data). Since health care spending depends on the number of services provided (quantity) and the price of each service (price), health economists have scrutinized both factors, concluding that high *prices* explain most of the difference in health care spending between the United States and its peers. Nevertheless, these same experts have also concluded that **up to a third of health care services are of little to no benefit** to patients receiving them.[1] Ironically, medical overuse occurs at the same time as medical underuse.[2] Thus, the failures of our health care system might best be summarized as an *allocation problem*, or what Enthoven and Kronick have called "*a paradox of excess and deprivation.*" **Some patients are overtreated at the same time that other patients (sometimes even the same patients) are undertreated.** The result is scattershot quality of care and shameful health disparities.

While high prices need to be addressed (and there are plenty of health economists and policymakers working ardently to do so), misallocation seems like a more appropriate target for the clinicians and future clinicians reading this book. For one thing, allocation (and misallocation) of health care resources is largely under the control of physicians, advanced practice nurses, and physician assistants. For another, cutting drug prices and physicians' salaries by even 50% would result in no more than a 15% one-time reduction in total health care expenditures.[3] Most importantly, **improving allocation of health care services has the potential to improve quality of care and reduce disparities.**

The causes of over- and under use of health care are many, but they can be divided into systemic, organizational, clinician, and patient factors. A health care system that fails to cover 10% of the population yet uses fee-for-service reimbursement will tend to deliver too few cancer screenings to the uninsured and too many coronary stents to those with "Cadillac" insurance plans. Health care organizations can influence under- and overuse through economic incentives, practice guidelines, reminders or defaults encoded into electronic medical record systems, and culture as expressed through formal and informal social networks. Individual clinicians retain significant control, however, and research has shown clear effects of individual physician practice patterns or "style" on use of health care resources [4] Finally, **patients themselves are a relatively unheralded but important influence on what physicians do.** This presents an important opportunity, since patients' advocating for themselves ("patients as agents for quality")[5] can help assure that they receive necessary services, while making it less likely that they will receive unnecessary or inappropriate care.

Clinicians and patients operate together in a process of mutual influence. Ideally, this exchange facilitates better understanding of the problem, the plan, and anticipated challenges. In *theory*, the process proceeds in a linear fashion, as illustrated in Figure 7-1.

In *practice*, the process is less linear and more recursive, with patients and clinicians exerting mutual influence at multiple stages of the encounter. For example:

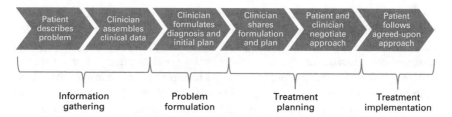

Figure 7-1. A linear model of patient-clinician negotiation.

> Patient: *I've been feeling tired lately, and I wonder whether my testosterone might be low.*
>
> Clinician: *Oh? Is there anything else that makes you think that might be the case?*
>
> Patient: *I saw an ad on TV, and they said "low T" can cause symptoms just like mine.*
>
> (doctor nods, encouraging patient to go on)
>
> *I'm tired all the time, I never want to go out at night, and I'm not gaining any muscle at the gym despite working out a lot.*
>
> Clinician: *Well, low testosterone is certainly one thing we should consider. Before I ask you more questions, is there anything else you can think of that might account for your fatigue?*
>
> Patient: *Not really. I've been working late quite a bit and my girlfriend isn't happy about that, but we've been through stuff before. I never felt like this. Can't we just do a blood test and see?*

In this exchange, the patient makes an oblique request for a blood test and possible androgen-replacement therapy. In so doing, he influences the physician both to consider a new diagnosis (hypotestosteronemia) and to probe more deeply for other causes of fatigue. In turn, through questioning, the clinician helps the patient consider related symptoms and alternative mental representations of illness. The patient accedes to the exercise, but ultimately expresses directly what may have been his underlying goal from the beginning.

In this chapter, we first take up the different ways clinicians and patients influence each other in ways that matter. Equipped with this taxonomy of mutual influence (which builds on material in Chapter 2), we can proceed to describe the importance of request fulfillment and nonfulfillment for patient outcomes and the role of trust in mediating how request fulfillment and denial are received. We conclude with specific advice about how to negotiate effectively about diagnostic tests, referrals, and treatments.

SECTION 7.2: THE PAS DE DEUX OF MUTUAL INFLUENCE

The pas de deux has been a versatile metaphor in many different fields.[6–8] The analogy to the patient-clinician encounter is of course limited. Patients and clinicians approach the clinical encounter with their own knowledge base, predispositions, attitudes, and concerns. But as in other forms of communication, patients and clinicians also support and influence each other. Active patient participation (expressing opinions, concerns, and questions) predicts physician partnership-building (verbal acts that encourage patients to express their opinions, talk about feelings, ask questions, and participate in decision making). But the reverse is also true: roughly one-sixth of patient participation is prompted by physician partnership behavior.[9]

Patients' influence has direct and practical consequences. Within the gray zone of medical practice, where several different diagnostic or treatment options are reasonable, patients (or parents of patients) have been shown to influence physician test-ordering, referrals to specialists, and prescribing of everything from antibiotics to antidepressants.[10,11] At the same time, clinicians not only direct patients' treatment but also shape attitudes and behaviors.

But how does this process of mutual influence take place? Table 7-1 displays several potential mechanisms by which patients might influence clinicians (and vice versa), organized according to stage of encounter.

In the early stages of the encounter, the clinician's first task is to *establish rapport* as a prelude to information gathering. Clinicians can encourage patient disclosure by conveying warmth and openness and being alert to verbal, paraverbal, and nonverbal clues. If the clinician seems rushed or tense, the patient may clam up, reluctant to impose on the clinician's time or fearful of having their concerns ignored. If on the other hand the clinician greets the patient warmly, sits down, makes eye contact, and listens attentively, the patient will be more inclined to share information they consider worrisome or embarrassing. By the same token, clinicians who allow the patient to complete their opening statement without interruption will find that they have not only successfully elicited the patient's agenda and gained valuable insight into the patient's experience of illness, but they will have done so (in the vast majority of cases) within the first 3 minutes of the encounter.[12]

Patience is similarly rewarded during the *information gathering* stage, particularly in the taking of the history of the present illness. Novice clinicians will be tempted to direct the patient to answer specific questions about the presenting complaint (e.g., duration, intensity, aggravating and alleviating factors, associated symptoms, etc.) or conduct a stereotyped review of systems. Following Osler's maxim to "listen to the patient," expert history-takers will allow the patient's story to unfold more naturally in a chronological framework, reserving closed- ended questions for later. In fact, as noted in Chapter 6, the time course of illness is so vital to diagnosis that medical educator Kelley Skeff has persuasively advocated for a more chronologically structured method of clinical documentation.[13] This documentation structure may facilitate not only the primary care provider's clear understanding of the patient's history, it can also support the understanding of others, like consultants, who use the documented history to contribute to patient care.[14]

Of course, patients are not passive recipients of care. Not only are they responsible for sharing their story, they are capable of directing clinicians towards—or away from—a therapeutically useful problem formulation. On rare occasions, misdirections are intentional, as when a patient with chronic pain on opioids provides misleading information about her use of nonprescription controlled substances. More often, they reflect the patient's struggles to categorize, organize, and express their experiences in terms the clinician can understand.

In the *problem formulation* stage, the clinician's task is to conceptualize the problem in terms that support a working differential diagnosis while conveying to the patient that he or she is understood. Here clinicians influence patients by eliciting and interpreting patients' mental representations of illness; patients influence clinicians by sharing their mental models. Sometimes the clinician will elicit patients' mental representations directly by asking, "What do *you* think might be going on?" Just as often, the patient will reveal their concerns indirectly through requests for tests, referrals, and treatments. For example, "I've been so tired, I was thinking I might need some kind of brain scan," might imply concern about a brain tumor, multiple sclerosis, or early-onset dementia. The clinician will never know unless she asks, using language like, "You do seem more worn out than usual. What do you think might be going on?"

At the *treatment planning* stage, clinicians may attempt to educate patients about their condition and make recommendations for diagnostic and therapeutic interventions. At the same time, patients influence clinicians by making explicit or implicit requests. Patients in the United States—and increasingly around the world—are exposed to massive amounts of health information in the mass media, online, and through interactions with family, friends, and acquaintances. The "prepared patient"[15] is well-equipped to use hints, conjecture, questions, requests, and even outright demands to obtain what they need or desire. As indicated in Table 7-1, these communication strategies can be applied prospectively (before the clinician makes initial recommendations) or retrospectively (after the clinician has done so).

During the *treatment implementation* phase the balance of power shifts back to the patient. Physicians can advocate, prescribe, recommend, warn, or abjure, but as autonomous human beings, patients have control over what they do or don't do. Sometimes this works to the patient's advantage, as in cases where patients have noted important side effects, leading them to discontinue prescribed medications before serious damage is done. But often, nonadherence impedes disease management.[16,17]

In summary, a linear view of the clinician-patient encounter inadequately incorporates mutual influence—the ways in which clinicians and patients shape the behavior of the other. Clinicians influence patients by asking questions,

Table 7-1 Mechanisms of Mutual Influence Enacted During Each Stage of the Clinical Encounter

Stage of Encounter	Possible Mechanisms of Mutual Influence	
	Clinicians Influencing Patients	Patients Influencing Clinicians
Establishing rapport	• Conveying warmth and openness • Noticing clues (verbal and nonverbal)	• Telegraphing emotions • Amplifying and masking reactions
Gathering information	• Asking questions • Choosing what to pursue	• Assembling and disclosing an agenda • Telling their story • Emphasizing and withholding details
Formulating the problem	• Eliciting mental representations of illness • Suggesting alternative representations or expressions	• Sharing mental representations of illness
Treatment planning	• Recommending for or against diagnostic interventions • Recommending for or against referrals to specialists • Recommending for or against therapeutic interventions	• Making explicit requests for care (tests, referrals, medications, procedures) • Making implicit (veiled) requests for care • Expressing agreement (or disagreement) with the treatment plan

Treatment implementation	• Monitoring of treatment adherence
	  • Questioning
	  • Laboratory tests
	  • Digital surveillance
	• Encouragement to adhere
		• Adherence to clinician treatment recommendations
		• Adherence to clinician monitoring recommendations

making recommendations, and encouraging adherence. Patients influence clinicians by choosing when and how to disclose information, making requests, and deciding whether to adhere to recommendations. **In an important sense, clinical negotiation is a matter of influencing and being influenced in ways that simultaneously support the patient's health and reinforce professionalism.**

SECTION 7.2: EPIDEMIOLOGY OF PATIENTS' REQUESTS

In ordinary life, when we want to know something (need information), or when we wish for someone to do something (want action), we *ask*. Requests can range from direct ("Could you please turn on the light?") to subtle ("My, it's dark in here."). Either way, it is now the responsibility of the other party to respond—in ways that may or may not be perceived as helpful. For example, a person near the light switch might say to the man quietly sitting in the dark, "You're right, I can't see anything either, let me get the light." Or, if that person were feeling night-adapted, ecologically minded, and surly, he might say, "I can see just fine. Besides, we're trying to reduce our power usage. Why don't you wait a few minutes and see if your eyes adjust?"

Similar dynamics operate during the clinical encounter. Patients' requests during office visits are common, diverse, and influential in shaping clinician behavior. To understand the frequency and distribution of patients' requests in clinical practices, researchers have adopted a number of approaches, including patient surveys, clinician surveys, audio- and video-recording, and direct observation by a third party.

Requests for Information

One definition of a request is "a question, command, statement or conjecture that a native speaker would recognize as an expression of desire for information or action."[18,19] Applying this definition to 270 audio-recorded visits in primary care and cardiology, we sorted patient requests into 21 categories (Table 7-2). The leading categories of *requests for information* were questions about medications and nondrug treatments (27%), physical symptoms or problems (19%), and diagnostic investigations (11%). Patients made direct requests for information an average of 4.3 times per visit. *Requests for action* were less common, averaging just under one request per visit. The most common action request category was for medications and other treatments (9%), followed by administrative requests (e.g., completing paperwork for insurance or disability purposes) (3%).

Requests for Action and the Shadowy Territory of "Veiled Requests"

In a related study of 45 physician practices, we looked specifically at requests for action.[20] The results were remarkably similar: 559 patients made 545 explicit audio-recorded requests for physician action—again, an average of about one per visit. About a quarter of patients requested at least one diagnostic test, specialty referral, or new prescription. And just like the man sitting in the dark, patients often buried "requests for action" within "requests for information." Table 7-3 gives examples drawn from the 74 camouflaged or "veiled" requests for action. The patient with the red face and a sick cousin (Table 7-3, first row) was not

Table 7-2 Audio-Recorded Requests for Information and Action Across 270 Visits in Internal Medicine (210 Visits) and Cardiology (60 Visits)

Request Type	Number of Requests	Percentage (of 1436 total requests)
Requests for information		
Physical symptoms or problems	271	18.9
Psychosocial problems	12	0.8
Physical examination	40	2.8
Tests or diagnostics	153	10.6
Medications/treatments	384	26.7
Prevention	63	4.4
Patient-clinician relationship	47	3.3
Other clinicians	18	1.2
Administrative issues (including managed care and financial issues)	82	5.7
Other requests for information	98	6.8
All requests for information	1168	81.3
Requests for action		
Physical examination	29	2.0
Laboratory tests, imaging studies, other diagnostic investigations	23	1.6
Referral to physician	19	1.3
Referral to nonphysician	9	0.6
Medications/treatments	128	8.9
Administrative requests (including paperwork)	44	3.1
Other requests for action	16	1.1
All requests for action	268	18.7

just story-telling; he wanted the physician to examine his skin and "listen to his arteries." The patient who asked, "Do you think a sonogram would show us anything?"(third row) was not merely curious about the optic resolution of medical sonography; she wanted the doctor to order an ultrasound.

But what about patients who do not articulate their needs at all? In after-visit surveys, 10% of patients reported that they wanted something of the clinician but refrained from asking. These patients with *unvoiced desires* had lower visit

Table 7-3 **Veiled Requests for Action in a Study of 559 Office Visits**

Information Request Category	No. of "Veiled Requests for Action"	Verbatim Example
Questions about physical symptoms, problems, or diseases	2	You notice how red my face is? My cousin who is four years younger than me went for a checkup ... and they checked her arteries and she eventually had to go have them reamed out because they were 99% closed and nobody's ever listened to my arteries.
Questions about the physical examination	2	Did you look at ... They are kind of going away now. They were, and I can't show you one on my head, it itches like ...
Questions about tests or test results	17	Do you think like a sonogram would show us anything?
Questions about medication	35	What I want to know is since you know I'm on this [acetaminophen with codeine] ... why I'm not getting extra refills that I have to come in for month after month?
Questions about nondrug therapies	8	Then I seen some new stuff coming around on hearts. Where they go in with the laser blaster, what about that?
Questions about other health care providers	10	Would it be worth seeing a podiatrist for this?

Source: Reproduced with permission from Kravitz RL, Bell RA, Azari R, Kelly-Reif S, Krupat E, Thom DH. Direct observation of requests for clinical services in office practice: what do patients want and do they get it? Arch Intern Med. 2003;163(14):1673–1681.

satisfaction, less symptom improvement, and more effortful visits (as reported by clinicians).[21]

In summary, patients' requests for *information* are ubiquitous; requests for *action* are less frequent but still common. Action requests are often "veiled" and sometimes unspoken altogether. **Requests that are not recognized cannot be addressed and may lead to worse patient and clinician satisfaction and outcomes.** In the next section we take up what happens when patients voice requests that clinicians can't or won't fulfill.

SECTION 7.3 REQUEST FULFILMENT AND PATIENT-REPORTED OUTCOMES

Most people are pretty good at using language to express themselves. **However, the clinical encounter is a special situation with its own set of rules.**

There is an imbalance of knowledge (the patient knows more about their own circumstances, the clinician knows more about diseases and their treatment), of power (the clinician makes the ultimate decision as to what is recommended or prescribed), and of familiarity with the clinical setting (the clinician works in the medical office or hospital, the patient does not). Whether by dint of education, experience, or personal or family background, patients are variably equipped to deal with what is essentially foreign territory. We therefore see an impressive variety of communication behaviors aimed at getting the clinician to listen, speak, act, and emote in various ways. Patients can express their desires and expectations directly and explicitly, implicitly (as "veiled requests"), or tacitly (e.g., through body language).

Deeper Dive 7.1: Defining Effective Clinical Communication

Researchers have worked hard to identify different dimensions of effective clinical communication.[63-66] The absence of consensus reflects not only the complexities of human communication but also the perspectives of different evaluators. Consider the following scenario.

A patient is worried about persistent headaches, is afraid she may have multiple sclerosis, goes to her primary care doctor (a resident at a teaching center), and requests a magnetic resonance imaging (MRI) study of the brain. The physician reports her blood work is normal and recommends watchful waiting and symptom management for a few weeks to see if the headaches subside. The patient is insistent, questions why the doctor is withholding a diagnostic test, and once again asks for an MRI. The two go back and forth until the physician suggests that he could refer her to a neurologist who could provide more expertise on whether the test is needed. The patient reluctantly agrees, and the physician makes the referral. [67,68]

Does this encounter represent effective clinician-patient communication? *It depends on who you ask.* For example, the patient may think she was an effective communicator because through her assertiveness and refusal to take no for an answer, she was able to make an insensitive doctor provide a referral to a specialist who could approve the MRI. The clinician may think he effectively reached a compromise with a demanding and uncooperative patient. Finally, after watching a video-recording of the encounter, an attending physician may rate the resident as communicating poorly by not averting a medically unnecessary referral.

As revealed in this scenario, what counts as effective clinician-patient communication depends on who you ask. For example, the patient believes in the idea that patients need to speak up by asking questions, expressing their concerns, and stating their preferences. [69] The physician embraces the tenets of shared decision-making, whereby the best decisions are supported by the evidence, consistent with patient preferences, and feasible to implement.[70] Hence, a referral to a specialist best satisfies those criteria. Finally, the attending physician believes that good communication must balance efforts to make patients happy with the organizational goals of achieving a more efficient workflow and wise use of resources. Three different perspectives, each using different sets of criteria, produce different judgments of communication quality.

While differences in perspective in part reflect the parties' individual motivations and criteria for communication success, there are also fundamental differences in the way self, interlocutor, and observers evaluate a communication encounter. For example, the interactants (clinician and patient) are engaged in a *cooperative* activity—creating a conversation. That is, to have a successful encounter they must work together to meet their individual and mutual goals. However, observers who are judging quality of communication are conducting an *evaluative* activity and have no responsibility for the conduct of the encounter. Thus not surprisingly, interactants tend to make more positive evaluations of their partners in general,[71] and in clinician-patient encounters in particular,[72,73] than do observers of an interaction. While little research has compared patients' ratings of themselves and clinicians with clinicians' ratings of themselves and patients, there is some evidence for differences. For example, one study reported that physicians are more critical judges of communication quality than are patients,[74] whereas another study found that first- and second-year residents rated their own communication higher than did the faculty or standardized patients.[75]

There is no gold standard for effective clinician-patient communication. There are, however, scores of different communication assessment measures used in training, certification, and research. These measures differ in many ways, including their assumptions about what constitutes effective communication, who decides, and what features of communication are being assessed (e.g., information-giving, relationship building, shared decision-making).[76,77] In studies that have compared different communication ratings systems focusing on the same construct (e.g., patient-centeredness), different measures often lead to different conclusions.[78,79]

The panoply of existing measures might be harmless were they merely used as tools to advance communication science and to improve clinician-patient dialog. However, in practice, several specific evaluation instruments have been applied as if they represented a gold standard. For example, Press-Ganey surveys of patient satisfaction are used in some health systems to compare clinician performance and to set annual bonuses. Others have proposed the use of patient satisfaction measures to identify and divert clinicians with low ratings into remedial communication training programs.[80]

The approaches advocated in this book, including the negotiation framework advanced in Chapter 6 and the "Five Rules" promoted here, are evidence-based and experience-based options for effective clinical negotiation, not gold standards for performance. Our recommendations are grounded in the scientific evidence for what works and for what clinicians and patients can do as communicators to make this happen—sharing perspectives and beliefs, finding common ground, reconciling differences, creating shared understanding, and reaching agreement on next steps. The breakdown of negotiations in the case of the patient requesting an MRI was not in the values or the well-intentioned efforts of the different parties. It was that they communicated singularly as individuals and not collaboratively as partners.

Whatever the means of expression, it takes psychic energy to make a request. What happens when patients' requests are not fulfilled?

In general, just what you would expect. Patients whose requests are fulfilled incompletely or not at all tend to be less satisfied with their care, less likely to recommend the clinician to a friend, and (for acute conditions) less likely to report symptom resolution at follow-up.[22] **However, as we will see, the *way* in which clinicians deflect patients' requests matters a great deal.**

How might this work? The answer has substantial practical importance. As professionals, clinicians cannot and should not accede to every patient request. **Sometimes, "getting to no" is just as important as "getting to yes."**[23] But how?

In a field experiment examining the effects of patients' requests on physician prescribing, we sent actors posing as patients into clinicians' offices.[24] The actors portrayed patients suffering from major depression (a serious condition requiring expeditious evaluation and treatment) or adjustment disorder (a less serious condition often successfully addressed by providing psychological support and watchful waiting). The portrayals were assigned at random, but considering only the visits in which actors requested an antidepressant prescription, clinicians who peremptorily denied those requests received lower ratings of interpersonal quality of care. On the other hand, those who offered psychosocial support ("It sounds like you've been under a whole lot of stress—can we talk about that?"), an alternative treatment ("Would you consider counseling?"), or a contingency plan (e.g., "Let's hold off on antidepressants for now but see you back very soon to make sure you are feeling better") received significantly higher ratings.

Analogous findings have emerged from critical care settings, where the request (often coming from family members) is to continue care that the medical team considers potentially inappropriate or futile.[25] Clinician statements offering reassurance about the primacy of the patients' comfort, a promise of non abandonment, and support for the family's decision were associated with more rapid conflict resolution and higher family satisfaction.[26]

The common thread is that relationships count. The corollary is that time invested in building relationships can provide valuable returns. Clinicians who are able to successfully communicate genuine interest and compassion will have an easier time "getting to no." As Peabody might have said, *the secret of the care of the (request-making) patient is in caring for the patient.*

SECTION 7.4: TRUST AND ITS DISCONTENTS

Healers have enjoyed a special place in human history. This was true even when shamans, traditional healers, and physicians had little to offer clinically, and it is true today. Nonetheless, **trust between patients and clinicians is fragile,** subject to easy disruption by socioeconomic, interpersonal, and psychological forces that are often beyond the control of the parties involved. Consider this case:

> *Mrs. Ettinger is a 76-year-old African-American woman who comes to see Dr. Patchett, her primary care physician (PCP), after a recent COPD exacerbation requiring a 5-day hospital stay. Mrs. Ettinger is very upset that Dr. Patchett did not come to see her in the hospital. Several facts appear to be at play:*
>
> * *Forty years prior: The US Public Health Service completed the Tuskegee experiment, in which African-American men were left with untreated syphilis in order to observe the natural history of the disease.*
> * *Five years prior: Dr. Patchett was asked by his primary care group to stop seeing his own patients in the hospital in the interests of efficiency. Instead, he was to leave inpatient duties to the newly affiliated hospitalist group.*
> * *Six months prior: Mrs. Ettinger's new Medicare Advantage plan required that she switch to Dr. Patchett's group from Dr. Alford, her previous PCP.*
> * *Two weeks prior: The hospitalist admitting Mrs. Ettinger promised the patient he would call Dr. Patchett, but in the heat of a busy day (eight admissions, one code), she forgot to do so.*
> * *One hour prior: Mrs. Ettinger arrived for her appointment with Dr. Patchett on time. The receptionist asked her about her recent hospitalization loudly enough that she could be heard across the waiting room. Then Mrs. Ettinger was kept waiting for more than 45 minutes with no explanation.*

In this scenario, history does not dictate the lines but it does help set the stage. African-Americans were surely the objects of discrimination by White physicians and other health care providers long before Tuskegee,[27] but that seminal experience remains a central narrative in the lives of many African-Americans today. This is manifested in diminished trust in the health care system and in health care professionals,[28] attitudes that have been reinforced by ongoing structural and interpersonal racism.[29] But in our scenario, both yesterday's history and today's disparities are prelude. For reasons that are not entirely clear to Mrs. Ettinger, her own physician was not available to take care of her in the hospital; instead, she was seen by a team of unfamiliar and arguably overworked hospitalists, one of whom failed to follow through on a promised phone call. Making matters worse, Mrs. Ettinger had only recently switched to Dr. Patchett's practice (leaving a physician she liked) due to insurance requirements. When she recovered sufficiently to attend her first outpatient visit following the hospitalization, Mrs. Ettinger was treated in what she considered a disrespectful manner.

Scholars have identified four broad dimensions of patient-clinician trust: 1) fidelity (acting in the patient's best interests); 2) competence (technical capacity to serve those interests); 3) honesty (telling the truth and not withholding desired information); and 4) confidentiality (not disclosing sensitive information to third parties without permission).[30] Little is known about how patients assess and weigh up these dimensions to say, in the end, "I trust (or do not trust) this doctor to take care of me." But it seems clear that individual clinician behaviors and the structure of health care systems are both influential.[31] **Doctors can build a reservoir of trust by explaining to patients how their recommendations serve the patient's interests; by demonstrating thoroughness and skill in history taking, physical examination, and technical procedures; and by disclosing information in a manner concordant with the patient's preferences.** Clinicians should strive to bolster trust when they can, as trust is not only a contributor to healing but also the foundation of successful clinical negotiation about tests, referrals, and treatments.

SECTION 7.5: TALKING ABOUT RISKS, BENEFITS, AND COSTS OF DIAGNOSTIC TESTS

When one of us was a medical resident in the 1980s, the chair of medicine declared that "diagnosis is becoming trivial." The chair, a superb diagnostician, based this conclusion on the rapid development of diagnostic imaging technologies. Computed tomography (CT) was maturing, magnetic resonance imaging (MRI) was nascent, and positron emission tomographic (PET) scanning was making some very early forays into clinical medicine.

The chair's prediction of the demise of diagnosis was premature. New imaging and other diagnostic advances (including now routine biomarkers like brain natriuretic peptide [BNP], procalcitonin, D-dimer, and high-sensitivity troponin) have opened new diagnostic windows, but they have, if anything, complicated the picture. Does a 1.2-cm adrenal adenoma, detected on an MRI scan for other reasons, need to be investigated? Does a normal D-dimer level rule out venous thromboembolism in a patient recovering from hip surgery? Does the CT finding of a tree-in-bud appearance in the left lower lobe mean this inpatient with altered consciousness has aspirated? These are important questions that, at least in the present moment, require clinical judgment and cannot be answered with technology alone.

Informational and Signaling Value of Diagnostic Tests

From the standpoint of clinical negotiation, diagnostic tests (a term we will use broadly to include examination of body fluids or tissue as well as imaging studies) serve two purposes. The first—which we call *"informational"*—is derived from Bayes' Theorem, which says that the probability of having a given disease after completing a diagnostic test is a function of both the test result and the "pre-test probability of disease"—the likelihood of the condition based on the patient's epidemiologic and clinical characteristics. In this frame, tests are useful to the extent that they support accurate diagnosis or prognosis.

The other purpose of diagnostic tests is arguably more relevant to clinical negotiation. From this perspective, tests are important less for the diagnostic information they provide[32] than for their ability to signal the clinician's interest in the patient's problem and to help clinician and patient shape a more coherent narrative of the illness experience. By ordering tests and imaging studies, the clinician conveys to the patient that the clinician takes their situation seriously; believes their condition may have an organic basis; is intent on finding a cogent explanation; and (implicitly) believes that identifying a cause may lead to more effective treatment. At the same time, laboratory and imaging findings can often help wrap a more compelling narrative around the proposed diagnosis, causal factors, and prognosis associated with the patient's illness.

> *Ms. Higa is a 48-year-old project manager for a technology company. Over the past 6 months, she has experienced irregular menses (sometimes missing a period) and intermittent hot flashes and night sweats. After taking a careful history, her primary care nurse practitioner, Patricia Charles, thinks the most likely explanation is menopause. Ms. Higa, however, is skeptical. "How would you know that? Isn't there a blood test you can order?" Ms. Charles obtains a serum FSH, which returns elevated, confirming her suspicion of menopause.*

Was this FSH test necessary? Was it likely to add sufficient value to Ms. Higa's care to justify the modest cost ($50-$100), the small immediate risk (hematoma or infection from phlebotomy), the possibility of sampling error (FSH levels fluctuate markedly and can sometimes be normal in the perimenopause), and the potential for downstream "cascade effects"?[33] In the case of Ms. Higa, a reasonable clinician (such as Nurse Practitioner Charles) might conclude that it is prudent, not to mention expeditious, to order the test. But another, equally reasonable clinician, might decide to negotiate.

Ms. Higa: *Isn't there a blood test you can order?*
NP Charles: *Well, yes there is one, and it would be easy to do. But it may not be necessary, because your symptoms—the irregular periods, the hot flashes—are all so consistent. You know the saying, "if it looks like a horse and runs like a horse, it's probably not a camel."*
Ms. Higa: *I see what you mean. But aren't I a little young for menopause?*

Here Ms. Higa is providing an important clue. Her comment suggests that she is less worried about diagnostic alternatives (like cancer—a common concern) than about the implications of menopause. But this needs to be explored.

NP Charles: *Actually, you're right at the age when we would expect to see this. But I was wondering what you've heard or read about menopause.*

The clinician could have jumped in and asked directly whether the patient found the idea of menopause threatening. But she wisely follows a more oblique approach.

Ms. Higa: *Oh, the usual stuff in all the magazines, you know, "how to be sexy after 50" (smiles). But to be honest this whole thing is a little hard to accept.*
NP Charles: *It can be hard, for sure, to deal with a changing body. But as I know you've read in the magazines, this is just another life phase, and what you're experiencing is completely normal. How about we hold off on the lab tests but have you keep track of your cycles over the next 3 months? Then let's check in and make sure you're not having any unusual symptoms that would need more testing.*
Ms. Higa: *That sounds ok. See you in 3 months.*

This clinical negotiation was successful in the sense that an unnecessary test was averted and the patient was placated, if not fully satisfied. However, it did take time. Given the relatively low stakes, many clinicians would have opted to order the requested test. But what about more complex situations?

Edgar Martinez is a healthy-appearing 45-year-old political lobbyist. His father (age 73) had a heart attack in his late 60s. Five years ago, Mr. Martinez was noted to have an LDL cholesterol of 150 (with no other risk factors) and was placed on a low-dose statin. Two years ago, he saw a direct-to-consumer ad for CT calcium scanning; he decided to obtain the test, which returned a score of 86 (0 is very low risk; anything higher than 0 suggests the presence of calcified atherosclerosis, with higher scores indicating greater calcium burden). When Mr. Martinez brought the result to his primary care physician Dr. Lopez, he was advised to "repeat the test because a lot of these fly-by-night companies are not accurate." The repeat score was 130, and Dr. Lopez advised the patient to switch to a high-dose statin regimen (atorvastatin 40 mg daily). Now it is 2 years later, and Mr. Martinez is asking for a repeat calcium scan "in order to see whether things are getting better or worse."

Addressing a case like this starts with a thorough understanding of the relevant medical facts. To convincingly dissuade a patient from

unnecessary or low-value testing, the clinician needs to be secure in his or her knowledge of the patient's history, to have conducted pertinent parts of the physical exam, and to have sufficient knowledge of the relevant pathophysiology and differential diagnosis to develop a reasonable clinical assessment leading to a safe and effective therapeutic plan. In the case of Ms. Higa, this might have been relatively easy: the vasomotor symptoms were classic, there was nothing suggestive of more ominous causes, and the patient was squarely in the age range when menopause is expected to begin. With Mr. Martinez, however, many nonspecialists would lack the top-of-head knowledge to credibly reject the request. In that case, depending on the clinical urgency, it might be possible to defer the decision briefly in order to consult reference material or a colleague. It is never a good idea for clinicians to stake out a position that they cannot defend, medically and ethically.

However, even with the relevant clinical facts and medical knowledge in hand, the clinician is unlikely to conclude the negotiation successfully without also understanding something about the patient's underlying motivation. Has Ms. Higa been burned by misdiagnosis in the past? Is she worried because her great aunt (a recent immigrant) was recently hospitalized for tuberculosis after several months of night sweats? Is Mr. Martinez, upon learning that his wife is pregnant with their second child, worried that he might leave his growing family in the lurch if he were to die suddenly of coronary heart disease? Has he misinterpreted the increase in calcium score over the past 2 years as indicating a higher risk of heart attack? What does he imagine is happening to his body? As we saw in Chapter 2, understanding patients' mental representations (mental models) of illness is a critical prerequisite to effective negotiation.

Maintaining Receptivity to Clues: A Comparison of Two Dialogs

Consider the two clinician-patient dialogs in Table 7-4. Both are heavily slanted towards the biomedical; there is lots of information transfer. But in Dialog 2, Dr. Lopez notices a change in the patient's facial expression, accompanied by a short verbal pause. The change is subtle, and Lopez might not have noticed were his attention focused on the computer screen. But he does notice, and he uses the opportunity to show empathy and inquire about the patient's emotional state. This leads to an important revelation, which in turn allows Dr. Lopez to address the patient's fears more directly. Both dialogs conclude with a "victory" for Dr. Lopez, in that an arguably unnecessary repeat CT calcium score is not ordered. However, the resolution of Dialog 1 is arguably pyrrhic, as the patient, his underlying concerns skirted, leaves the office fearful and disgruntled.

In summary, requests for diagnostic tests are often a plea for clarity, a way of signaling distress, or an effort to evaluate the depth of the clinician's commitment to find answers. Successful clinical negotiators know that such requests are not to be taken wholly at face value. A little bit of questioning can go a long way.

Table 7-4 **Two Parallel Conversations**

Speaker	Dialog 1	Dialog 2
Mr. Martinez	I'd like to get another scan to see whether things are getting better or worse.	Same as Dialog 1.
Dr. Lopez	We could certainly do that, but you're on a high-dose statin already, so as long as you're not having chest pains, the results really wouldn't change our treatment.	That's an interesting possibility. If we got a repeat scan, how do you imagine we might use the information?
Mr. Martinez	Ok, but I'd still like to get the test.	I have no idea. You're the doctor. But I assume it would tell us if my arteries are getting closed off.
Dr. Lopez	Again, the calcium scan is not likely to show us anything that we don't already know. I would encourage you to keep up with plant-based diet you talked about, continue to exercise, and take your statin. We'll keep a close eye on your cholesterol and blood pressure, and periodically reassess. And of course, if you have any heart-related symptoms—things like chest pain with exercise, fainting, or shortness of breath—let me know right away. And in an emergency of course, call 911.	Yes, the amount of calcium on the scan correlates with the amount of hardening of the arteries. But the real problem is when that plaque becomes hard and brittle and ruptures, causing a sudden blockage which then leads to a heart attack. That's why we have you on that statin drug—to soften and stabilize the plaque so it doesn't cause problems, and to keep new plaque from forming. And your cholesterol has been doing really, really well.
		(Pauses, notices patient's worried look.)
		This whole thing can be scary though, right?
Mr. Martinez	Ok, I see your point; I guess I don't have much choice. What about my knee?	You better believe it's scary. I have a family to support.
Dr. Lopez		So you're worried about something happening to you, leaving your family to struggle alone?
Mr. Martinez		(gazing downwards)
		That's a big part of it.

(Continued)

Table 7-4 **Two Parallel Conversations** (Continued)

Dr. Lopez	That's a really serious concern. But I have to tell you, I'm optimistic. Your blood pressure is controlled, your cholesterol is good, you don't smoke, and you're reasonably physically active. When we plug your numbers into the formula, your 10-year risk of a heart attack or stroke is less than 7%. That means that over the next decade, out of 14 men like you, 1 will have an event—most of which are survivable —and 13 will be just fine. Pretty good odds, I'd say.
Mr. Martinez	Ok then. I guess I'll keep doing what I'm doing.

SECTION 7.6: TALKING ABOUT CONSULTATIONS, REFERRALS, AND SECOND OPINIONS

Technically, consultation refers to a time-limited evaluation of a specific problem, whereas referral implies a request for assistance in ongoing care. Second opinions are consultations requested by the patient. From a practical standpoint, however, consultation, referral, and second opinions all start the same way: a question is posed to a specialist, the patient sees them, and a revised plan of care is developed based at least in part on their impressions. In this chapter we will adopt the term "referral" to incorporate requests for both focused consultation and ongoing care.

A Model of Referral Decisions

Health care systems want to get their referral rates "right."[34] *Under-referral* can result in medical error, failure to deploy beneficial procedures, and suboptimal patient care. *Over-referral* can generate unnecessary health care costs and lead to overuse of specialty-based tests and procedures. However, measuring appropriateness of referrals is challenging.[35] Part of the reason is that **the threshold for appropriate referral depends not only on the patient's medical condition and psychosocial status but on the practitioner's own knowledge, skills, and self-efficacy** (Figure 7-2). While one might argue that all primary care practitioners should be able to perform a skin biopsy, if the clinician has no experience with this procedure it would be unwise to simply "give it a go"; the dermatology referral is appropriate, leaving continuing medical education for another time.

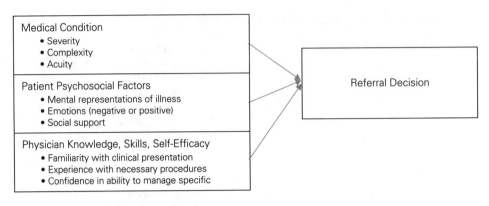

Figure 7-2. A simple model of referral decisions.

Similarly, resistant (refractory) hypertension is common enough in primary care that most primary care clinicians are comfortable initiating a search for secondary causes and treating the elevated blood pressure. However, clinicians lacking experience in this area would be justified in seeking consultation from a hypertension specialist.

In practice, it is assumed that requests for specialty consultation originate with the requesting clinician. After all, it is the clinician (or clinician's office) that must call the specialist's office, complete the referral form, or place the consultation order. However, patients can and do ask for referrals; physicians report that patient requests are a factor in referral decision making about one-third of the time.[36] As discussed previously, patients make referral requests both directly ("I want to see a dermatologist for my acne") and obliquely ("I heard there are some new drugs the dermatologists are using for this.") When asked for a referral, what is the clinician to do? Consider this dialog between Dr. Mills, a young internist, and Mr. Wallis, a 56-year-old industrial foreman with hypertension, prediabetes, and a remote history of smoking.

> Dr. Mills: *Hi Mr. Wallis, what brings you in today?*
> Mr. Wallis: *I've been having chest pains and thought I should see a cardiologist.*
> Dr. Mills: *So you came in for a referral?*
> Mr. Wallis: *That's right.*
> Dr. Mills: *Well, if it's ok with you, I'd like to understand the problem a bit better, and then maybe we can work out a plan together. But before we do that, have you had any chest pains in the past few days?*
> Mr. Wallis: *No, the last one was over the weekend.*

In this encounter, Mr. Wallis does not equivocate; he's had some worrying symptoms that he ascribes to possible heart problems, and he wants to see a cardiologist. In the initial moments of the encounter, Dr. Mills needs to simultaneously rule out a medical emergency and quell her own emotional reaction to Mr. Wallis' request. After all, Dr. Mills has been treating Mr. Wallis for hypertension for more than 2 years, and some part of her can't help but interpret his request for referral as a negation of her own skills. She easily rules out acute chest pain with a simple question, buying herself time. But dealing with her own psychological reactivity is more difficult. The first step is to recognize that **patient requests for referrals can sometimes provoke a spectrum of negative emotions in clinicians, including anxiety, anger, guilt, and sadness.** Even more than requests for tests or treatments, requests for referrals may be heard as if they imply a vaguely disguised message: "I'm afraid you won't be able to handle my problem, so I want to see someone else."

In the heat of the moment, there is little time for rational reflection. For this reason, seasoned clinicians engage in explicit *affective forecasting*,[37] anticipating their *internal* reactions to patients' requests and planning their *external* responses. Another robust defense against succumbing to emotional reactivity is *curiosity*: asking not "why doesn't the patient trust me?" but rather, "what has stirred up the patient's anxieties to such a degree that he wants a referral for a problem that, so far, seems quite manageable?"

After shaking off her initial defensiveness, Dr. Mills enlists the patient's cooperation in exploring his symptoms. Indeed, Mr. Wallis has been having exertion-related central chest pains several times per week over the past 3 months that, except for an occasional sharp stabbing component, are fairly classic for chronic stable angina. Blood pressure is well-controlled, physical examination is unremarkable, and a lipid panel from 2 years ago showed total cholesterol 215 mg/dl and HDL 45 mg/dl. His 10-year risk of heart attack, stroke, or cardiovascular death is 7.6%. He is not currently on a statin.

> *Dr. Mills: Based on what you've told me, I agree with you that we need to be concerned about heart disease.*
>
> *Mr. Wallis: Yeah, I was afraid of that.*
>
> *Dr. Mills: Hearing that there might be something wrong with your heart would be a big deal for anyone. (Mr. Wallis nods.). But there's some things we can do right now to evaluate the problem further and start treatment. First, let's do an EKG in the office. Then, if the EKG is ok, we'll send you for an exercise stress test. That will give us a lot of information about the severity of the problem as well as the longer-term prognosis—which, by the way, I suspect is good—mainly because you continue to be healthy and active. Finally, I'd like to start three medications, one to control your cholesterol, one to prevent a heart attack, and the third to help with your chest pains.*
>
> *Mr. Wallis: That all sounds fine, but what about seeing a cardiologist?*
>
> *Dr. Mills: Well, I was thinking of getting these preliminary studies together before deciding whether we need to go that route, but I wonder if there are some things you're still concerned about.*

Here Dr. Mills invites Mr. Wallis to share the underlying drivers of his referral request. Mr. Wallis may not accept the invitation. Some patients are naturally more expressive, others more reticent.

Mr. Wallis: I don't know, I just thought it might be good to get a specialist involved.

Now Dr. Mills is at a crossroads. She can put in the referral, reasoning that if the stress test is negative it can always be cancelled. She can try to defer consultation for now, suggesting to Mr. Wallis that if the stress test suggests a problem that is more serious than expected, referral can occur then. Or she can squash the request altogether.

Why Not "Just Say No"?

We do not recommend this last approach. **When the clinician denies requests outright without addressing patients' underlying concerns, research suggests that trust and satisfaction suffer.** Offering an *alternative or contingency* is much more effective.[24]

> *Dr. Mills: Well, that's certainly reasonable; sometimes it can be very helpful to get a specialist's opinion. On the other hand, we want to get a cardiologist involved at the right time, when he or she could be of the most help. And right now I think we should concentrate on getting that stress test and starting some medicines that will help with the chest pains and prevent any further narrowing of the arteries. How about if we try that and have you back here in 1 or 2 weeks?*
>
> *Mr. Wallis: That sounds good. I just didn't want to miss anything. I don't think I told you, but my grandfather dropped dead of a heart attack at 68.*

This is crucial information, and it would have been helpful if Dr. Mills had inquired about the patient's family history earlier in the visit. Nonetheless, the visit concludes satisfactorily, Mr. Wallis undergoes his stress test (it is mildly positive, with 1 mm of ST segment depression but good endurance and a heart rate approaching 90% of maximum), he takes his prescribed statin and beta blocker assiduously, and when seen in follow-up, his chest pains have diminished markedly. Dr. Mills mentions that she ran his case by a cardiology colleague earlier in the week, and everyone agreed that if medical therapy successfully suppressed his symptoms, further evaluation would not be needed at this time.

Reasons for Referral Requests

Few studies have examined patients' reasons for requesting specialty referral. In one such study, 45% of 860 patients surveyed in primary care waiting rooms had definite or possible desires to see a specialist. The most common reasons for referral requests were need for reassurance (67%), having seen a specialist before (56%), and believing the primary care physician lacked expertise (49%).[38]

Although each of these reasons are superficially distinct, they revolve around the belief that the primary care clinician may not be prepared to take on the problem at hand. Sometimes this belief arises from the misperception that a particular problem is outside the domain of primary care. Other times patients may recognize that the condition can be handled in primary care but believe that their own case is too unusual, complex, or multifaceted to be manageable without assistance from a specialist. Having seen a specialist before may be reason enough to want to see them again.

Finally, there is the quest for reassurance. A systematic review suggests that for many patients, cognitive reassurance (changing patients' perceptions and beliefs through education) is more effective at promoting positive outcomes (reduced anxiety, improved satisfaction) than affective reassurance (attempting to reduce worry and enhance rapport).[39] Through this lens, specialty referral can be viewed as supporting cognitive reassurance by providing the patient with access to a professional with special knowledge of the symptom complex or condition that is most troubling to the patient. **However, when reassurance is the goal, medically equivocal referral should be selective.** Such referrals are most likely to provide reassurance when the problem is sufficiently well-defined to fall into a single specialty domain. Every clinician can recall patients with vague or undefined symptoms who were sent on endless, and ultimately counterproductive, ventures to see multiple subspecialists, each of whom ordered a battery of tests, yielding both true positive and false positive results, and generating more diagnostic ambiguity than clarity.

Thus, the rationale for selectively resisting patients' requests for referrals is not simply a matter of avoiding excessive costs; unnecessary referrals are associated with other forms of unnecessary care. **It is simply not true that "it never hurts to get a second opinion."** Sometimes the price—in terms of inconvenience, cascade effects, and confusion as to who is in charge—is too high.

SECTION 7.7: TALKING ABOUT TREATMENT: PRESCRIPTION DRUGS, THERAPEUTIC PROCEDURES, AND DURABLE MEDICAL EQUIPMENT

Licensed physicians, nurse practitioners, and (in some states) physicians' assistants are endowed by the government with unique authority to mete out (or deny) a medley of therapeutic interventions, including prescription drugs, therapeutic procedures, and durable medical equipment. In the usual case, the practitioner evaluates the patient, suggests a diagnosis, and recommends a slate of therapeutic interventions. Patients will almost always accede to these recommendations, although they may adhere with less-than-perfect fidelity.[40–42] But as we have seen in prior chapters, patients frequently bring with them well-formed expectations for treatment, often a prescription drug but sometimes a procedure, medical device, or piece of durable medical equipment. These expectations are communicated as requests.[21]

Media Influences on Requests for Treatment

It is impossible to contend seriously with patients' requests for treatment without understanding the media environment in which patients live, work, and socialize. The average American television viewer watches up to nine drug advertisements per day,[43] and pharmaceutical companies spent over $6 billion on direct-to-consumer advertising in 2016.[44] Though small by comparison, advertising efforts by hospitals and physicians plying specialized procedures such as robotic surgery, proton beam radiation, and micro-discectomy have been increasing rapidly.[45] Add to this the dozens of health-related stories appearing every day in print, broadcast, and social media, many of which tout new therapies without adequately weighing the evidence.[46,47] **Given this barrage of exposure, it is no wonder that many patients arrive at their doctor's doorstep intently curious about, if not adamantly demanding, new drugs, devices, procedures, and equipment.** As we saw in Chapter 3, the media is but one of many influences on patients' illness representations (mental models of illness) and expectations for care. However, in surveys of physicians and several observational studies in outpatient settings, media-driven requests for treatment seem poignant, impactful, and—from the doctor's perspective—often unwelcome.[48,49]

Consider the following dialog between Mrs. Pearl, a 73-year-old retired attorney, and Dr. Chen, a recent graduate of the local internal medicine residency program.

> Mrs. Pearl: *[near end of visit]. There's one more thing, Dr. Chen.*
> Dr. Chen: *Sure, what is it?*
> Mrs. Pearl: *This is kind of embarrassing, but I've wet myself a couple of times when I couldn't get to the bathroom fast enough. I saw this ad for Vesicare® and I wondered if I could try it.*

Dr. Chen is aware that solifenacin (Vesicare) reduces urgency modestly (by about one episode per day, according to a meta-analysis she remembers from journal club) but causes bothersome anticholinergic side effects in some older patients.[50] After obtaining additional history, performing a urine dipstick (negative for blood, nitrates, and leukocyte esterase), and noting that the patient had a normal gynecological exam 6 months ago, she decides she will encourage Mrs. Pearl to try behavioral approaches first. But she is aware that abruptly shutting down Mrs. Pearl's request could backfire. She is also mindful that her next patient is waiting.

> Dr. Chen: *I'm so glad you told me about this trouble you've been having. How were you hoping Vesicare® could help?*

This is a critical question that generalizes to many different kinds of patient requests.

> Mrs. Pearl: *Well, like I said, I don't like wetting myself. It's embarrassing and inconvenient. I'd like it to stop.*

Mrs. Pearl is clearly annoyed by the question. But it's an important starting point.

> Dr. Chen: *I can understand how distressing this must be. Based on what you've told me, as well as your office urine test and prior pelvic exam, I'm thinking you probably do have overactive bladder, a very common problem in middle aged (and older) women.*

> Mrs. Pearl: *[Smiles]*

Dr. Chen makes an empathetic statement, summarizes the clinical facts, and proposes a diagnosis.

Dr. Chen: Medicines like Vesicare® do work, but the truth is they're not a cure—studies show they reduce episodes of needing to use the bathroom urgently by about one episode per day. So if you're rushing to the bathroom four times a day now….

Mrs. Pearl: I can expect to only rush three times?
Dr. Chen: That's right, at least on average. I'm happy to write a prescription for Vesicare® or another similar medicine, but there's another approach that works better and has no side effects. However, it does require some work on your part.

Because there is no strict contraindication to prescribing an anticholinergic medicine, Dr. Chen sets the patient at ease by telling her, in effect, "I'm willing to comply with your request. But first let's talk."

Mrs. Pearl: Not those Kegel exercises!
Dr. Chen: No, not Kegels, though they might help you hold on a little longer when you get the urge. What I was talking about is behavioral therapy. I can ask our nurse to go over the details with you, but basically it involves going to the bathroom at specific times so that you gradually retrain the bladder—and the brain—to fall in line.

Dr. Chen is fortunate to work in a practice where the nurse:clinician ratio is 1:1 and where the nurse is skilled in educating patients about a variety of topics. This level of support in primary care is still rare, despite evidence that it may improve efficiency and reduce burnout.[51]

Mrs. Pearl: Ok, but I'd still like to try the medicine.
Dr. Chen: Well, how about this? I'll write a prescription for Vesicare® and will "pend" it for the nurse I'm working with today. You go over the behavior therapy with her, and if you still want the prescription at the end of the session, she'll release it. Just be prepared for some dry mouth and possibly some fatigue. If you get too tired or your thinking seems muddled, stop the meds and give me a call.

At this point in the negotiation, Dr. Chen offers a contingency plan: at least hear about behavior therapy, then decide whether to take a medicine where the benefits are closely balanced by risks.

Mrs. Pearl: Alright, thank you, Doctor.
Dr. Chen: I'll see you in a month.

Strategies for Addressing Requests for Treatment

Table 7-5 outlines several strategies for addressing patient's requests for treatment, many of them illustrated in the dialog between Mrs. Pearl and Dr. Chen. The first two strategies lay the groundwork for the negotiation. The clinician needs to connect with the patient and demonstrate genuine interest in the problem. The second two strategies emphasize "blending with the force."[52] **Overt refusals, though sometimes necessary, are often counterproductive.**[24] Offering a contingency plan can be satisfying to both parties.

Table 7-5 Strategies for Addressing Patients' Requests for Treatment

Strategy	Sample Language
Show empathy or support	*I can understand how distressing this must be. You are doing an amazing job coping with this problem.*
Demonstrate interest in the problem	*Can you tell me more about this problem? Start at the beginning.* *Let's take a look. (prelude to physical examination)*
Deflect, don't repel	*The medicine you saw advertised is definitely an option.* (But there are other, safer options.) *Robotic surgery has been advancing rapidly.* (But the jury is still out on whether patients actually benefit.) *I can see how additional hours of home health services could be useful to you.*
Consider a contingency	*I'll put in a prescription for Vesicare®, and you can fill it if behavior therapy doesn't work for you.*

Negotiating Over Therapeutic Procedures

Although the majority of the literature on clinical negotiation addresses prescription drugs, other categories of treatment deserve attention. Requests for procedures within primary care are often conflated with requests for referral, because the specialized procedures most avidly marketed to patients are generally provided in specialized settings. For example, "I was hoping I might get a referral to the back clinic downtown" could be a thinly disguised request for the microdiscectomy procedure the patient had seen advertised in the local newspaper. Our focus here is on direct requests for procedures.

Contested procedures tend to fall into three groups: 1) *purely elective* (such as cosmetic surgery); 2) *innovative but incompletely vetted* (such as intravenous ketamine for depression or autologous platelet-rich plasma for tendonitis); or 3) *mainstream but not necessarily appropriate* in light of the patient's personal circumstances (such as elective coronary angiography for a patient with chronic stable angina who has not yet tried medical therapy). In the first instance, the primary care clinician (PCC) encourages discussion of procedural risks and benefits but is spared the role of gatekeeper, because most third-party payers do not cover purely elective procedures lacking medical indications. As the clinician most familiar with the patient's biopsychosocial circumstances, the PCC is also in a good position to ask questions about the patient's underlying motivation. Patients' responses to a few probing questions ("How long have you been thinking about liposuction?" "I guess ever since my divorce") can sometimes illuminate deeper problems that require further exploration.

In the case of promising but unproven interventions, the PCC should acknowledge the patient's initiative ("That's a very interesting idea"), highlight areas of uncertainty ("My understanding is that this procedure has not been around very long; we would really need to do our homework"), and arrange for some form of follow-up after the patient has had a chance to investigate further ("Send me a message through the patient portal after you've seen the surgeon. I'd be happy to work through the decision with you.").

Finally, with regard to mainstream procedures, the primary care clinician's role is not to supplant the specialist, but to implement whatever evidence-based therapies he or she is comfortable providing, direct the patient to a qualified specialist, and keep channels of communication open. Assuming that they are clinically stable, patients with chronic angina, nonmorbid obesity, or migraines do not need stents, gastric bypass, or Botox injections until they have been tried on evidence-based lifestyle interventions or medications.

Negotiating Over Durable Equipment, Medical Supplies, and Disability Forms

Over the past decades, an expanding array of specialized medical equipment, assistive devices, and supplies have made patients' lives easier and more functional. Figuring in this category are walkers and wheelchairs, electronic scooters and hospital beds, CPAP machines and insulin pumps, syringes and incontinence supplies. To assure public and private payers that these items are medically necessary and likely to deliver functional benefit, clinicians are required to complete mountains of paperwork. Failure to do so—and to do so meticulously—results in interminable delays and unhappy or angry patients. Distinguishing between patients' *wants* and patients' *needs* is a physically, mentally, and morally taxing enterprise. The moral hazard derives from two dilemmas: 1) asking payers to subsidize items of marginal value threatens to deplete the medical commons and 2) the availability of certain types of equipment (e.g., motorized scooters) may, in rare instances, discourage behavior (e.g., walking) that would actually be beneficial to the patient's health. Until clinicians are relieved of the requirement to police the dispensing of these items, we recommend that they focus on advocating for their patients. These steps will make it easier:

- Try to keep up with the evidence on indications for the most common types of durable equipment and supplies.[53]
- Proactively recommend equipment and supplies when supported by evidence or clinical judgement.
- Ask patients regularly if they "have what they need at home to manage their health conditions."
- Get to know a good physical therapy department and a home health agency; work with them to assess the need for specialized equipment and supplies.
- Train someone in your practice to handle most of the correspondence with DME companies and third-party payers, leaving the clinical decision making to you.

Clinicians may incur similar moral distress from requests for long-term disability certification. Here it is important to stay focused on the patient's best interests (which may or may not align with the patient's current perceptions). At the same time, unless employed as formal adjudicators, the physician's role is to document the patient's medical conditions and resultant functional limitations—nothing more or less.

SECTION 7.8: NEGOTIATING TOWARD ADHERENCE

So far, we have emphasized negotiations in which patients make requests and clinicians respond. But it is important to acknowledge that there are just as many occasions where clinicians make requests, offer suggestions, or order interventions—and patients explicitly or implicitly disagree. Mountains of literature have been published on the problem of patient nonadherence.[54]

However, in our view, the problem is incompletely understood. Patient adherence to clinical directives may or may not benefit the patient's health, depending on the evidence supporting the recommendation, the "fit" of the evidence with the patient's individual characteristics, and the patient's social and environmental circumstances. Furthermore, the relationship between adherence to evidence-based care and health outcomes is more complex than is often acknowledged.[55] As illustrated in Figure 7-3, the relationship may be dichotomous (no benefit below a certain adherence threshold, near-maximum benefit above that threshold), linear (increasing adherence leads to increasingly good outcomes), curvilinear (slope of the relationship changes at different adherence levels), or S-shaped (little benefit

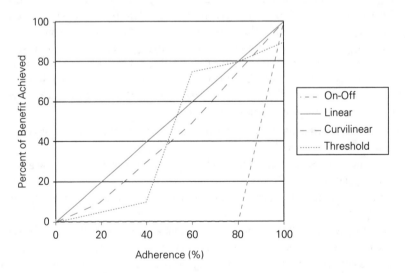

Figure 7-3. Linear and nonlinear models of adherence. *Source:* Reproduced with permission from Kravitz RL, Melnikow J. Medical adherence research: Time for a change in direction? Medical care. 2004;42(3):197–199.

below a certain threshold, rapid increase in benefit with modest adherence increments, then little gain above a second, higher threshold).

Acknowledging these complexities, assume that the clinician has recommended evidence-based care modified to fit the patient's individual circumstances and preferences. What can clinicians do to maximize the likelihood that these care plans will be carried out as intended? Schaffer and Yoon have summarized a set of practical, evidence-based strategies that can be implemented, to one degree or another, by every clinician (Table 7-6). These strategies are grouped into affective,

Table 7-6 Affective, Behavioral, and Cognitive Strategies for Enhancing Patient Adherence to Clinician Recommendations

Affective Strategies	Behavioral Strategies	Cognitive Strategies
Establish patient relationships that allow free discussion of adherence. Preface adherence questions with "Other patients have difficulties with…"	Ask the patient about adherence at every visit and continue until treatment is no longer needed.	Clearly state the purpose of the drug and how to take it.
Allow the patient to express concerns without interrupting.	Call the patient if an appointment is missed.	Tell the patient what to do if doses are missed.
Treat the patient as an equal partner.	Ensure that the patient has the physical ability (hand strength, coordination, vision) to adhere.	Reinforce instructions in writing (be certain that the patient can read and that information is on the appropriate reading level).
Involve spouses or intimate partners in identifying strategies to help with adherence.	Prescribe medication in concert with the patient's daily schedule. Consider asking the patient to take medication in association with regular daily activities.	Keep patient information simple and succinct; avoid medical jargon. State the most important information first.
	Advise the patient to keep medicines where they will be remembered.	
	Keep the medication regimen simple (e.g., once daily if possible). Consider using pill containers that can be prefilled for 1 week.	
	Endorse the potential benefit of the prescribed medication during all patient contacts.	
	Ask the patient how medication will be remembered if his or her schedule is interrupted.	

Source: Reprinted with minor changes from Schaffer SD, Yoon S-JL. Evidence-based methods to enhance medication adherence. *Nurse Pract.* 2001;26(12):44–50. with permission.

behavioral, and cognitive categories.[56] **The main points are to engage the patient by listening to their concerns, ask about adherence at every visit, simplify the treatment regimen as much as possible (e.g., by prescribing once-a-day drugs), and provide written directions.**

SECTION 7.9: FIVE RULES FOR NEGOTIATING ABOUT TESTS, REFERRALS, AND PRESCRIPTIONS

Talking with patients about tests, referrals, and treatments is something most physicians do dozens of times every day. Most of the time these conversations go so smoothly as to be entirely unnoticed. But sometimes things veer rapidly off course. The patient with tension headaches demands an MRI. The patient with garden-variety osteoarthritis wants to see a rheumatologist. The patient with long-standing irritable bowel syndrome presents to the emergency department with chronic pain, has an abdominal ultrasound showing a single gallstone, and now wants his gallbladder out.

In cases like these, there is no foolproof method for finding common ground between the patient's expectations and desires and the clinician's medical judgement. But that doesn't mean there is nothing clinicians can do. The five rules listed in Table 7-7 and elaborated upon below can ease the way from conflict to conciliation.

Table 7-7 Five Rules for Negotiating around Tests, Referrals, and Treatments

1. Create space at the beginning.
2. Talk less, listen more.
3. Respond to patients' emotions.
4. Be self-aware.
5. Give something to get something.

Deeper Dive 7.2: The Communicative Power of Requests

Patients who make requests of clinicians are engaging in a powerful form of interpersonal communication. For one thing, given conversational norms, a patient making a request, whether for information or action,[81] obligates the clinician to respond. In the case of a request for antibiotics, for example, the clinician could respond by granting, denying, or deflecting the request. (Deflection is often accomplished with a question, e.g., "How were you thinking antibiotics might help?")[82]

Furthermore, when the interactants have an established and/or coopera-tive relationship, as is often the case with clinicians and patients, there is considerable pressure on the person being asked to comply with the request (e.g., to avoid feelings of guilt, to make the other happy, or to sustain the relationship).[83] These reasons in part explain why clinicians struggle with how to handle patient requests that are unsupported by evidence or oth-erwise conflict with the clinician's professional judgement. For similar rea-sons, patients who harbor doubts about physicians' recommendations for medical treatment or lifestyle changes may be reluctant to say so directly.

Request making and granting often unfold in stages, especially when the request is one the responder is reluctant to accommodate (or is perceived that way by the requester). In such situations, the request maker may engage in a process of sequential requesting where the first request (which is not the real ask) creates a more favorable setup for the second request (the pri-mary ask). Research on communication and compliance-gaining identifies several strategies for sequential request making, two of the most prominent being the "door in the face" and "foot in the door" approaches.[84,85]

The door-in-the-face approach involves making a big request that is likely to be rejected. That sets up a second request that is more tolerable and more likely to be accepted than the original ask. The foot-in-the-door takes the opposite approach. The initial request is small and thus easy to accept. An incrementally bigger asks comes later after the responder has granted the first request.

Evidence from experimental and field research indicates both approaches can be effective at gaining compliance.[85] Savvy patients could use the "door in the face" approach to convince clinicians to grant their requests. For example, a patient concerned that a clinician wants to taper his opi-oid prescription might ask for an *increase* in opioid dose, knowing it will be rejected, with the expectation that the second request, *maintaining* the current prescription, will be accepted. Another example might be where a patient asks for a medical note allowing time off work for a trivial injury. The patient expects this request to be rejected, but the primary ask, a note requesting exemption from heavy lifting, would be granted. Patients' use of the "foot in the door" approach is probably less common, but one example would be when the patient with a chronic illness wants to extend the time interval between follow-up visits because travelling to the physician's office is costly and inconvenient. In this case, rather than asking up-front for annual revisit intervals, the patient might negotiate for extending 3-month visits to every 4 months. Then after demonstrating clinical stability, the patient might ask for every-6-month and then every-12-month follow-up.

Clinicians trying to convince patients to accept potentially effective but risky interventions will occasionally deploy a variation of the "door in the face approach." For example, a surgeon might say to her diabetic patient with osteomyelitis of the big toe unresponsive to antibiotics, "a below the knee amputation would be the safest approach and the one that I generally prefer, but we could try just removing the toe and continue to watch you very closely." However, in this variation it is the clinician, not the patient, who proposes the less invasive compromise. The standard door in the face dynamic is not generally a practical negotiating tactic for clinicians, because few patients feel comfortable talking a clinician down from their initial recommendation even if they find it unreasonable—for fear of making the physician upset or being labeled a "difficult" patient.[86] For example, a patient may be absolutely opposed to colonoscopy because of fear, modesty concerns, or the belief that she is not at risk for colon cancer. Nevertheless, the patient may not actively question her doctor's recommendation in the interest of not causing offense.[87]

The "foot in the door" approach, on the other hand, has considerable intuitive appeal as a negotiation strategy for clinicians, especially in situations where patients' resistance to treatments may be due to denial (e.g., substance abuse), learned helplessness (e.g., obesity), or stigma (e.g., depression). Here the clinician could make a small ask that is not threatening but achievable (e.g., try an online counseling program, a modest change in diet and exercise, or meditation). A patient who successfully achieves that may then be more confident or amenable to a larger ask, such as enrolling in a substance abuse program, obesity clinic, or psychotherapy. In many ways, the small ask is similar to goal-setting approaches to managing chronic disease, where success in achieving realistic, smaller goals incrementally can ultimately lead to achievement of more ambitious goals.

Rule 1: Create space at the beginning. Much of the work of clinical negotiation occurs before the negotiation actually begins. Clinicians tend to interrupt patients within seconds of soliciting the chief complaint.[12,57] However, when patients are allowed to continue uninterrupted, few speak for more than 3 minutes. Furthermore, patients encouraged to unpack their full agenda have fewer last-minute requests.[58] Exceptions notwithstanding (e.g., the manic or extremely anxious patient), in most cases little is lost by letting the patient have their say. This lesson is easily ignored by clinical trainees as they struggle to construct a coherent narrative out of a rambling opening statement. However, the payoff from attentive listening and planful agenda setting can be immense.

Rule 2: Talk less, listen more. Primary care clinicians have invested countless hours (and often, thousands of dollars) in their own education and training. Clinicians know things. And they are often eager to convey what they know to patients. This is honorable and fitting. But it is sometimes counterproductive. **When patients ask questions or request interventions (directly or indirectly), it is easy to assume that they want information, action, or both.** However, this assumption is sometimes wrong. People do not always know exactly how they feel or what they want, and a few moments of exploration will help them clarify their concerns and obtain such psychological relief as comes from feeling better understood. Taking time for reflection and exploration is especially important when differences in language, race/ethnicity, culture, or socioeconomic status create social distance between clinician and patient. Table 7-8 provides examples of patient statements (column 1) that commonly trigger the kinds of instinctive responses (column 2) generated by what cognitive psychologist Daniel Kahneman might call "System 1."[59] However, both clinician and patient will be better off if the clinician slows down, invokes "System 2," and explores the sources and implications of the patient's statement.

Rule 3: Respond to patients' emotions. Patients' requests for services may reflect underlying anxiety about a serious disease, potential loss of control, or fear of abandonment by the treating clinician. It is clearly impossible for PCCs to fully explore a patient's motivations for requesting clinical services, let alone their reactions to illness or to the threat of illness, during a short office visit. However, patients may provide clues that provide opportunities for giving empathic support. In a study of 116 office visits to primary care physicians and surgeons, Levinson et al. found that patients provided clues ("direct or indirect comments about their lives or emotions") in over 50% of encounters. Physician responses classified as "helpful" included acknowledgement; encouragement, praise, or reassurance; and support (Table 7-9). Potentially harmful responses included inadequate acknowledgment, inappropriate humor, denial, or premature termination. If anything, visits in which patient clues were met with helpful responses tended to be shorter than visits in which such clues were ignored or brushed off.[60] The bottom line is that patients experience powerful emotions in relation to symptoms or illness; they frequently offer clues regarding their emotional states; and they are grateful when clinicians pick up on clues and encourage disclosure and exploration. Disclosure and exploration can, in turn, increase the likelihood of finding common ground.

Rule 4: Be self-aware. Negative or unnerving emotions arising in the course of clinical negotiation are not the sole province of patients. The struggle to hear, understand, and respond to patients' requests for clinical services can provoke a range of emotions in clinicians themselves, including defensiveness, anger,

Table 7-8 Instinctive (System 1) versus Reflective (System 2) Clinician Responses

Patient Statement	Clinician's Instinctive Response (System 1)	Better Response (System 2)
I take my blood pressure medicine when I need it.	That's not how it works. Blood pressure medicines have to be taken every day.	1. How do you know when to take the medicine? 2. How do you know it's working? 3. What do you imagine might happen if you took the medicine every day?
I want an MRI so we can find out the cause of my back pain, not just treat the symptoms.	You have what we call non-specific mechanical low back pain. Although I know your pain can be quite severe, you don't have other symptoms (like fever, weight loss, or weakness) that would make us worry about something more serious. So, an MRI is not likely to help us.	1. What do you think might be happening inside your back right now? 2. What do you imagine an MRI might show? 3. What will we do if the MRI comes back negative? What if it comes back positive, and shows some arthritis or a slipped disc?
I'm due for my annual visit with Dr. King (my cardiologist).	You know, that's probably not necessary anymore. Your heart attack was years ago.	1. Oh—how long have you been seeing Dr. King? 2. What does he usually do for you? 3. Do you have any particular concerns about your heart?
I'm due for a refill on Ativan®. I take ½ milligram every night. Otherwise I can't sleep.	That's really not the safest thing to be doing, especially as you get older.	1. How long have you been on Ativan®? 2. What happens when you don't take it? 3. Do you ever feel drowsy or dizzy in the morning after you take the medicine? 4. Have you ever thought about tapering down?

anxiety, sadness, and guilt. Defensiveness can emerge as the clinician comes to believe that their judgment has been questioned. ("Who does this patient think they are? I'm pretty sure I am the one who went to medical school.") Anger can follow. If the conversational temperature rises, patients and clinicians may make provocative statements that only escalate the conflict. Clinicians may experience anxiety as they wonder whether the requested service is actually needed. ("What

Table 7-9 Helpful and Harmful Responses to Patient Clues

Type of Response	Definition	Example
Positive Response		
Acknowledgment	Physician names patient's feelings or acknowledges life concerns	Ph: I'm very frustrated, so I'm sure that your frustration is much more than mine. ...
Encouragement, praise, reassurance	Physician encourages, praises, or offers reassurance	Ph: I think people like you, who care enough about your diabetes control, that you'll hang in there. ...
Supportive	Physician is supportive of patient's concerns	Ph: I think it's really important you get second opinions for the complicated problems ... you want the best for yourself
Missed Opportunity		
Inadequate acknowledgment	Physician acknowledges clue, but does not respond to patient's underlying concerns	Pt: I just am so tired. ... Ph: I would like you to do as much as you feel like doing ... I used to encourage you to get out and walk, I can't really tell you anymore, you know. ...
Inappropriate humor	Physician jokes or laughs inappropriately	Ph: I guess, we're just gonna have to, you know ... you're getting so old ... we're gonna have to shoot ya ... that's all there is to it ...
Denial	Physician denies patient's concerns	Ph: This really isn't a big deal.
Termination	Physician terminates discussion of emotions	Pt: Hhhh, I'm a wimp, heh heh, I'm imagining. ... Ph: All right ... We'll see you Friday, do you have any questions?

*Ph indicates physician; Pt, patient.
Source: Reproduced with permission from Levinson W, Gorawara-Bhat R, Lamb J. A study of patient clues and physician responses in primary care and surgical settings. *JAMA.* 2000;284(8):1021–1027.

if I'm missing something?") Anger and anxiety can evolve into sadness, as the clinician realizes that he or she is perceived to be less than fully competent, knowledgeable, or trustworthy. Finally, regardless of the clinical decision, clinicians can feel guilty: if they accede to the request they may wonder if they are wasting resources while scurrying down a clinical rabbit hole; if they reject the request they may worry about shutting down patients' legitimate requests in the interest of preserving their own authority.

There is little that clinicians can do to ward off these emotions, but self-aware-ness can mitigate some of the destructive consequences. Sometimes it is enough to pause, reflect, and step back from the brink, asking "what can I do to de-escalate the situation and allow cooler heads to prevail?" And, as psychiatrists have long realized through their study of countertransference, the clinician's emotions can also provide clues to the patient's psychological state. Feeling angry? Perhaps the patient is feeling out of control. Feeling disrespected? Perhaps the patient feels threatened by a loss of autonomy. Just acknowledging the possibility of these connections can help clinicians focus on finding common ground.

Rule 5: Give something to get something. When responding to patients' requests for tests, referrals, and treatments, the main thing to remember is to never lead with "no." Even if the patient's request is for the most risible, far-fetched, clinically inappropriate service one can imagine, the clinician will advance the conversation more effectively if she acknowledges the legitimacy of the request ("I'm glad you asked about that") and makes an effort to understand the patient's point of view ("That's an interesting idea. How did you come upon it?"). Then, should the clinician decide that acceding to the request is not in the patient's best interest, we recommend following one or more of these three strategies:

- *Substitution* involves offering an *alternative diagnosis* ("I doubt that restless legs syndrome explains your insomnia, but I suspect you've been under a lot of stress lately") or an *alternative approach* ("Let's get a serum iron and also teach you some behavioral techniques that many people find very helpful."). The substituted diagnosis should be defended credibly and framed provisionally. For example, a patient with knee pain is concerned about arthritis. The clinician thinks a mechanical problem (patellofemoral syndrome) is more likely. A credible but provisional response might run something like this:

Arthritis is always a possibility in cases of joint pain, but your pain is just in one knee not both, the pain gets worse with prolonged sitting, there's no swelling, your knee has great range of motion, and I can bring on the pain by pressing down on your kneecap. [Patient nods.] So I think it's far more likely you have something called patellofemoral syndrome, which should respond to physical therapy. If you're willing to try PT, let's see how you do with that—I'd like you to come back in about 6 weeks—and we can always do x-rays later.

The clinician in this case assembles and organizes evidence, using the patient's own words and experience. He provides a provisional diagnosis as an alternative to the patient's view. But he also indicates an openness to revising his opinion based on new evidence, while at the same time signaling commitment to work with the patient over time.

- Offering a *contingency* involves putting off provision of the desired service for a period of time, allowing for other treatments to take effect or for the natural history of illness to unfold. This strategy is particularly effective in primary care, where many illnesses are self-limited and can safely be followed expectantly. Contingencies have been used with positive effect in pediatrics, where withholding antibiotics for a few days in children with suspected otitis media results in similar clinical outcomes compared with immediate antibiotics.[61] When offering a contingency, however, it is important to be explicit about the algorithm that is on offer: what the patient or parent should look for, when they should look, what will happen next, and how the contingency will be implemented. For example, a pediatrician might say: "I think Luca will feel much better just with acetaminophen and a humidifier, but if he's still uncomfortable in 3 days, here's a prescription for amoxicillin which you can fill and give to him. If anything changes or you have any further concerns, you know our number."

- *Availability* means reassuring the patient that they will be able to reach you (or a colleague) in the event that their symptoms progress, fail to improve, or simply trigger unendurable anxiety. Patients are much more likely to accept more conservative treatment (especially when the safety advantages are explained) if they know that—should things go wrong—there is a back-up plan. In many large health systems, patients have to fight their way through a centralized triage system that is often overburdened and may sometimes overprioritize protecting clinicians from unnecessary calls. Therefore, in high-stakes situations, clinicians should consider providing patients with their personal pager or cell phone number. Most patients (although certainly not all) will safeguard the privilege (and not abuse it) if carefully instructed on parameters, and they will be very grateful to have been entrusted in this way. In lower stakes, less time-sensitive clinical situations, tools like secure electronic health portals can be a very convenient way to keep tabs on an evolving clinical situation.

SUMMARY POINTS:

- Allocation of health care resources is important from both a clinical and policy perspective.
- Resource allocation is largely under the control of clinicians, but clinicians are influenced by practice structures, financial incentives, and patients themselves.
- Medical decision-making is best described as a process of mutual influence.
- Patients frequently make requests of clinicians for both information and specific action, including ordering tests, making referrals, and prescribing treatments.
- Patient request fulfilment has been associated with greater visit satisfaction, higher likelihood of recommending the clinician, and faster symptom resolution.
- Some requests cannot reasonably be fulfilled. How patients react to request nonfulfillment depends in part on how the request denial is communicated: flat-out rejection is rarely appreciated.
- Patient trust in the clinician is a fundamental driver of how patients respond to request nonfulfillment. While most patients trust their doctor, many—particularly

those from excluded or disadvantaged groups—have good reason to distrust the systems and personnel charged with their care.

- Diagnostic studies serve both an instrumental and relational purpose. To some patients, test ordering signals that the clinician is interested in their condition, takes the situation seriously, and is committed to finding a specific cause. For this reason, request denial should occur in a context where the clinician's commitment is already clear.

- Patients' requests for referrals are generally routine but on occasion can trigger resentment or self-doubt in the clinician. Understanding the reason(s) for the patient's referral request is a prerequisite for an appropriate response.

- Two strategies for responding to patients' requests for treatment are 1) deflect, don't repel and 2) offer a contingency.

- The flip side of managing patients' requests for treatment is encouraging patient adherence. Several evidence-based affective, behavioral, and cognitive strategies are available.

- Five rules for negotiating around tests, referrals, and treatments are:
  - Create space at the beginning
  - Talk less, listen more
  - Respond to patients' emotions
  - Be self-aware
  - Give something to get something

QUESTIONS FOR DISCUSSION:

1. Dr. Khouri moves from his fee-for-service practice to a group-model health maintenance organization (HMO), and his patient Mr. Tabat switches insurance so that he can retain Dr. Khouri as his primary care physician. What new pressures might Dr. Khouri experience in his new practice environment? What changes might Mr. Tabat expect in Dr. Khouri's readiness to approve Mr. Tabat's many requests for tests and referrals?

2. What is the distinction between requests for information and requests for action? In the study summarized in Table 7-2, what were the most common requests of each type?

3. Aside from the positive outcomes discussed in Section 7.3, what are some other reasons clinicians might be inclined to fulfill patients' requests, even when the service is at the margin of clinical appropriateness (balance of risk and benefits)?

4. Psychologists have identified "agreeableness" as one of the Big Five Personality Traits. Agreeableness relates to a person's general concern for maintaining social harmony. How do you think physicians typically score in this domain (higher or lower than the average member of the population)? How does agreeableness

relate to the propensity to fulfill patients' requests? (Hint: Some insight can be gained from this article.)[62]

5. A growing literature suggests that patients are more comfortable with clinicians who speak their native language; patients in language-concordant dyads may also experience better outcomes. (This is as true of monolingual English-speaking patients as anyone else, but in the United States the problem is most acute for patients with limited English proficiency.). Three possible policy approaches are to recruit more diverse clinicians who are demonstrably bilingual/bicultural; require fluency in a second language as a prerequisite for medical school; or fully fund programs to help new immigrants achieve English language fluency as quickly as possible. What do you see as the advantages and disadvantages of each proposal?

6. How does systemic racism in the United States influence the clinician-patient negotiation over tests, referrals, and treatments?

7. A 27-year-old woman whose grandmother just succumbed to breast cancer at age 78 requests testing for the BRCA genes. What questions would you ask to understand the nature of her request? How might you best reach a reasonable clinical accommodation?

8. A 48-year-old former middle manager is now homeless, living in his minivan, which he parks in a friend's driveway at night. He successfully applies for Medicaid insurance. At his first visit to a new physician, he worriedly states that he thinks he has been exposed to scabies and would like a referral to a dermatologist. How might you approach this patient?

9. A 44-year-old health care administrator sees an ad for Requip® (ropinirole) and wonders whether her sleeping difficulties could be due to restless legs syndrome. After taking a complete history and performing a brief physical and neurological examination, you conclude that she most likely has anxiety and insomnia related to recent disturbing news events. How would you negotiate her request?

10. (For practicing clinicians) Which of the "FIVE RULES" do you already routinely apply in your own practice? Which (if any) do you believe might need more attention?

References:

1. Cutler DM. What is the US health spending problem? *Health Aff*. 2018;37(3):493-497.
2. Kravitz RL, Laouri M. Measuring and averting underuse of necessary cardiac procedures: a summary of results and future directions. *Jt Comm J Qual Improv*. 1997;23(5):268-276.
3. Jha A. Unique US solution needed to tackle high health spending. In: Writer ASN, ed. *AMA State Advocacy Summit*. Available at https://www.ama-assn.org/practice-management/economics/dr-jha-unique-us-solution-needed-tackle-high-health-spending: American Medical Association; 2019.
4. Cutler D, Skinner JS, Stern AD, Wennberg D. Physician beliefs and patient preferences: a new look at regional variation in health care spending. *Am Econ J Econ Policy*. 2019;11(1):192-221.
5. Kravitz RL. Beyond gatekeeping: enlisting patients as agents for quality and cost-containment. *J Gen Intern Med*. 2008;23(10):1722–1723.

6. Berridge MJ, Lipp P, Bootman MD. Signal transduction. The calcium entry pas de deux. *Science*. 2000;287(5458):1604-1605.

7. Chenette EJ. Cancer: A Ras and NF-kappaB pas de deux. *Nat Rev Drug Discov*. 2009;8(12):932.

8. Stearns T. Centrosome duplication. a centriolar pas de deux. *Cell*. 2001;105(4):417-420.

9. Street RL, Krupat E, Bell RA, Kravitz RL, Haidet P. Beliefs about control in the physician-patient relationship. *J Gen Intern Med*. 2003;18(8):609-616.

10. Mangione-Smith R, McGlynn EA, Elliott MN, McDonald L, Franz CE, Kravitz RL. Parent expectations for antibiotics, physician-parent communication, and satisfaction. *Arch Pediatr Adolesc Med*. 2001;155(7):800-806.

11. Kravitz RL, Epstein RM, Feldman MD, et al. Influence of patients' requests for direct-to-consumer advertised antidepressants: a randomized controlled trial. *JAMA*. 2005;293(16):1995-2002.

12. Beckman HB, Frankel RM. The effect of physician behavior on the collection of data. *Ann Intern Med*. 1984;101(5):692-696.

13. Skeff KM. Reassessing the HPI: the chronology of present illness (CPI). *J Gen Intern Med*. 2014;29(1):13-15.

14. Skeff KM. Restructuring the patient's history: enhancing the consultant's role as a teacher. *Gastroenterology*. 2014;147(6):1208-1211.

15. Hu X, Bell RA, Kravitz RL, Orrange S. The prepared patient: information seeking of online support group members before their medical appointments. *J Health Commun*. 2012;17(8):960-978.

16. Ho PM, Magid DJ, Masoudi FA, McClure DL, Rumsfeld JS. Adherence to cardioprotective medications and mortality among patients with diabetes and ischemic heart disease. *BMC Cardiovasc Disord*. 2006;6(1):48.

17. Eells SJ, Nguyen M, Jung J, Macias-Gil R, May L, Miller LG. Relationship between adherence to oral antibiotics and postdischarge clinical outcomes among patients hospitalized with Staphylococcus aureus skin infections. *Antimicrob Agents Chemother*. 2016;60(5):2941-2948.

18. Kravitz RL, Bell RA, Franz CE. A taxonomy of requests by patients (TORP): a new system for understanding clinical negotiation in office practice. *J Fam Pract*. 1999;48(11):872-878.

19. Kravitz RL, Bell RA, Franz CE, et al. Characterizing patient requests and physician responses in office practice. *Health Serv Res*. 2002;37(1):217-238.

20. Kravitz RL, Bell RA, Azari R, Kelly-Reif S, Krupat E, Thom DH. Direct observation of requests for clinical services in office practice: what do patients want and do they get it? *Arch Intern Med*. 2003;163(14):1673-1681.

21. Bell RA, Kravitz RL, Thom D, Krupat E, Azari R. Unsaid but not forgotten: patients' unvoiced desires in office visits. *Arch Intern Med*. 2001;161(16):1977-1984.

22. Kravitz RL, Bell RA, Azari R, Krupat E, Kelly-Reif S, Thom D. Request fulfillment in office practice: antecedents and relationship to outcomes. *Med Care*. 2002;40(1):38-51.

23. Fisher R, Ury WL, Patton B. *Getting to yes: Negotiating agreement without giving in*. Penguin; 2011.

24. Paterniti DA, Fancher TL, Cipri CS, Timmermans S, Heritage J, Kravitz RL. Getting to "no": strategies primary care physicians use to deny patient requests. *Arch Intern Med*. 2010;170(4):381-388.

25. Bosslet GT, Pope TM, Rubenfeld GD, et al. An official ATS/AACN/ACCP/ESICM/SCCM policy statement: responding to requests for potentially inappropriate treatments in intensive care units. *Am J Respir Crit Care Med*. 2015;191(11):1318-1330.

26. Stapleton RD, Engelberg RA, Wenrich MD, Goss CH, Curtis JR. Clinician statements and family satisfaction with family conferences in the intensive care unit. *Crit Care Med*. 2006;34(6):1679-1685.

27. Gamble VN. Under the shadow of Tuskegee: African Americans and health care. *Am J Public Health*. 1997;87(11):1773-1778.

28. Halbert CH, Armstrong K, Gandy OH, Shaker L. Racial differences in trust in health care providers. *Arch Intern Med*. 2006;166(8):896-901.

29. Bailey ZD, Krieger N, Agénor M, Graves J, Linos N, Bassett MT. Structural racism and health inequities in the USA: evidence and interventions. *Lancet*. 2017;389(10077):1453-1463.

30. Hall MA, Zheng B, Dugan E, et al. Measuring patients' trust in their primary care providers. *Med Car Res Rev.* 2002;59(3):293-318.

31. Levinson W, Gorawara-Bhat R, Dueck R, et al. Resolving disagreements in the patient-physician relationship: tools for improving communication in managed care. *JAMA.* 1999;282(15):1477-1483.

32. Siontis KC, Siontis GC, Contopoulos-Ioannidis DG, Ioannidis JP. Diagnostic tests often fail to lead to changes in patient outcomes. *J Clin Epidemiol.* 2014;67(6):612-621.

33. Mold JW, Stein HF. The cascade effect in the clinical care of patients. *N Engl J Med.* 1986;314(8):512-514.

34. Mehrotra A, Forrest CB, Lin CY. Dropping the baton: specialty referrals in the United States. *Milbank Q.* 2011;89(1):39-68.

35. Thom DH, Kravitz RL, Kelly-Reif S, Sprinkle RV, Hopkins JR, Rubenstein LV. A new instrument to measure appropriateness of services in primary care. *Int J Qual Health Care.* 2004;16(2):133-140.

36. Donohoe MT, Kravitz RL, Wheeler DB, Chandra R, Chen A, Humphries N. Reasons for outpatient referrals from generalists to specialists. *J Gen Intern Med.* 1999;14(5):281-286.

37. Wilson TD, Gilbert DT. Affective forecasting. *Adv Exp Soc Psychol.* 2003;35(35):345-411.

38. Lin C-T, Albertson G, Price D, Swaney R, Anderson S, Anderson RJ. Patient desire and reasons for specialist referral in a gatekeeper-model managed care plan. *Am J Manag Care.* 2000;6(6):669-678.

39. Pincus T, Holt N, Vogel S, et al. Cognitive and affective reassurance and patient outcomes in primary care: a systematic review. *Pain.* 2013;154(11):2407-2416.

40. Liaw S, Young D, Farish S. Improving patient-doctor concordance: an intervention study in general practice. *Fam Pract.* 1996;13(5):427-431.

41. Staiger TO, Jarvik JG, Deyo RR, Martin B, Braddock CH. Brief report: Patient-physician agreement as a predictor of outcomes in patients with back pain. *J Gen Intern Med.* 2005;20(10):935-937.

42. Tamblyn R, Eguale T, Huang A, Winslade N, Doran P. The incidence and determinants of primary nonadherence with prescribed medication in primary care: a cohort study. *Ann Intern Med.* 2014;160(7):441-450.

43. Parekh N, Shrank WH. Dangers and opportunities of direct-to-consumer advertising. In: Springer; 2018.

44. Horovitz B, Appleby J. Prescription drug costs are up; So are TV ads promoting them. *USA Today.* March 16, 2017, 2017.

45. Larson RJ, Schwartz LM, Woloshin S, Welch HG. Advertising by academic medical centers. *Arch Intern Med.* 2005;165(6):645-651.

46. Moynihan R, Bero L, Ross-Degnan D, et al. Coverage by the news media of the benefits and risks of medications. *New Engl J Med.* 2000;342(22):1645-1650.

47. Schwartz LM, Woloshin S, Baczek L. Media coverage of scientific meetings: too much, too soon? *JAMA.* 2002;287(21):2859-2863.

48. Mintzes B, Barer ML, Kravitz RL, et al. How does direct-to-consumer advertising (DTCA) affect prescribing? A survey in primary care environments with and without legal DTCA. *CMAJ.* 2003;169(5):405-412.

49. Weissman JS, Blumenthal D, Silk AJ, et al. Physicians Report On Patient Encounters Involving Direct-To-Consumer Advertising: Doctors see both positive and some negative effects on their patients and practices. *Health Aff.* 2004;23(Suppl1):W4-219-W214-233.

50. Luo D, Liu L, Han P, Wei Q, Shen H. Solifenacin for overactive bladder: a systematic review and meta-analysis. *Int Urogynecol J.* 2012;23(8):983-991.

51. Shipman SA, Sinsky CA. Expanding primary care capacity by reducing waste and improving the efficiency of care. *Health Aff.* 2013;32(11):1990-1997.

52. Walter A, Chew-Graham C, Harrison S. Negotiating refusal in primary care consultations: a qualitative study. *Fam Pract.* 2012;29(4):488-496.

53. Bradley SM, Hernandez CR. Geriatric assistive devices. *Am Fam Physician.* 2011;84(4):405-411.

54. van Dulmen S, Sluijs E, van Dijk L, de Ridder D, Heerdink R, Bensing J. Patient adherence to medical treatment: a review of reviews. *BMC Health Serv Res.* 2007;7(1):55.

55. Kravitz RL, Melnikow J. Medical adherence research: Time for a change in direction? *Med Care*. 2004;42(3):197-199.

56. Schaffer SD, Yoon S-JL. Evidence-based methods to enhance medication adherence. *Nurs Pract*. 2001;26(12):44-50.

57. Marvel MK, Epstein RM, Flowers K, Beckman HB. Soliciting the patient's agenda: have we improved? *JAMA*. 1999;281(3):283-287.

58. Baker LH, O'Connell D, Platt FW. "What else?" Setting the agenda for the clinical interview. *Ann Intern Med*. 2005;143(10):766-770.

59. Kahneman D. *Thinking, fast and slow*. Macmillan; 2011.

60. Levinson W, Gorawara-Bhat R, Lamb J. A study of patient clues and physician responses in primary care and surgical settings. *JAMA*. 2000;284(8):1021-1027.

61. McCormick DP, Chonmaitree T, Pittman C, et al. Nonsevere acute otitis media: a clinical trial comparing outcomes of watchful waiting versus immediate antibiotic treatment. *Pediatrics*. 2005;115(6):1455-1465.

62. Duberstein P, Meldrum S, Fiscella K, Shields CG, Epstein RM. Influences on patients' ratings of physicians: Physicians demographics and personality. *Patient Educ Couns*. 2007;65(2):270-274.

63. Rodin G, Zimmermann C, Mayer C, et al. Clinician-patient communication: evidence-based recommendations to guide practice in cancer. *Curr Oncol*. 2009;16(6):42-49.

64. Duffy FD, Gordon GH, Whelan G, et al. Assessing competence in communication and interpersonal skills: the Kalamazoo II report. *Acad Med*. 2004;79(6):495-507.

65. Langberg EM, Dyhr L, Davidsen AS. Development of the concept of patient-centredness - A systematic review. *Patient Educ Couns*. 2019;102(7):1228-1236.

66. McCormack LA, Treiman K, Rupert D, et al. Measuring patient-centered communication in cancer care: a literature review and the development of a systematic approach. *Soc Sci Med*. 2011;72(7):1085-1095.

67. Gallagher TH, Lo B, Chesney M, Christensen K. How do physicians respond to patient's requests for costly, unindicated services? *J Gen Intern Med*. 1997;12(11):663-668.

68. Street RLJr. How clinician-patient communication contributes to health improvement: Modeling pathways from talk to outcome. *Patient Educ Couns*. 2013;92(3):286-291.

69. Street RLJr, Gordon HS, Ward MM, Krupat E, Kravitz RL. Patient participation in medical consultations: why some patients are more involved than others. *Med Care*. 2005;43(10):960-969.

70. Epstein RM, Gramling RE. What is shared in shared decision making? Complex decisions when the evidence is unclear. *Med Care Res Rev*. 2013;70(1 Suppl):94S-112S.

71. Street RLJ, Mulac A, Weimann JM. Speech evaluation differences as a function of perspective (participant vs. observer) and presentational medium. *Hum Commun Res*. 1988;14(3):333–363.

72. Pass M, Belkora J, Moore D, Volz S, Sepucha K. Patient and observer ratings of physician shared decision making behaviors in breast cancer consultations. *Patient Educ Couns*. 2012;88(1):93-99.

73. Gordon HS, Street RL. How Physicians, Patients, and Observers Compare on the Use of Qualitative and Quantitative Measures of Physician-Patient Communication. *Eval Health Prof*. 2016;39(4):496-511.

74. Hall JA, Stein TS, Roter DL, Rieser N. Inaccuracies in physicians' perceptions of their patients. *Med Care*. 1999;37(11):1164-1168.

75. Joyce BL, Steenbergh T, Scher E. Use of the kalamazoo essential elements communication checklist (adapted) in an institutional interpersonal and communication skills curriculum. *J Grad Med Educ*. 2010;2(2):165-169.

76. Zill JM, Christalle E, Muller E, Harter M, Dirmaier J, Scholl I. Measurement of physician-patient communication--a systematic review. *PLoS One*. 2014;9(12):e112637.

77. Street RLJr, Mazor KM. Clinician-patient communication measures: drilling down into assumptions, approaches, and analyses. *Patient Educ Couns*. 2017;100(8):1612-1618.

78. Rimal RN. Analyzing the physician-patient interaction: an overview of six methods and future research directions. *Health Commun*. 2001;13(1):89-99.

79. Mead N, Bower P. Measuring patient-centredness: a comparison of three observation-based instruments. *Patient Educ Couns*. 2000;39(1):71-80.

80. Fullam F, Garman AN, Johnson TJ, Hedberg EC. The use of patient satisfaction surveys and alternative coding procedures to predict malpractice risk. *Med Care*. 2009;47(5):553-559.

81. Kravitz RL, Bell RA, Franz CE. A taxonomy of requests by patients (TORP): a new system for understanding clinical negotiation in office practice. *J Fam Pract*. 1999;48(11):872-878.

82. Robinson JD. Asymmetry in action: Sequential resources in the negotiation of a prescription request. *Text*. 2001;21(1/2):19-54.

83. Feeley TH, Anker AE, Aloe AM. The Door-in-the-Face persuasive message strategy: A meta-analysis of the first 35 years. *Commun Monogr*. 2012;79(3):316-343.

84. Dillard J, Hunter J, Burgoon M. Sequential-request persuasive strategies: Meta-analysis of foot-in-the-door and door-in-the-face. *Hum Commun Res*. 1984;10:461-488.

85. Pascual A, Gueguen N. Foot-in-the-door and door-in-the-face: a comparative meta-analytic study. *Psychol Rep*. 2005;96(1):122-128.

86. Frosch DL, May SG, Rendle KA, Tietbohl C, Elwyn G. Authoritarian physicians and patients' fear of being labeled 'difficult' among key obstacles to shared decision making. *Health Aff (Millwood)*. 2012;31(5):1030-1038.

87. Denberg TD, Melhado TV, Coombes JM, et al. Predictors of nonadherence to screening colonoscopy. *J Gen Intern Med*. 2005;20(11):989-995.

CHAPTER 8

Clinical Negotiation and Controlled Substances

With Stephen G. Henry, MD

Clinical Take-Aways

- Controlled substances (opioids, sedative-hypnotics, stimulants, and testosterone replacement therapy) are defined legally, not medically. Most have the potential for addiction, serious side effects, or both.
- Many clinicians worry that encounters with patients taking opioids for chronic pain will be conflict-ridden. In reality, most such patients defer to clinicians' recommendations for pain management, agree with clinicians' treatment recommendations, and try to be responsible users of pain medicines.
- The approach to the clinical negotiation is different for opioid-naïve patients requiring treatment for severe acute pain (limit the treatment course); patients on long-term opioids for chronic pain (focus on functional goals); and patients who exhibit signs of a substance use disorder (taper opioids and refer for SUD treatment).
- In negotiating with patients taking other (nonopioid) controlled substances, the governing principles are to do a good intake exam; inform the patient about risks and benefits of treatment; and monitor the patient's progress closely.
- Clinicians should:
  - Be mindful of their own emotions, attitudes, and prejudices when providing care to patients using controlled substances.
  - Show that they take the patient's distress seriously through careful history-taking, elicitation of the patient's perspective, and empathic statements.
  - Assess the patient's risk for harms related to controlled substance use.
  - Work collaboratively to establish treatment goals.
  - Develop a goal-directed treatment plan that emphasizes functional progress rather than pill-counting.

229

SECTION 8.1: INTRODUCTION

Categories of Controlled Substances

Controlled substances are drugs that are monitored and regulated by the federal government due to their potential for abuse and physical dependence. A wide variety of medications are classified as controlled substances, including opioids, sedative-hypnotics, stimulants, and androgens. They can be effective for managing symptoms that impact patients' quality of life (e.g., pain, fatigue, insomnia) but also are associated with substantial side effects and risks for dependency and abuse. As a result, clinician-patient communication about the use of controlled substances presents a number of challenges for effective clinical negotiation. Much of what we say in this chapter will focus on clinician-patient communication and decision-making related to opioid use for pain management. However, we will also discuss negotiation related to other controlled substances. We conclude with suggestions for effective communication regarding controlled substances, coupled with examples of both "good" and "bad" communication specific to pain management.

In the United States, controlled substances are classified by the FDA into one of five different categories or schedules, ranked according to medical indications, safety, and potential for abuse and dependence. The FDA periodically adds new drugs to these schedules and moves drugs from one schedule to another. Schedule I medications are those deemed by the FDA to have no legitimate medical use and so cannot be legally prescribed by clinicians or dispensed by pharmacies. The most commonly used Schedule I drug is cannabis, which is now legal in many individual states but cannot be prescribed by clinicians. In contrast, Schedule V drugs are deemed to have minimal potential for abuse. The most commonly prescribed Schedule V drugs are combination medications prescribed for cough that contain low doses of opioids. Medications within a certain schedule may serve very different purposes. For example, both hydrocodone and methylphenidate are Schedule II drugs, but the former is prescribed for pain control and the latter for attention deficit disorder. Within the context of clinical negotiation, effective ways to talk about controlled substances vary depending on the patient's health conditions, symptoms, and risks for abuse. In this chapter, we focus on controlled substances in Schedules II-IV, particularly opioids, sedative-hypnotics, stimulants, and androgens. Table 8-1 gives clinical indications; major risks and side effects; and abuse potential for each category of drug.

Controlled Substances in Practice: Opioids, Sedative-Hypnotics, and Androgens

Opioids. Opioids are substances that act on opioid receptors in the central nervous system and are prescribed primarily for pain relief (Table 8-1). Other medical uses

Table 8-1 Major Categories of Controlled Substances

Drug Category	Common Clinical Indications	Major Risks/Side Effects
Opioids	Pain relief; suppression of cough or diarrhea; treatment of opioid use disorder	*Expected*: physical dependence, tolerance with medium-long term use *Common*: constipation, fatigue, nausea *Common with long-term use*: sexual dysfunction, hyperalgesia *Less common*: opioid use disorder, respiratory depression, death
Sedative-Hypnotics	Insomnia; second-line treatments for anxiety, panic disorder	*Expected*: physical and psychological dependence, tolerance with long-term use *Common*: Somnolence, fatigue, confusion, impaired fine and gross motor coordination *Less common*: respiratory depression unusual except in combination with alcohol or other CNS depressants.
Stimulants	Attention deficit-hyperactivity disorder, narcolepsy; used in past for appetite suppression (obesity)	*Expected*: tolerance, physical dependence *Common*: agitation, insomnia, hypertension *Less common*: cardiac arrhythmias and ischemia, stroke, and (with chronic use) psychosis
Androgens	Androgen deficiency syndromes ("hypogonadism"), female-to-male gender transitions	*Expected*: (in men receiving physiologic replacement): none (in women): virilization *Common*: hypertension, acne *Less common*: increased risk of ischemic heart disease and stroke; polycythemia

include treating diarrhea, suppressing cough, and treating opioid use disorder. **Regular opioid consumption reliably produces physical dependence (withdrawal symptoms when opioids are discontinued) and tolerance (the need for higher doses to produce the same analgesic effects).** For some patients, opioid consumption also produces euphoria that can result in opioid use disorder (loss of control over opioid consumption with continued use despite adverse consequences). In excess, opioids can cause respiratory depression and even death. Opioids are the most commonly prescribed controlled substance in the United States, accounting for approximately half of controlled substance prescriptions.[2]

Relative to other controlled substances, negotiation around opioids presents some unique challenges due to recent dramatic shifts in clinical practice. From the late 1990s through the mid-2010s, physicians were encouraged to prescribe opioids liberally for chronic pain, which led to a large number of patients being prescribed long-term, high-dose opioids. Starting in the 2010s, a surge of opioid-related overdose deaths, together with recognition that opioids were much riskier and less beneficial for chronic pain than previously believed, prompted a reversal in clinical practice. Opioids are now used less frequently for both chronic and acute pain.[3]

Sedative-hypnotics. Sedative-hypnotics are a class of drugs that suppress central nervous system function (Table 8-1). Benzodiazepines were widely used for sleep and anxiety in the 1970s as a safer alternative to barbiturates; however, their use has declined in recent decades as their abuse potential was better understood. They are not considered first-line treatments for chronic anxiety or insomnia. Sedative-hypnotics (i.e., benzodiazepine and benzodiazepine-like medications) account for approximately 30% of controlled substance prescriptions.

Stimulants. Stimulants are drugs that increase activity of the central nervous system and produce pleasurable and invigorating responses (Table 8-1). Common stimulants include dextroamphetamine, methylphenidate, and lisdexamfetamine. As with opioids and benzodiazepines, ongoing use can lead to tolerance and physical dependence. Stimulants constitute approximately 10% of controlled substance prescriptions.

Androgens. This category of controlled substance comprises mostly testosterone supplements, which are prescribed as "testosterone replacement therapy," principally for men with hypogonadism (Table 8-1). Anabolic steroids (congeners of testosterone) have a few legitimate medical uses but are most commonly used illicitly to build muscle or enhance athletic performance. Testosterone naturally declines in men once they reach middle age. This in turn can contribute to poorer sexual function, fatigue, loss of muscle mass, and lower bone density. Since 2000, there has been a significant increase in use of testosterone supplements due in part to patient demand prompted by direct-to-consumer advertising.[4]

SECTION 8.2: CLINICIAN-PATIENT COMMUNICATION ABOUT PAIN AND OPIOID USE

There have been a number of investigations of clinician-patient communication about legally prescribed controlled substances. However, the bulk of these studies have focused on communication about pain control and opioids. We review some of this research, as many insights about communication patterns and outcomes in the context of pain management apply to communication about other controlled substances as well. **A common source of disagreement animating discussions about controlled substances is whether the medication is delivering sufficient clinical benefit to justify the established risks.** For example, a clinician may recommend tapering or stopping diazepam because it does not seem to be reducing the patient's anxiety. The patient, on the other hand, may wish to continue using the medication because it helps with sleep. Disagreements about a medication's relative risks and benefits is prominent during discussions about controlled substances but are sometimes a point of contention for noncontrolled substances that provide symptomatic relief (e.g., use of diuretics to treat leg swelling). **Negotiations involving controlled substances are also often difficult because patients' experience of symptom relief are sometimes due to physical dependence or substance use disorder. This dynamic is unique to negotiations involving controlled substances and is a common source of disagreement during discussions involving opioids, especially when the presence of dependence or opioid use disorder is contested.**

Pain is a major contributor to patient suffering and utilization of health care services.[5-7] Thus, it is not surprising that pain, and particularly chronic pain, is frequently discussed in primary care.[8-10] Clinician-patient communication about pain management is often difficult for both patients and clinicians,[11,12] especially when opioids are involved. Physicians may be quick to assume they are dealing with a "narcotic-seeking" patient (i.e., a patient whose primary goal is to obtain narcotics rather than to achieve better pain control), whereas patients may think doctors are dismissing their pain-related concerns.[13,14] On the other hand, some patients may unnecessarily endure pain that could be more effectively managed using more aggressive prescribing. For example, patients with advanced cancer may try to be stoic about their pain, assume pain is just part of having cancer, or fear they will become "addicted."[15] Thus, the success of clinical negotiation will depend on the extent to which both patients and clinicians are open and honest when discussing pain symptoms and analgesic use, including their concerns and fears about the possible causes of pain and risks of opioid medication.

Ingredients for Effective Communication Around Chronic Pain

In a recent review of clinician communication about pain, the authors identified four domains posited to promote effective, patient-centered communication: information exchange, decision-making, responding to emotions, and relationship-building.[16,17] **Contrary to the conventional wisdom that discussion of pain management often produces clinician-patient disagreement and conflict, most patients in fact defer to clinicians' recommendations for pain management, are likely to agree with clinicians, and work to present themselves as responsible users of pain medication.**[18,19] This is not to paint conflict in pain management as rare. Disagreement about pain medications appears to be more frequent than disagreement about other common clinical topics, occurring in up to 10% of primary care visits with patients on long-term opioids. Thus, it is important to understand the factors that mitigate or intensify conflict. For example, there is less conflict when patients present themselves as responsible users of pain medications,[18] when patients believe their clinicians genuinely care about their well-being,[20] and when clinicians and patients are on the same page about treatment preferences.[21,22]

Another study conducted an in-depth analysis of the "talk" of pain-related discussions in clinical encounters and the relationship between communication and both patients' and physicians' perceptions of the encounter.[23] The data of interest included video-recordings of 86 consultations with patients who were long-term users of opioids for musculoskeletal pain. Notably, on average over half of the talk in these conversations was specifically focused on pain-related issues. In these encounters, patients made an average of five requests for physician action (e.g., refill medications, make a referral) and asked a mean of almost six pain-related questions. Most patients made at least one negative assessment about their pain (e.g., "pain is driving me crazy," "I can't walk"). In turn, physicians made a mean of more than 15 pain-related recommendations per visit, and all visits contained at least one instance of "patient-centered" communication (e.g., asking about the patient's perspective, making empathic statements, etc.).

These communication patterns are in many ways not surprising. Patients suffering from chronic pain ask questions, share their pain control problems and issues, and make requests for pain relief or management. Physicians in turn make efforts to understand the patient's pain experiences, be supportive, and make pain-related recommendations. However, three specific communication patterns were observed to degrade the patient experience: 1) patient requests for increased opioid dose; 2) patient-physician disagreement about pain management; 3) increased time spent discussing opioid risks and side effects. These statistically significant associations were driven largely by two highly contentious "outlier" visits (representing 2/86, or 2.3% of the total). All three negative communication patterns may be tapping into the same overarching narrative: patients are convinced that more opioids are needed, physicians resist, and both engage in (possibly fruitless) information exchange that arguably focuses too much on the medical facts and not enough on the patient's distress.

Contentious visits in the context of pain management may indeed be outliers. But they nonetheless take up outsize prominence in clinicians' collective consciousness, and as such, they pose a challenge for clinical negotiation. Merely spotting the name of a potentially disagreeable patient with pain on one's schedule can heighten clinician vigilance. Furthermore, such visits may highlight the stigma associated with opioid use in pain management,[24] leading clinicians to project stigma onto other patients—many of whom are at low risk for opioid-related harms or are willing to talk about opioid alternatives. In a similar vein, clinicians' experience with highly contentious encounters may reinforce clinicians' stereotypical view that patients who request pain medications tend to be "drug-seeking" and should therefore be regarded with suspicion.[23] **Several studies have shown that this opioid-related stigma is more common and more severe for minority patients, and particularly Black patients, compared to White patients, due to racial stereotypes and biases common in American culture.** For example, in a national study of veterans, Black patients with moderate or severe pain were less likely to be prescribed opioids than White patients with similar levels of pain.[25]

Role of Emotions

Whether resulting from chronic pain itself, opioid dependence, or the stigma associated with either, patients' communication about pain often reveals clues to the patients' underlying emotions and concerns that can range from obvious to subtle. This is especially true when pain and pain management are discussed.[16] As mentioned in Chapter 5, clinicians often fail to recognize and respond appropriately to subtle emotional clues. For example, one study of patients with fibromyalgia found that clinical nurse specialists typically noticed and empathically responded to patients' negative feelings when they were explicitly articulated, but not when communicated nonverbally or vaguely, expressed as physiologic correlates of unpleasant emotional states (e.g., "I broke out in a cold sweat"), or buried within "neutral utterances that stand out from the background narrative and refer to stressful life events."[26]

Nonverbal clues to emotions—both positive and negative—may be especially salient in clinician-patient communication about pain. For example, Henry and Eggly[27] analyzed the affective tone of 133 video-recorded consultations of mostly low-income, African-American patients. Raters blind to the study watched and listened to several 30-second clips ("thin slices") of the recordings in which pain was or was not discussed and then marked their impression of the physician's and the patient's displayed emotions (e.g., engagement, hostility, sadness). The observers' ratings of both patient unease (tense/anxious, upset/distressed) and positive connection (warm/friendly, engaged/attentive) were greater when pain was being discussed as compared with other topics during the same visit. In addition, greater pain severity was associated with significantly more patient and physician unease.

Perhaps these findings should not surprise us. Pain has special salience to those who experience it, and humans have evolved to detect the experience of pain in others.[28] However, how clinicians respond to patients' expressions of pain is variable: sometimes with empathy, often with "detached concern," and occasionally with callousness.[29]

Influence of Patients' Requests on Opioid Prescribing

As noted in Chapter 7, there is a substantive body of research on how patients' requests for medication influence clinicians' prescribing behavior. As with requests for other medical tests, treatments, or medication, patients ask for opioids because of their belief that opioids will effectively reduce pain or at least limit misery. **However, during discussions about opioids and other controlled substances, clinicians are often focused on determining the extent to which patients' requests for opioid initiation or dose increases are driven by a need for better pain control versus physical dependence or an underlying opioid use disorder. To make things more complicated, these categories are not mutually exclusive.**

As mentioned at the beginning of this chapter, opioid prescribing is a matter of national concern. Current guidelines suggest curtailing opioid initiation, limiting duration of therapy when possible, titrating doses cautiously, and using risk reduction strategies (including tapering) with selected patients deemed to be at high risk of opioid-related complications. However, new evidence suggests that tapering patients who have been on long-term opioids for chronic pain can increase their risks of opioid-related overdose and emergency department visits.[30] These new findings have prompted additional guidelines urging caution when reducing opioid doses and emphasizing the need to secure patient agreement before doing so.[31]

Applying these guidelines to patients who make direct requests for opioids can be difficult. As discussed in Chapter 7, clinicians often experience the tension between wanting to accommodate patient preferences and being reluctant to initiate therapies that are contraindicated, are of uncertain benefit, or have the potential to cause harm. There is indeed good evidence that patients' requests for opioids can, all else equal, vastly increase the likelihood that an opioid prescription will be provided.[32]

A Deeper Dive 8.1: Vignette Studies

Lord Kelvin, inventor of the eponymous temperature scale, is quoted as saying, "when you can measure what you are speaking about... you know something about it." Investigators interested in the clinician-patient relationship have a limited number of tools available for observing and measuring clinical interactions. They can ask patients and clinicians for their views on the content and quality of the interaction, they can access archival data (like medical records or billing data), and they can directly observe the interaction (e.g., by audio- or video-recording the visit). But there is one additional trick. *They can try to anticipate clinicians' and patients' actual behavior in real clinical encounters by observing their reactions to experimentally manipulated stimuli.* These stimuli can be presented as announced or unannounced standardized patients, as real audio- or video-recorded clinical encounters, or as clinical "vignettes."

Vignette studies present textual, audio, visual, or audio-visual depictions of hypothetical situations that are shown to research participants in order to elicit their judgments or reactions.[59] Vignette studies are experimental research designs where investigators manipulate a theoretical variable(s) of interest. Vignette studies can manipulate the behavior of patients, clinicians, or third parties and in turn recruit any of these groups as "subjects." For example, one could randomly assign patients to read about *clinicians* exhibiting (or eschewing) patient-centered behaviors and then register their liking for and/or satisfaction with the practitioner. Or one could randomly assign clinicians to view videos of *patients* displaying various levels of assertiveness and then assess the clinician's diagnostic impressions, clinical recommendations, and visit satisfaction.

In the study by McKinlay et al.,[32] four video scenarios were created depicting a patient presenting one of two health conditions (sciatica or knee osteoarthritis) and either specifically requesting strong pain medication or not requesting pain medication at all. Other than whether the patient had sciatica or knee osteoarthritis and requested pain medication or not, the content and actors in the scenario were exactly the same. After watching one of the four scenarios, physicians who participated in the study were asked how they would manage the case and what medications they would prescribe. In videos depicting patients with sciatica, those in which patients made a request for oxycodone were much more likely to trigger a "prescription" from the physician-subject than those in which patients made no request (20% versus 1%). Similarly, in videos depicting patients with knee osteoarthritis, patients requesting Celebrex® were much more likely to receive it compared to those making no request (53% versus 24%). In short, all else equal, patients requesting specific medications were significantly more likely to have them prescribed.[32]

Vignette studies offer some important advantages when investigating clinician-patient communication. For one thing, they allow for manipulations that are generally infeasible in clinical practice. It would be difficult, not to mention ethically suspect, to instruct *real* patients to make specific requests or use specific language within a real encounter. Using vignettes, researchers can carefully control variables of interest in order to explore how clinicians and patients respond to different situations. Here are some examples of how a clinician's behaviors are manipulated to garner patients' reactions. When disclosing a medical error, do different levels of a physician's nonverbal expressiveness predict whether patients forgive the error?[60] Which of three ways of presenting health information improves patients' recall of the information?[61] Do patients report less stigma about obesity when a clinician's explanations for weight focus on genetics rather than on diet and exercise?[62] When presented with a video of a clinician's communication style, does a patient's level of anxiety affect his or her preferences for more doctor-centered vs. more patient-centered communication?[63]

Other vignette studies manipulate the patient's behavior and/or characteristics to see how clinicians react. The McKinlay study is one such example. Here are two others. Is a physician's intent to disclose a medical error to a patient affected by the seriousness of the error and whether the physician was personally responsible for the error?[64] Does physician initiation of preventative care discussions depend on the type of clinical condition presented (e.g., diabetes, depression, or COPD)?[65]

Vignette studies also have limitations, most related to poor or unknown *external validity*. The degree to which findings derived from vignettes apply to real life is limited in at least five ways.

First, vignettes are hypothetical, not real. The real-world prevalence of behaviors depicted in vignettes is often unknown.

Second, to examine different levels of the variables of interest, investigators must control for other potential influences. For example, in the study where investigators were interested in the effect of nonverbal expressiveness in how patients respond to admission of a medical error,[66] the scenarios kept constant the verbal content of the physician's communication, the type of error (surgical sponge retained in the abdomen), as well as the age, sex, and race of the physician, all of which could affect how a patient responds to the error disclosure. By focusing attention on one or a few variables of interest, vignette studies in effect ignore other "real life" influences that also may affect the outcome.

Third, the extent to which vignettes simulate real life varies considerably. For example, a video vignette using trained actors enacting a scene based on an actual medical encounter is a much more realistic depiction of a clinical event than a five-sentence written paragraph.

Fourth, as is true in most experiments, including many randomized clinical trials, respondents frequently do not fully represent the population of interest. For example, in a study examining patients' reactions to the disclosure of a surgical sponge left in their body, respondents were actual hospitalized patients. However, none had experienced the medical error described.[66] Other studies use "analogue" patients where research participants (e.g., people without cancer) are asked to respond to the vignette as if they were cancer patients.[61] Although the judgments of real patients to a simulated encounter may be modestly correlated with the judgments of analogue patients,[67] the experiences of those who actually have had the health condition represented in the vignette are no doubt different from those who have not.

Finally, participants in vignette studies are not participating in a medical encounter, but observing those who are. As noted in Deeper Dive 7.1, participants in an encounter often have different judgments of the interaction of the same interaction.[68]

As a result of these limitations, vignette studies need to be interpreted in light of collateral information from other studies, such as those employing direct observation of real clinicians and patients, medical records, and clinician and patient surveys. As a case in point, consider the evidence of racial disparities in cardiovascular care. Epidemiological studies indicate that African-American patients are less likely to have cardiovascular procedures (e.g., revascularization) than Whites.[69] Explanations for the disparity include Black patients are more likely to decline these treatments, Black patients may be overrepresented at hospitals that underperform with regard to high-quality cardiac care, or clinicians have unconscious bias against using certain procedures for Black patients.[70] To explore the possibility of bias, Schulman et al.[71] conducted a vignette study where a group of physicians were presented with one of four video scenarios and were asked how they would treat the patient. Each scenario contained the same scripted information of a patient presenting chest pain symptoms. The only difference in the scenarios was whether the patient was White or Black, and male or female. One finding was that, even when presenting with the exact same symptoms, Black patients were less likely to be referred for cardiac catheterization than Whites, with the biggest differences associated with being a Black woman.

While this vignette study certainly raises suspicion for physician bias, one could argue that judgments made when viewing a video do not necessarily mean similar judgments would be made in real clinical encounters.[72] The main reason for discrepancies is that video studies simply can't account for the many contextual effects that may influence patient and physician behavior.

In summary, one might think of vignette studies as an important but relatively narrow window into clinician-patient communication. Taken together with epidemiological, survey, observational, and intervention studies, vignette studies play a unique and important role in shaping our understanding of clinician-patient communication processes and outcomes.

Challenging Situations in Negotiations Around Opioids

The clinician's goal during clinical negotiation is to render high-quality pain care while meeting the patient's wishes and expectations to the extent possible. There can be a natural tension between the two. **There are at least three clinical scenarios that are often associated with challenging negotiations involving**

opioids: a) opioid-naïve patients with pain who request opioids; b) patients on chronic opioids who ask for an increase in their regular dose; c) patients on chronic opioids for whom the risks of continued opioid prescribing outweigh the benefits (e.g., because the patient shows evidence of opioid misuse or addiction, or because the patient has not demonstrated improved pain-related functioning on high-dose opioids). The approach to effective clinical negotiation will differ for each. With opioid-naïve patients (e.g., those with acute pain following an injury or surgical procedure), clinicians should educate patients about the potential harms of opioids and limit the dose and duration of any opioid prescription.[1] With patients on chronic opioids requesting a dose increase, the clinician should strive to organize the conversation around the patient's functional goals ("let's talk about how to help you get parts of your life back") and how to best achieve them. Sometimes the solution is cautious up-titration of opioids, but sometimes not. Finally, with patients for whom continued opioid use poses unacceptable risk (e.g., patients who regularly cross boundaries or appear to be at risk for abuse), clinicians should be prepared to clarify and explain risks, negotiate with the patient to begin a voluntary opioid dose taper (which may have to be done very slowly), and refer for substance use disorder treatment if indicated.[31] Given the risks associated with dose reduction among patients who are physically dependent on opioids, involuntary or unilateral dose reduction should be reserved for patients who are at imminent risk of harm. In all these scenarios, clinicians should make liberal use of nonopioid pain control strategies.

SECTION 8.3: COMMUNICATION CHALLENGES IN DEALING WITH PATIENTS ON OTHER CONTROLLED SUBSTANCES

While there has been a considerable body of research on clinician-patient communication and decision-making around opioids, much less work has focused on communication involving other controlled substances. As with pain management, shared decision-making on whether to prescribe, continue, or taper off other controlled substances can be complicated by the need to balance patients' interests in receiving the medication against the expected risks and benefits associated with its use.

Communication about sedative-hypnotics. As discussed earlier, sedative-hypnotics are most commonly used to treat sleep and anxiety disorders. Although their use has declined in recent decades, some patients with complicated anxiety disorders, such as PTSD, do benefit from sedatives. On the other hand, patients who take sedative-hypnotics, particularly benzodiazepines, often develop physical dependence. Weaning or tapering patients off benzodiazepines must be done gradually to avoid seizures and other harmful effects of acute withdrawal. In our experience, negotiating dose reduction of benzodiazepines can sometimes be more challenging than negotiating reduction of opioids, in part because common opioid-related side effects (constipation, pruritis) and safety concerns (overdose) tend to be more salient to patients than the side effects and risks associated with benzodiazepines. Few studies have empirically examined clinical negotiation involving benzodiazepines.

Communication about stimulants. Stimulants are prescribed to both adults and children. Of the limited research on clinician-parent-child communication about treatment for ADHD, studies indicate a number of communication challenges, including lack of concordance between clinicians' and parents' priorities for the goals of treatment. For example, from an analysis of the communication between 11 psychiatrists and 32 parents of patients who had ADHD (and either one other psychiatric condition or learning disability), the authors observed that visits focused primarily on medication management and school performance, with much less attention to managing mood and behavioral problems.[33] Psychiatrists and parents couldn't even agree on what they identified as the child's "most concerning behavior." Parents most often reported concerns about consequences of ADHD for school or social functioning or about comorbid behavioral health issues such as hyper-aggression and depression. Psychiatrists, in contrast, focused on the core symptoms of ADHD (inattention, hyperactivity, impulsivity). The difference highlights one of the more important ways communication can fail. **When clinicians and patients (or parents) lack understanding of each other's perspective on the goals of therapy, finding common ground on treatment becomes nearly impossible.**

Shared understanding promotes adherence to stimulant regimens. For example, college students often misuse stimulants such as Adderall (amphetamine/dextroamphetamine) by sharing or selling their medications to other students. In a study of 200 college students, the communication between users of prescription stimulants and their clinicians predicted illegal-distribution practices. Specifically, students were less likely to distribute when they reported that their physician frequently asked (1) if they ever "share" their medication with others and (2) if they understand the dangers associated with sharing medical stimulants with people to whom they are not prescribed. By inquiring in a nonjudgmental way about unauthorized medication sharing, these clinicians signaled both vigilance ("I know this happens and I'm watching you") and concern ("I know you wouldn't want to harm a friend or acquaintance.")[34] Despite its importance, comprehensive health education in this setting is inconsistent at best. A recent survey of over 800 child/adolescent psychiatrists, neurologists, and developmental-behavioral pediatricians (DBP) found that fewer than half of the respondents reported that they "often' or 'very often" educated their patients about the harms and legal consequences associated with stimulant misuse.[35]

Communication about testosterone replacement therapy. As noted earlier, testosterone replacement may benefit men with hypogonadism, leading to improvements in sexual function, bone density, muscle mass, body composition, mood, and quality of life. Some men with clear indications for testosterone replacement therapy (e.g., unequivocal clinical symptoms plus two subnormal serum testosterone levels) have not been offered treatment or are not taking it consistently.[36,37]

On the other hand, patients may request testosterone replacement therapy even when they do not have clinical evidence of hypogonadism. Patient requests for treatment have been spurred by direct-to-consumer advertising, in which testosterone supplements are promoted as improving male performance in "the bedroom and the boardroom."[4,38,39] However, very little research has examined how clinicians and patients talk about testosterone replacement therapy and the circumstances within which clinical negotiation takes place.

SECTION 8.4: STEPS FOR EFFECTIVE CLINICAL NEGOTIATION ABOUT CONTROLLED SUBSTANCES

The suffering borne by patients taking controlled substances is compounded by the stigma clouding their use. Controlled-substance-related stigma creates a disorienting communication hall of mirrors. The clinician, under fierce regulatory scrutiny, worries the patient might misuse the medicine. The patient senses, and may resent, the clinician's suspicion. The government, meanwhile, requires database checks, urine tests, signed agreements, and limitations of quantity and duration of prescriptions. Actual evidence for effectiveness of these interventions is limited; they clearly avert some adverse events, but heightened regulatory scrutiny can also lead clinicians to avoid or stop prescribing controlled substances to patients who are receiving benefit from them.[40,41] On occasion, clinicians may find it useful to hide behind the law ("I wish we didn't have to do these urine tests, but they are a requirement.").[42] However, in general, this regulatory apparatus contributes little to healing.

> Janice Pearce is a 57-year-old woman with a long history of anxiety and chronic musculoskeletal pain. Until recently, her symptoms were controlled with a combination of a serotonin-norepinephrine reuptake inhibitor, intermittent nonsteroidal anti-inflammatory drugs, and occasional use of hydrocodone-acetaminophen. However, 6 weeks ago she hurt her back while lifting a package out of her car trunk, and since then she has called twice for early refills of hydrocodone-acetaminophen. In addition, she has been experiencing periodic panic attacks and asks for a prescription for lorazepam (which she has taken before, with good results).

Mrs. Pearce's situation will be familiar to many clinicians. She suffers from a complex mix of conditions, acute and chronic, medical and psychiatric. Her clinician wants to alleviate suffering without taking undue risks or otherwise violating standards of professional practice. But how should the clinician proceed?

Table 8-2 summarizes a five-step process for negotiating with patients on controlled substances. These steps are adapted from educational materials developed at the University of California, Davis to assist clinicians in negotiating with patients with chronic pain on opioids.[43] Many of the suggestions parallel other recommendations we have made in Chapter 4 (How Communication Fails) and Chapter 6 (Strategies for Clinical Negotiation).

Table 8-2 **Framework for Discussing Controlled Substances**

Step	Suggested Communication Strategies
1. Mentally prepare for the visit	• Be mindful of negative emotions • Approach the visit with an open mind
2. Show that you take the patient's distress seriously	• Ask open-ended questions • Elicit patient's perspective • Build rapport and convey commitment
3. Assess patient's risk for harms related to controlled substance use	• Identify features of low-, medium- and high-risk patients based on behaviors, dose, comorbidities
4. Set treatment goals	• Identify realistic goals based on patient function • Focus on treatment effectiveness
5. Develop a goal-directed treatment plan	• Emphasize improving pain, not counting pills • Be flexible, commit to working with the patient long term

Step 1: Mentally Prepare for the Visit

For any consultation, particularly those where potential communication challenges are anticipated, clinicians should reflect briefly on the situation (the patient, condition, and other relevant information) before starting the visit. Two suggestions are "be mindful" and "be curious."[44,45] Mindfulness refers to monitoring one's own feelings, perceptions, and judgments in an effort to limit implicit biases and modulate the effects of emotion (e.g., liking or disliking a patient) on the tone, content, and outcome of the consultation.

Curiosity refers to having genuine interest in the patient's perspective about a particular aspect of health or well-being. The curious clinician is on the lookout for anomalies: facts that don't fit, nonverbal expressions that seem discordant with what is being said, vague generalities that beg for more detail. For example, a clinician who presumes that a patient's request for testosterone gel is just another reflection of "cosmetic pharmacology" may miss the downcast eyes and subtly quickened breathing that when explored, reveals the patient's suspicion that his wife may be having an affair.

Being mindful and curious is particularly important when discussing controlled substances, especially since some clinicians are too quick to judge a patient who requests medications or procedures the clinician regards as not medically indicated. Clinicians may unjustifiably assume that patients seeking controlled substances merely want a pharmacological "Band-Aid" for problems rather than engaging in the hard work of evidence-based behavioral therapies for pain, anxiety, insomnia, or relationship problems. Furthermore, clinicians may interpret a patient's recurring requests for controlled substances as direct challenges to their medical authority. Being mindful and curious helps clinicians to leave their biases outside the exam room and to remain open to learning about the patient's needs and concerns during the visit. Clinicians who can stay mindful and not get distracted by their own emotions are also more likely to see patients' requests for controlled substances as springboards for exploring patients' concerns, goals, and values.

A mindful and curious clinician also will be less likely to underestimate a patient's capacity for undertaking treatment with controlled substances responsibly. For example, in an analysis of 86 video-recorded clinical visits with adults taking opioids for chronic pain, Henry et al.[46] observed that in over half the visits, patients made at least some negative assessment of opioid use, including concerns about analgesic effectiveness, effects on function, or opioid safety. **These negative assessments represent potential conversational openings that clinicians can exploit to start discussions about opioid tapering, adjunctive pharmacotherapy, or nonpharmacologic interventions.**

A Deeper Dive 8.2: Clinician Explicit and Implicit Bias

Several chapters in this book have discussed problems associated with clinician bias. There are three forms of social bias toward a group and its members: (a) prejudices, which are attitudes reflecting an overall evaluation of a group (e.g., liking or disliking); (b) stereotypes, which are associations and attributions of specific characteristics to a group (e.g., these kind of people act and believe this way); and (c) discrimination, which is biased behavior toward, and treatment of, a group or its members (e.g., avoidance, hostility, inattention, favoritism). Dovidio and colleagues[73] have adapted these concepts to explain how clinician bias manifests in clinical encounters. The authors contend that interactions with certain types of patients may activate stereotypes about members of that group (e.g., beliefs about their friendliness and competence) as well as emotional prejudices (e.g., disgust, envy, pride). These in turn produce a discriminatory favorable or unfavorable response (active or passive neglect, help). Although Dovidio et al. focused their analysis in biases with respect to social categories (e.g., race, gender, education, employment status, religion, age), clinician bias can also be activated by health-related factors such as the patient's weight and mental health status.[74,75]

Clinician bias is a particularly important issue when examining communication about controlled substances because clinicians might be prone to two kinds of biases, explicit and implicit.

Explicit bias refers to beliefs and attitudes people are aware they hold and can control deliberately and strategically.[73] For example, some clinicians are quite aware of how they feel towards patients who ask for opioids or who request being placed on permanent disability, and they have ideas for managing these "difficult" patients (and may even offer advice to others on how to do so).

Implicit biases, on the other hand, are more insidious because they cut across educational and socioeconomic levels, represent learned cultural associations of affective reactions, are difficult to change, and are hidden from conscious awareness.[73,76] Implicit bias has been listed as one possible reason for undertreatment of pain among non-White patients,[77] although other factors could also come into play, including problems of adherence, fear of addiction, and poor clinician-patient communication.[78]

Although clinician bias toward patients may manifest across a number of patient characteristics, racial bias has by far received the most academic and public attention. To examine this issue, we need to unravel some ways racial bias may (or may not) contribute to poorer communication and lower quality of care for non-White patients. First, a clinician's prejudicial or stereotypic bias in part determines his or her cognitive and affective orientation toward a patient in a medical encounter. This is akin to what we referred to in Deeper Dive 4.2 as part of the clinician's "representation of the interaction," which activates a mental model of presumed patient attributes, plausible communication strategies to use in the interaction, and emotional reaction to the patient. For example, if a clinician assumes Black patients are more passive, less educated, and have less healthy lifestyles, he or she may approach the consultation in a more directive way by doing most of the talking, offering simple and limited explanations, and making recommendations with little effort to assess the patient's preferences and values. If this cognitive frame also activates some affective aversion, the clinician may nonverbally interact with the patient in a less friendly way.[79] The patient may sense subtle verbal and nonverbal expressions of these attitudes, especially if the patient has past experiences of being disrespected and feeling not cared for.[73] Indeed, one study[80] reported that Black patients who interacted with clinicians who had scored more highly on a measure of implicit bias (Implicit Attitude Test) rated their interactions with clinicians less positively than those patients seeing clinicians with less implicit bias. Furthermore, a patient who is having a less than positive encounter (e.g., being treated in a less friendly manner, feeling patronized) may respond reciprocally by feeling less respect and liking for the clinician.[73] These feelings in turn generate a communicative response that is more cautious and serious (e.g., reticent, not smiling) which, ironically, reinforces the clinician's original expectations of Black patients, thereby creating a classic self-fulfilling prophecy.[81]

However, as mentioned earlier, there are many other factors that affect clinician-patient communication that may moderate or even override racial bias. A review of implicit racial bias in studies using vignettes found mixed results for significant effects of racial bias on clinician decision-making and communication.[82] While some of the investigations reviewed in that study reported main effects of bias on outcomes, the majority did not because, as mentioned earlier, a number of other factors come into play to influence clinician judgment and behavior. Consider, for example, in the Schulman et al. study[71] that presented clinicians with a video of a patient present-ing chest pain symptoms, researchers only manipulated the patient's race and gender—everything else was the same. Yet what would happen if, in addition to race, researchers also varied the way the patient talked? Burgess et al.[83] did exactly that. Physicians were presented with vignettes of an encounter with either a White or Black male patient. Each vignette featured pictures of the patient accompanied by written dialogue in which the patient's communication varied in one of two ways. The "challenging patient" was one who was aggressive about his need for stronger pain medi-cation and was highly expressive about his pain and his need for relief. By contrast, the "non-challenging patient" was stoic, underplayed his pain, and did not demand stronger pain relief. The authors did not find a main effect for race, but rather an interaction between communication style and race—physicians were more likely to switch to a stronger opioid dose for the "challenging" Black patient and for the "non-challenging" White patient. In effect, both the patient's communication and race had an effect on physi-cian behavior. The authors speculated that the "challenging" Black patient communication alerted the clinician to urgency of needing pain relief, yet it raises the question of why the communication effect was opposite for the White patient. In another vignette study, Krupat et al.[84] also demon-strated the importance of the Black patient being a more active communica-tor to receive better care. In that study, a Black woman's assertive behavior was more likely to prompt physicians to recommend full staging of breast tumors than when the Black woman was not assertive. The patient's asser-tiveness did not affect staging decisions for the White patient.

These findings are in line with observational studies by Gordon and col-leagues. In one study,[85] the researchers found that, while Black patients with lung cancer received less information than did White patients, the disparity was nullified when the patient's communication behavior was taken into account. Patients received more information when they expressed more concerns and asked more questions, and White patients produced more of these behaviors than the Black patients. Gordon et al. observed a similar pattern in an analysis of post angiogram consultations.[86] Furthermore, in both studies, physician utterances that provided information were divided into those that were "prompted" (in response to the patient asking a question, expressing a concern, or being assertive) from those that were "self-initiated" (information giving not prompted by the patient's communication). There was no effect for race on self-initiated information-giving; the difference was associated with the "prompted" information.

In summary, racial bias can have deleterious effects on communication and decision-making in medical consultations, especially under circumstances when a clinician's way of thinking and approaching race is not challenged by information contradictory to the stereotype (e.g., a highly educated Black patient) or a patient communicating in a way that prompts the clinician to be more responsive to the patient's concerns. The power of a patient's communication style is an important theme in this book because it can have powerful effects on what clinicians and patients accomplish in medical encounters, and thus is a critical element of effective clinical negotiation.

Step 2. Show That You Take The Patient's Distress Seriously

One of the easiest ways to lose a patient (figuratively and literally) is to come off as dismissive of their complaints. Like our hypothetical Mrs. Pearce, patients on controlled substances often suffer from multiple somatic and psychological symptoms. Patients want to be taken seriously, and they have various ways of determining whether the clinician measures up. A critical criterion for many is whether the clinician is treating them as an individual and not a "number" or generic "pain patient." The clinician's task is to demonstrate genuine interest and respect for the patient as a person. This is true for all patients but may require special effort when working with patients who—by virtue of race, ethnicity, or class—may have experienced mistreatment by the health care system in the past.[47]

Clinicians can communicate sincere interest by (a) asking questions, listening carefully, and performing a directed physical examination; (b) actively eliciting patient concerns and perspectives; and (c) making empathetic statements.

Because the history and physical are so closely interwoven into routine practice, clinicians often underestimate the importance patients place on being *questioned and examined carefully*. Asking questions and performing a physical examination communicates to the patient that the clinician is willing to invest in characterizing the problem correctly and develop a therapeutic approach tailored to their circumstances. In a qualitative study of 21 opioid-using patients, Henry et al.[48] reported simple open-ended questions "How are the pain medicines working for you?" and "What problems are you having?" facilitated productive information exchange. By the same token, if the patient is tired, has already provided the history multiple times, or senses that the clinician's questions belie an ignorance of what the doctor should have learned from the medical record, some forms of questioning can backfire.

Before making inferences about patients' underlying motives for requesting controlled substances, clinicians must address the patient's illness experience, striving to understand their *concerns and perspectives*. One study[20] found that primary care physicians who demonstrated genuine concern for their patients' well-being were more highly regarded by patients, who in turn were more likely to accept a reduction or denial of opioid medications by their physicians. Two studies of patients with back pain found that patients were more responsive to clinicians they perceived as taking their pain seriously.[49] These studies suggest that patients' perceptions of clinicians can influence both the process of communication and patient-centered outcomes.

Asking patients to "walk me through your day" can be a particularly effective way of entering the patient's world. At the same time, clinicians should be mindful of patients' well-founded fears of uncontrolled pain and withdrawal resulting from forced tapering of controlled substances. As one patient told us, "I have that fear that if I stop, things are going to go to hell."[48]

Making empathetic statements is a third way to demonstrate concern. For example, the clinician caring for Mrs. Pearce might have said:

> *Wow, this has been a really hard time for you. I want to make sure I understand the sequence of things, and then let's do a careful physical exam. After that I hope we can put together a reasonable plan. How does that sound?*

The order in which we say things matters. With the opening sentence, the clinician demonstrates empathy; if delivered sincerely these kinds of statements are an important step in establishing rapport. The clinician then outlines a proposed course of action. Finally, the clinician checks in with the patient about their agreement with the plan. This is a critical maneuver signaling partnership and respect. Of course, the clinician must be prepared to suggest an alternative plan should the patient show resistance, either verbally or nonverbally.

Patients who need or want controlled substances often experience negative emotions before and during visits with clinicians, whether arising from physical pain, an underlying psychiatric condition, self-stigma, or fear that the clinician will reject or ignore their prescription needs.[50,51] Addressing these emotions is critical to achieving successful visit closure. The primary care clinician need not master psychotherapeutic theory. Instead, we recommend a return to the basics: listen carefully, elicit concerns actively, and make empathetic statements when appropriate.

Yet clinicians frequently miss the opportunity to apply these tools. Among the reasons are failure to prepare adequately for the visit, feeling rushed, or having

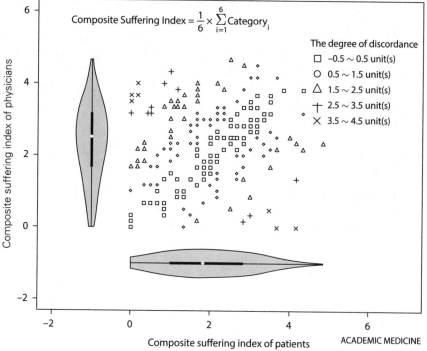

$$\text{Composite Suffering Index} = \frac{1}{6} \times \sum_{i=1}^{6} \text{Category}_i$$

The degree of discordance
- □ −0.5 ∼ 0.5 unit(s)
- ○ 0.5 ∼ 1.5 unit(s)
- △ 1.5 ∼ 2.5 unit(s)
- + 2.5 ∼ 3.5 unit(s)
- ✕ 3.5 ∼ 4.5 unit(s)

Figure 8-1. Composite suffering index.

Source: Reproduced with permission from Lesho E, Foster L, Wang Z, et al. The accuracy of physicians' perceptions of patients' suffering: findings from two teaching hospitals. Acad Med. 2009;84(5):636–642.

inadequate support from other members of the health care team. An additional reason is that clinicians are surprisingly bad at estimating the extent of patients' suffering. In one study, correlations between doctor and patient reports of suffering severity (on a 1-5 scale) ranged from 0.12 to 0.35 (i.e., not strong). Using a composite index across six domains of suffering, only 30% of doctor-patient pairs matched up within one point on the five-point index (Figure 8-1).[52]

The clinician who consistently overestimates suffering might be prone to overprescribe controlled substances. Conversely, a clinician who underestimates suffering might be more likely to dismiss a patient's concerns.

In the specific case of opioids, it can be difficult to distinguish the suffering caused by uncontrolled pain from the (sometimes severe) discomfort of opioid withdrawal. One approach is to ask: "What happens if you miss or are late for a dose of your pain medication" and "Walk me through a typical day, including how and when you take your medication."[53] Answers that are suggestive of uncontrolled pain would be taking more pain medications before intense physical activity and less when patients are more sedentary, and having stable opioid use over time. Conversely, taking opioids to get up in the morning, to alleviate restlessness, or "calm nerves" suggests withdrawal. The distinction matters, because uncontrolled pain requires more intensive pain management (whether pharmacologic or nonpharmacologic), whereas opioid withdrawal demands intensive patient education, adjustment of dosing schedules or use of longer-acting agents, and perhaps opioid tapering or referral for evaluation and treatment of a substance use disorder. Clinicians can use an analogous approach to distinguish uncontrolled anxiety from benzodiazepine withdrawal for patients taking chronic sedative-hypnotics.

Step 3. Assess the Likelihood of Benefit Versus Harm in Prescribing Controlled Substances.

By effectively eliciting the patient's perspectives, concerns, and preferences for managing health conditions, clinicians are in a better position to assess the likelihood of benefit versus harm from prescribing controlled substances. Clinicians should gather the information they need to assess patients' side effect burden and potential risk of harm from controlled substance use (e.g., physical dependence and substance use disorder), the likelihood of clinical benefit, and whether alternatives to controlled medications should be pursued. Once clinicians have this information, they can better communicate and negotiate with patients regarding treatment goals and plans. Of course, part of this communication involves making sure patients understand the potential risks and benefits of controlled substances themselves.

Evaluating a patient's risks and benefits related to controlled substances can be a tricky business. To some patients, the benefits of controlled substances are almost immediately manifest in less pain, better sleep, greater (or less) alertness, and significant (albeit transient) euphoria. The potential harms are often either less personally salient or hypothetical, so patients can interpret a discussion of side effects as indicating physician mistrust and a poorly disguised ruse to discourage use of needed medication. Therefore, it is almost always best to begin with the patient's perspective, by asking (for example): "What has been your experience with [name of medication]? What issues or problems are you having with this medication? What do you know about some of the long-term problems we've been seeing with these medicines?"

With these caveats in mind, when prescribing stimulants, benzodiazepines, and opioids, it is important to inform patients about the potential for physical dependence and risks of developing substance use disorders, particularly when long-term use is anticipated. Education on the potential adverse health effects of misuse and legal consequences is important not only for the sake of informed decision-making but also because this information may prevent patients from diverting medication to others. For example, a study by Colaneri et al.[54] found a large portion of doctors did not educate patients on health risks and legal consequences of stimulant misuse and diversion. This was particularly true for physicians with limited experience in stimulant prescribing.

Patient factors associated with risk of opioid-related harm (especially opioid over-dose) have been relatively well-studied compared to risks of stimulants and benzo-diazepines. In comparison, data on the adverse effects of testosterone, particularly long-term use, are the least well understood. The spike in opioid-related overdose deaths prompted a substantial amount of research on factors associated with risk of overdose, so that we now know much more about safety concerns related to opi-oid use (especially chronic use) compared to the use of other controlled substances. Table 8-3 shows the practical approach that we use to classify patients on chronic opi-oids as low, medium, or high risk of opioid-related overdose.[43] **We have found that**

Table 8-3 A Practical Approach for Classifying Patients' Risk of Opioid Overdose

Absolute risk of opioid overdose	Low Risk	Intermediate Risk	High Risk
Definition	Meets ALL of the following criteria: • Taking ≤50 mg morphine equivalents per day • No history of substance use disorder or PTSD • Not taking benzodiazepines or other sedatives • No medical comorbidities that seriously impair lung function or respiratory drive • No behaviors concerning for opioid misuse or abuse	All patients who are not high or low risk	Takes >50 mg morphine equivalents per day AND has one or more of the following: • Active substance use disorder • Persistent evidence of impaired opioid control (e.g., early refill requests, obtaining opioids from multiple clinicians) despite remedial discussions • Severely impaired lung function or respiratory drive
Treatment priorities	Focus on treating pain and improving function. Monitor patient's opioid use. Do not press dose reduction if the patient feels opioids are helping.	Continually assess patient's benefits and risks. Consider tapering opioids if they do not appear to be helping. Do not initiate tapers without patient buy-in.	For patients with suspected opioid use disorder, focus on getting patient evaluated for substance use disorder. Tell the patient about your concerns for their safety and explain the need to taper down or off opioids. Initiate tapering without patient consent only if the patent is at imminent risk of harm.

classifying patients based on their absolute risk of opioid-related overdose (low, medium, or high) works well in practice and helps us to determine how we approach challenging negotiations around opioids. This classification is consistent with existing evidence and federal guidelines related to opioid prescribing; however, we do not claim that it is definitive and acknowledge that evidence about the benefits and risks of chronic opioid use is an active and evolving area of research.

Step 4: Set Treatment Goals

Treatment goal-setting is important for effective chronic disease management[55] and for improving patients' functional capacity and quality of life. Clinician-patient communication involving controlled substances frequently focuses on the latter (e.g., pain, attentiveness, anxiety, sexual function). Effective elicitation of the patient's perspectives and concerns, along with how their health affects everyday life, provides rich, detailed information that helps clinicians identify the appropriate treatment strategy and set realistic treatment goals that are functional in nature.[56] Goals should be objective, realistic, and meaningful to patients and tailored to their functional capacity. In the case of opioids, prescribing guidelines recommend that clinicians frame treatment goals in terms of enhancing patients' capacity to function (e.g., ability to walk, work, or fulfill family obligations) rather than in terms of reducing their numeric rating of pain intensity. **Notice how in this dialog the clinician subtly redirects the discussion from pain to function.**

> *Mrs. Pearce: If there was an 11 on that 0-10 scale that's where I'd be. I can barely get out of bed.*
>
> *Clinician: (empathetically) I can see how uncomfortable you are. I'd like to see if we can come up with a plan that helps you get back to your baseline—which we both know involves some level of pain, but nothing like this—as quickly as possible.*
>
> *Mrs. Pearce: That would be nice.*
>
> *Clinician: Ok, let's start with a few more questions followed by a good physical exam of your back.*
>
> *[Clinician completes focused history and physical, emphasizing normal findings but also registering attentiveness to the patient's complaints, e.g., "That spot is very tender."]*
>
> *Clinician: So your back pain is clearly worse after the injury, and you have some very tight muscle spots. But there's no bony tenderness and your neurologic exam is good.*
>
> *Mrs. Pearce: That's good, I guess. Are you going to refill my prescription?*
>
> *Clinician: Let's talk about short-term and medium-term goals. If all goes as well as it possibly could, what would you like to be doing in 2 weeks?*
>
> *Mrs. Pearce: What bothers me the most is not being able to keep up with my grandchildren. Sometimes when they come over to visit I am so worn out from the pain that I don't even want to see them. Also, it sure would be nice to garden again.*

[Patient and clinician engage in further discussion of specific circumstances surrounding family visits and recent gardening attempts.]

Clinician: Since you seem to start slow but your energy picks up by mid-morning, maybe you could arrange for short visits just before lunchtime. You might also take a half-dose of hydrocodone plus a 400 mg dose of ibuprofen about an hour before. The same thing might work for gardening, though I'd suggest starting out with very short sessions—maybe 10-15 minutes at a time. Then give it a day or two and see how you do.

Mrs. Pearce: Alright, I'll try. [Smiling.] Just don't cut off my pills.

In this exchange, the clinician helps the patient identify functional goals and avoids focusing exclusively on pain severity. The visit is over, but the dialog has by no means concluded. Clinical negotiation around chronic pain is a long game. In some cases, reassuring patients like Mrs. Pearce that you are not going to stop prescribing opioids in the short term can help relieve their anxiety and make them more receptive to discussions of dose reduction a few months' down the road.

Sometimes patients have difficulty identifying clear functional goals or simply don't want to participate in such discussions. In those instances, clinicians can shift the topic to effectiveness. **A small but significant proportion of patients with chronic, non-cancer-related pain receive steadily escalating doses of opioids but continue to have disabling pain. This is evidence that high-dose opioids are not working and may provide entrée to a discussion about tapering.** For patients who are physically dependent on benzodiazepines, clinicians can similarly point to uncontrolled anxiety or continued panic attacks as evidence that non-benzodiazepine treatments are needed to relieve the patient's symptoms.

Step 5. Develop a Goal-Directed Treatment Plan

Once functional goals have been established, the next step is to develop a goal-directed treatment plan. The approach depends in part on the patient's preferences for involvement in medical decision-making. Some patients want to run the show, while others prefer clear direction from the doctor. Furthermore, patients' decision-making preferences are fluid, depending on the situation.[57] In the context of opioids, research indicates that many patients with chronic pain readily defer to the clinician's authority or have their own, independent concerns about opioid-related side effects and risks.[18,46] Therefore, although clinicians may fear that patients are a hairbreadth away from demanding more opioids, this is often not the case. The same holds true for sedative-hypnotics; when older adults with insomnia were shown guidelines from "Choosing Wisely Canada" warning of the problems with "low value practices," 30% reported an intent to discontinue behaviors such as taking sleeping pills at higher than recommended doses or for prolonged periods.[58] **Wherever the patient falls along the continuum of participatory decision-making, clinicians can turbocharge their effectiveness as clinical negotiators by attending to three principles.** *First*, when tapering, stress better symptom control and functional improvement, not pill-counting. It is very easy to become immersed in discussions in which the patient wants 42 pills but the clinician is only comfortable prescribing 36. Clinicians should try not to get caught up in this conversational quicksand. Instead, they should emphasize their commitment to help the patient better manage their symptoms (pain, anxiety, inattention, etc.). *Second*, keep the focus on achieving patient treatment goals rather than on the risks and benefits of the controlled substance. We have seen visits where the entire negotiation focuses on the logistics and risks of opioid prescribing, with no mention of the clinical details of the patient's pain or functional status. Such visits are rarely productive and unlikely to contribute to better pain control down the line. Clinicians should keep bringing the conversation back to ways the care team can help the patient to accomplish more, be more active, and engage more meaningfully with friends and loved ones. *Third*, show a willingness to listen, be flexible, and persevere through adversity. To be heard, clinicians must first listen. What is the patient afraid of? What does he most want? The most successful clinical negotiators are willing to bend, compromise, experiment, and adjust. No one gets it perfect from the start, but in chronic pain (as in many chronic illnesses and conditions for which controlled substances are prescribed) clinical negotiation occurs over the course of an enduring relationship. **A key part of this principle is communicating to the patient that you are in this for the long haul and will continue working to help the patient heal and overcome setbacks or missteps that often occur when treating complicated conditions such as chronic pain or complicated anxiety.**

While there is less evidence to support specific negotiation strategies around controlled substances other than opioids (e.g., benzodiazepines, stimulants, or testosterone replacement therapy), it is still reasonable to frame treatment goals in terms of functional improvement using validated measures of sleep, anxiety, concentration, or other cardinal symptoms; to provide multiple options for addressing symptoms; and to be flexible within the limits of professional standards.

In summary, given that controlled substances are primarily used to address quality of life within the context of chronic conditions, it is hard to overemphasize the importance of aligning treatment with mutually agreed upon treatment goals. In other words, the treatment decision-making should focus most on functional goals, somewhat on symptoms, and least on the controlled substance per se. In the next section, we examine excerpts of clinician-patient conversations about pain control in order to provide examples of both good and not-so-good communication involving controlled substances.

SECTION 8-5: COMMUNICATION SUCCESSES AND MISSED OPPORTUNITIES: FOUR PATIENTS WITH CHRONIC PAIN ON OPIOIDS

In the prior section, we advocated taking a systematic approach to communicating with patients taking controlled substances. The five steps in Table 8-2 were derived from research on and experience with patients taking opioids for chronic pain, but they also apply to patients taking other classes of controlled substances. The rules themselves are simple: mentally prepare for the visit, show that you are taking the patient's complaints seriously, assess risks of treatment-related harms, set goals, and develop a goal-directed plan. But their application can be difficult, testing the skills of even expert clinical communicators. In this section we present segments of transcribed dialog from four real clinician-patient encounters, each occurring within primary care clinics at the University of California, Davis between 2014 and 2016. In presenting the cases we hope to achieve two things. First, using the five steps as an objective, albeit tentative standard, we can identify conversational forays exemplifying both communication successes and missed opportunities. Second, at least implicitly, we can evaluate the five steps in terms of their applicability, feasibility, and reasonableness within actual practice. Again, although the focus is on the use of opioids for management of chronic, noncancer pain, many of the issues apply more broadly to patients taking sedative-hypnotics, stimulants, and testosterone replacement therapy.

Scenario 1

In this first encounter, a middle-aged woman with Crohn's disease meets her new primary care physician shortly after undergoing multiple surgeries for Crohn's-related complications.

Speaker	Dialog	Comment
Clinician	My name is Dr. Jones, I'm your new doctor. Nice to meet you, too. How are you doing?	Open-ended question, creates space for patient to lay out concerns.
Patient	I'm surviving. Feeling kind of wrecked up.	
Clinician	What happened?	Another open-ended question.
Patient	Well, I just, you know I just went through some surgeries, about three or four surgeries for my Crohn's disease.	
Clinician	That must be tough.	An appropriate display of empathy.
Patient	And I've had a lot of pain. Hurt all over. Like, my hip be hurting, and feels a pinched nerve up in here, in my neck. I don't know.	
Clinician	So, how is the oxycodone and the Norco helping you with your pain? How's that going?	Arguably premature focus on medication rather than pain and functioning.

Patient	When I take my medication and the pain go away, I'm able to move around and function. When I'm on pain medication, I can function. You know, that's what keeps me going. I take my pain medication in the morning, I get up, I start walking. And I can cook and do most things I used to do.	Nonetheless, patient describes current level of functioning and also hints at activities she values (e.g., cooking). At the same time, the patient may also be building a case for remaining on opioids.
Clinician	And how about the Norcos? How many do you go through in a day?	Doctor returns to a focus on pill counts, perhaps prematurely. The patient's comment about cooking provides an opening for the clinician to explore pain-related function and potential treatment goals; however, the clinician does not take advantage of this opportunity.
Patient	I used to take four daily when he had me taking the 10s. But now I take like eight.	The patient seems to be asking for a return to using the 10-mg pills but is not asking for an increase in the total prescribed opioid dose.
Clinician	Oh, I see before you had Norco 10. So, how many were you taking with that?	Clarifying questions are almost always welcome, as they not only inform medical decision-making but signal interest in the patient. However, here the focus is on pill counts. Further exploration of the patient's daily activities and pain-related limitations would have been a more productive approach.
Patient	Sometime like three or four a day. They different. They different. They work. The 5s don't work better than the 10s. I took less pills when I was taking the 10s.	By now it is clear that the patient is unhappy with the lower potency, 5 mg hydrocodone pills.
Clinician	Do you think you would be able to take the 5s less than that? Maybe take five a day instead of eight?	We now seem to be entering an unplanned and unproductive "pill-counting war." While dose reduction may be medically appropriate, the clinician has not yet created a secure enough alliance with the patient to be confident in the success of this strategy.

Patient	Well, you know, it's like—in the evening time, in the morning time. It's pain. It just seems like how much I'm taking right now, I'm able to function. I'm able to take care of myself. I don't like living in pain cause I know if they take my pain medication it's gonna lead to another surgery	The patient frames her use in terms of functional goals but also registers fear of further surgery. It is unclear if this is a serious concern, a tactic to encourage the doctor to revert to the 10 mg pills, or both. Further exploration is warranted.
Clinician	Well, we do want you to function and be able to walk around, but you know, these medications do have risks. It would be best to see if you could take less, maybe 5 a day? Do any hard drugs? Any cocaine use?	Instead, the doctor fixates on reducing opioid consumption, followed by questions about illicit nonprescription drugs that seem to come out of nowhere and may rile the patient at a time when calm cooperation is needed.
Patient	No. Never ever. No hard drugs.	
Clinician	Okay. I think we should consider trying to minimize the number you take. I'm really glad that they're helping you, but you're taking a lot of Norcos. Way more than we would recommend.	The clinician persists in pushing dose reduction without sufficient exploration of the patient's pain or treatment priorities. Objectively, the patient is taking approximately 40 mg-equivalents of morphine daily. In the absence of any aberrant patient behaviors, this is "moderate risk" at worst. So tapering, while generally desirable, is not urgent for this patient.
Patient	But doctor, people don't understand my pain. I mean, I mean, they're gonna force me into another surgery.	Patient doubles down on argument that poor pain control will lead to further surgery.

In this scenario, the clinician misses several opportunities to express empathy and to elicit more detail about the patient's perspective on pain and how opioids help her function. For example, when the patient first raised her concern that inadequate pain control could lead to additional surgery, the physician could have responded with empathy by assuring the patient that the clinician and patient were on the same page: "Those surgeries must have taken a lot out of you, and it's understandable you'd want to avoid that situation if possible. (pause) So we will do everything we can to avoid that, including working together to make sure you have good pain control and can continue doing things that are important to you, like cooking." Instead, the clinician focuses on the opioid dose per se. Rather than being mindful of the patient's concerns, tuned in to her reflections on function ("I get up, I start walking...and I can cook"), and curious about the patient's treatment goals, the clinician seems to have gone into the visit with a predetermined goal of reducing the patient's opioid dose. As a result, what started out as an opportunity to explore strategies for more effective pain management shifted to a negotiation over opioid dosing, with each party progressively hardening their positions.

Scenario 2

In this second sample dialog, a middle-aged man with chronic pain describes a stressful situation at home. Unlike the first scenario, the patient and clinician have an ongoing relationship. The conversation starts off well enough, but quickly devolves into a heated negotiation over the value of incorporating multiple controlled substances (oxycodone and cyclobenzaprine [Flexeril®]) into his regimen on a long-term basis.

Speaker	Dialog	Comment
Clinician	So, how've things been going since we last I saw you?	
Patient	Uh, kinda stressed out lately.	
Clinician	What's going on?	Open ended question to explore patient's concern.
Patient	Well, just relationships with my father. You know, he's old guy that—older they get, the more like a kid they get. I gotta deal with him. Gotta help him, but I don't want to. So, it's stressful.	Patient is forthcoming about emotional stress.
Clinician	Yeah, that sounds really tough.	Appropriate empathetic response.
Patient	Yeah, just started, and I think it's going to be OK.	
Clinician	OK, well keep me posted, and let me know if I can help in any way.	Physician expresses interest and support.
Patient	And having this weigh on me, has just made my pain worse. I took a Flexeril®, and it just took care of everything. That's why I still take it. I don't want it to get bad.	Patient acknowledges relation of pain to stress, then reveals part of current agenda: to stay on cyclobenzaprine (Flexeril®).
Clinician	You were to go down off it, right?	In one sense the physician is stating the obvious. But she is also "poking the bear" by explicitly calling out the patient's nonadherence to a prior agreement.

Patient	I did but that was terrible, like I've always told you, I tried everything else, the physical therapy, the chiropractor. It didn't work. The medication, though, helps a lot. But I got a sense that you don't want me takin' it much more. What's gonna happen if I continue the oxycodone? As far as the other ones, you know, of course, I'm takin' those like I'm supposed to, but it's like it's just not quite enough.	Patient reacts defensively. But he also defends his status as a "good patient" who has tried multiple non-pharmacologic approaches to pain management and has adhered to "the other ones" (presumably including adjunctive medications for pain) as prescribed. Then, at the very end, he hints that he is also in pursuit increased opioids.
Clinician	But it's part of what we discussed before. As I've said before, one of the side effects is that over the long haul the meds don't manage the pain anymore. It creates dependence, addiction. And if people are taking these meds for other reasons than pain, like stress, then we're doing harm with these.	The clinician now becomes more confrontational. She is understandably frustrated that her previously expressed concerns about side effects, dependence, and addiction have not registered.
Patient	But I need it for the pain.	The patient clearly fears the clinician will deprive him of "needed" medication. This is a good opportunity to explore whether the medicines are in fact succeeding at improving function, perhaps by asking, "What have you noticed about your ability to do things that interest you or that you need to do, on different doses of the medication?"
Clinician	You can still stay on lower doses of pain meds, but we need to try to lower that and see how other things, a multidisciplinary approach—counselor, physical therapy, pain clinic—can help as well. Especially, physical therapy.	The clinician mixes reassurance (you can stay on the meds) with tacit scolding (but not the higher doses you're used to) and referral to therapies the patient just claimed have not worked in past.
Patient	Doc, I don't wanna do this. This meds are working. Nothing else is gonna work. I didn't wanna get on medication, but it worked.	Positions are hardening.
Clinician	Yeah, you know, again, for the same reasons that I've talked about, the direction we need to go is going down. I am your doctor, and my job is to give you the best care I can, and that care is titrating off this and using these other options. And so, I can write you the prescription to do it—to do the, um, 30 milligrams every 12 hours, okay, so twice a day.	Clinician draws on professional legitimacy and authority to draw the negotiation to a premature close.

| Patient | Fine. Fine, whatever. I'm highly upset with this decision. I do not agree with it at all. | From patient's perspective, negotiation concludes unsuccessfully. Undoubtedly the clinician is frustrated as well. |

In this example, the power dynamic surrounding controlled substance prescribing is glaringly explicit. The patient has undergone opioid tapering in the past and is adamant that the current dose "works" (although there is not much discussion of what this means). In any case, the patient does not want to taper further. The doctor is more concerned about reducing the patient's opioid dose and fails to engage with the patient's statements that opioids (along with cyclobenzaprine) are effective and that other treatment strategies (e.g., physical therapy) are not. The patient repeatedly states that he derives benefit from the medication, which "just took care of everything," "helps a lot," and "works." These are important but vague claims that should provoke clinical curiosity. "Can you explain what you mean by 'everything'? I'd really like to get a sense of what your life is like day-to-day." "How do the medicines seem to help? What do they allow you to do?" "I am glad to hear the medicines are working? Can you help me understand what they help you do?"

In asking questions like these, tone and nonverbal expression are important. If the patient perceives the approach as inquisitorial, he will clam up and resist. In contrast, conveying a spirit of genuine interest will put the patient at ease. Also, some patients will resent treatment recommendations that seem global, generic, or insufficiently customized, preferring statements that are tailored to their individual circumstances—because they, after all, are in pain and not at risk for adverse events like those "other people."[42] Clinicians can ward off these concerns by describing to patients how reducing or discontinuing opioids might benefit them personally (e.g., by accounting for their added risk of respiratory suppression due to chronic lung disease).

However, the physician in this scenario misses opportunities to explore the patients' concerns, establish functional goals, and develop an individualized and functionally oriented treatment plan. As a result, the consultation ends with both parties at odds and neither very satisfied with the outcome.

Assessing the patient's risk of controlled substance-related harms (Step 3) is particularly helpful in situations where negotiations appear to be reaching an impasse. Given the risks associated with unilateral tapering, federal guidelines recommend avoiding unilateral opioid dose reduction unless patients are at "imminent risk of serious harm."[31] In other words, clinicians should have a relatively high bar for reducing opioid doses when patients are actively opposed to the idea. As the patient and clinician in Scenario 2 make clear, clinicians have the ultimate authority to prescribe opioids. However, the clinician's actions seem to have damaged the therapeutic relationship and may make the patient more reluctant to follow the clinician's advice about other problems in the future. In the absence of serious concerns about the patient's immediate safety, a more productive approach would have been to defer discussion of dose reduction and instead use the visit to clarify the patient's functional status and treatment goals related to pain.

Scenario 3

In the next case, we enter the conversation as the clinician helps the patient complete a pain-related agenda for the consultation.

Speaker	Dialog	Comment
Clinician	And other pain issues?	With back pain already identified as a topic of interest, the clinician probes to see if there are other prominent concerns.
Patient	Besides the back pain? As you know, I also get headaches, migraines from time to time.	
Clinician	Okay, so with the Norcos, do you think it's doing you much good?	Clinician explores the patient's perspective on how well treatment is working.
Patient	If I didn't have the Norcos, I don't think I could get around the way I get around. I still don't get around that good but I wouldn't get around as good if I didn't have 'em.	Patient makes two somewhat contradictory statements: opioids aren't working all that well, but without opioids things could be worse.
Clinician	So it gives you some functionality. You can walk a little bit better with them?	The clinician confirms that he understands the patient's perspective while inviting the patient to elaborate.
Patient	Yeah, I can walk much better without the constant pain. Still hurts but not nearly as bad.	
Clinician	Does it work the way it used to for you?	Clinician deftly probes whether the effectiveness of current dose is waning.
Patient	Uh, not really. It don't work quite as well as it used to but like when I take it, it helps.	Patient admits to experiencing pharmacologic tolerance.
Clinician	Well what we want to work towards is a goal that makes you more functional. So right now, how far do you think you're able to walk?	Clinician focuses on attaining functional goals, steering away from a potential pill-counting war
Patient	I think I can go about a block. Not on the days I get off of dialysis, though.	

Clinician	Not the dialysis days but on days without dialysis, about a block?	The clinician paraphrases the patient's statement to convey that he is listening, confirm understanding, and offer an opportunity for elaboration
Patient	If I take my time, yeah, probably. Probably a little bit further than a block. But at the grocery store, I usually can't make it. Have to ride carts.	Cart-riding is another potential target for functional improvement.
Clinician	Okay, so in terms of reducing your pain, a goal that we're going to work on is maybe in 2 months, you can walk at the grocery store. Is that right?	The clinician picks up on the patient's function at the grocery store and proposes a treatment goal around cart riding. The clinician probes for patient buy-in to this goal.
Patient	Yeah. And I was going to say, I walk around the grocery store but it's like sometime when I go in there and I'm pushing the basket, and my legs, you know, start hurting real bad.	Patient seems okay with the proposed goal. One assumes that the clinician has ruled out correctable causes for symptoms resembling intermittent claudication.
Clinician	Okay. Maybe we can make a goal that in about a month you'd be able to spend 10 minutes in a grocery store walking around before you have to take a break. Does that sound reasonable?	
Patient	Yeah, and two blocks would be real good, too	The clinician and patient have mutually established goals for patient function. In addition to walking at the store, the patient also volunteers a goal of walking 2 blocks on non-dialysis days.
Clinician	Got it.	

This is an exemplary pain management dialog illustrating a clear focus on establishing functional goals. Of course, this truncated conversation leaves a lot out, since we are not privy to what happened before (e.g., how clinician and patient constructed such a seemingly warm relationship) nor what happened afterwards (e.g., how the parties negotiated a specific treatment plan). We can nonetheless reasonably conclude that having agreed on functional goals, clinician and patient are in a much better position to discuss specific management approaches. The focus on ends sets up a conversation about means. It is much harder to accomplish the reverse.

This conversation underscores the value of Step 4, setting treatment goals based on function. **By agreeing on these treatment goals, the patient and clinician in this scenario have implicitly established shared measures they can use to evaluate the success of pain treatment strategies at future visits.**

For example, if the patient tries physical therapy and a nonopioid pain medication, during future visits the patient and clinician can judge the effectiveness of these treatments by assessing how long the patient can walk at the grocery store before taking a break and how far the patient can walk on non-dialysis days.

Scenario 4

In this next encounter, the clinician responds to a patient with a myriad of pain-related complaints

Speaker	Dialog	Comment
Clinician	So before we fill this out, I guess I should ask—how is your pain?	Clinician launches conversation with open-ended question, although depending on the clinical situation, it is sometimes advantageous to begin even more broadly ("How have things been going with your health?")
Patient	It's not good. I've had to shorten my walks.	In describing impact of condition in terms of functional limitations rather than pain or misery, patient tosses clinician a "softball."
Clinician	Tell me more about that.	Clinician probes for additional details.
Patient	The pain is like, if I can get comfortable at night, enough to get some sleep, I can get sleep but it's like here and there sleep, not all night long. So I just don't know, you know, the pain might get worse and worse, I don't know how worse it can get, but yeah, it's just like...	Psychological distress and disrupted sleep emerge, to the point where it seems that patient may be starting to catastrophize. And yet, in the next passage, the patient shifts focus to a specific prescription request.
Clinician	I see.	
Patient	And I've always known I'm not going to be out of pain, just... just be able to deal with the pain, and I don't know if they were... maybe try that Voltaren® stuff, that gel?	Not obvious how the patient transitions from catastrophizing to a specific request for a nonopioid analgesic.
Clinician	Yeah, I can—I can write you for as much of that as you need. Does that take the edge off?	Clinician readily accommodates request, perhaps relieved that the patient did not ask for more opioids or some other controlled substance.
Patient	It does for some things, maybe it'll help with this.	Patient musters hopeful attitude.
Clinician	Because you know, when I first met you, we were starting to taper, but then you were having all this neck pain. So we put that on hold.	Clinician reaches back into history, reminding patient of a distant goal (tapering) that was interrupted by an intercurrent pain syndrome.

Patient	And that's the way I want to go, try to get off of it.	Absent any ancillary information (e.g., based on prior conversations), it is difficult to know whether statement represents a genuine commitment or an effort to co-opt the doctor. In the absence of ancillary information, the physician should generally give the patient the benefit of the doubt.
Clinician	I think that's awesome, and I commend you for sort of coming to that realization on your own, because at this point I don't know how the opiates are benefiting you necessarily.	However, based on prior knowledge, non-verbal behaviors, and intuition, the clinician offers praise, reinforcing the patient's desire to get off the medication
Patient	Thanks.	The patient appreciates the acknowledge-ment of effort.
Clinician	Do you feel like you have any side effects to it, negative ones, like being tired, when you take either the Norco or any other medications?	Clinician probes for other issues that might motivate patient to taper. Taken together, this question and the next are part of a "motivational interviewing" approach in which the patient is pitted against himself.
Patient	Uh, not really. Sometimes I feel like it's my balance is off, and but I still do my exercises. I feel that the balance thing has to do with the medicine too.	Patient introduces yet another issue, loss of balance, with an unclear connection to pain medication.
Clinician	Sure, what do you see as the ben-efits of being on the opiates?	Clinician prompts patient to reflect on the upside of opioids as well as the downsides.
Patient	It helps with the pain, for sure	
Clinician	The hydrocodone? Okay. So say your pain is at an eight, what does it bring it down to?	The virtues of the 0-10 pain scale in clinical practice are vastly overrated, mainly because the meaning of any given value varies so much from patient to patient and from day to day. An alternative might be to ask simply, "how much relief does Norco provide?"
Patient	I'd say it brings it down to a five or a six, cause that's when I do use it is for the pain.	
Clinician	What... what pain can you tolerate?	
	No more than 5 or 6. But if I'm hav-ing strong pain....	The patient implies that the hydrocodone brings the pain down to the point where it's just tolerable, perhaps signaling a reluctance to consider dose reduction at this visit.
Clinician	You take the Norco.	
Patient	Yes, it does help with the pain.	

Clinician	Ok, the Norcos help but you are also trying to get rid of medications. I think starting another medication will help us wean off the Norco.	Clinician follows another basic principle of communicating with patients on opioids for chronic pain: start something new before stopping or tapering something old.
Patient	Really?	
Clinician	It's called duloxetine. And it's a medication that has a lot of uses. We use it for mood, we use it for anxiety, we use it for people with sleep disorder, but we've found out that it actually is really good for pain.	When introducing this new medication option, the clinician mentions that it may help pain and sleep, both of which the patient has identified as problems.
Patient	Ok.	
Clinician	So it's really good at dampening that pain, and I know you're on gabapentin and you've had good success with the gabapentin, but this will I think augment that and it could help you with sleep as well.	
Patient	That'd be great, if it really works.	
Clinician	All right? Cause I think I would love to get you off of everything, and I know you would too.	By adding, "I know you would too," the clinician emphasizes the patient's status as a full partner in care.
Patient	Yeah, but what if I'm having really bad pain?	
Clinician	Yes, you might still need a little bit of Norco here and there to help when you're at the eight or higher.	The clinician reassures the patient that opioids will not be stopped "cold turkey."
Patient	Ok, just in case. That's makes me feel better.	
Clinician	We'll see how you do over the next 4 weeks. And then we come up with a taper schedule on getting you off the Norco.	Clinician wisely delays tapering until pain better controlled through use of duloxetine.
Patient	Ok, sounds good.	
	Now we have other options if that doesn't work, but I think today our goal should be let's start the duloxetine, let that kick in, and then we can start coming down on the Norco. It seems like you've already done a good job, because you were on Norco 10s before.	Clinician finishes by summarizing the plan, emphasizing partnership, and providing encouragement.
Patient	Thanks, Doc, thanks a lot	

In this example, clinician and patient work collaboratively to come up with a treatment plan that addresses the patient's pain, maintains function, and incorporates an eventual goal to start gradually decreasing the patient's opioid dose. The patient here brings up several different concerns, demonstrating that patient communication may proceed in ways that do not seem to follow logical or predictable sequences. The clinician consistently responds to the patient's statements in ways that demonstrate that the clinician is genuinely listening to the patient's concerns, shows that they are treating the patient as an individual (by, for example, referencing discussions and plans from prior visits), and seeks clarification when the patient expresses unclear or seemingly contradictory statements. These different techniques all help accomplish Step 2—showing the patient that you take their pain or distress seriously. While the patient and clinician in this case have a well-established relationship, the clinician's thoughtful approach early in the case also increases the chance that the patient will go along with the suggestion of adding a new medication. Without detracting from this clinician's formidable communication skills, the patient also deserves credit for being forthcoming about their concerns and for being flexible with respect to tapering.

In summary, clinical negotiations around controlled substances often require clinicians to cross treacherous conversational terrain and can present relatively unique challenges that stem from disagreement about the relative benefits and risks of prescribing and, in particular, concerns about physical dependence and substance use disorder. However, many of the strategies associated with successful negotiation covered in previous chapters—listening carefully to the patient's concerns and desires, recognizing and responding to patient distress, and working with the patient to build rapport and implement treatment plans—will also pay dividends when negotiating about controlled substances. During conversations about controlled substances, clinicians should take steps to guard against allowing prior unpleasant interactions or their own biases regarding controlled substance use to adversely influence their negotiation with patients. The five-steps presented in this chapter comprise a framework designed in part to help reduce clinician distress around patient encounters involving opioids and other controlled substances.

SUMMARY POINTS:

- Controlled substances are defined by law and regulation rather than by pharmacologic mechanism.
- The most commonly prescribed categories of controlled substances in the United States are opioids, sedative-hypnotics, stimulants, and testosterone replacement therapies.

- Chronic pain is a common syndrome that often requires a multimodal approach to therapy, including nonpharmacologic and pharmacologic treatments.
- In negotiating with patients with chronic pain on opioids, the approach depends on context:
  - For patients who have not been on opioids before, clinicians should educate patients and limit the dose and duration of any prescription.
  - For patients on opioids who ask for a dose increase, the clinician should try to organize the conversation around the patient's functional goals.
  - For patients at high risk of opioid-related complications, clinicians should explain risks, press for voluntary opioid tapering, and consider referal for treatment of substance use disorder.
- As a general rule, before attempting to taper down on opioids or other controlled substances, introduce new measures to achieve better symptom control: first add, and only then subtract.
- Although some of the same principles hold for negotiating with patients on sedative-hypnotics (e.g., benzodiazepines) and stimulants, the research base is much thinner for these medications relative to opioids.
- Our recommended approach for negotiating with patients taking controlled substances involves five steps: 1) mentally prepare for the visit; 2) show that you take the patient's distress seriously; 3) assess the patient's risk for controlled-substance-related harms; 4) set clear treatment goals; and 5) develop a goal-directed treatment plan.
- Clinicians who wish to encourage tapering of controlled substances should be alert to patient-supplied "clues" that they are having problems with or misgivings about the medication. These clues can provide openings into broader conversations about medication tapering and discontinuation.
- Clinicians should strive to keep the conversation focused on controlling the patient's symptoms and improving quality of life (including functional status), not on dispensing a particular number of pills.

QUESTIONS FOR DISCUSSION:

1. Mrs. G has chronic musculoskeletal pain treated with oxycodone 20 mg three times daily, supplemented by occasional nonsteroidal anti-inflammatory drugs and acetaminophen. She is not depressed, does not take sedative-hypnotics, and has never called the office requesting early refills.
   a. What is Mrs. G's risk for opioid-related complications (accidental overdose or suicide)? (low, intermediate, high)
   b. When asked to "walk me through your day," Mrs. G says if she doesn't take her oxycodone immediately on arising she can barely function. Sometimes, she admits, she takes a pill when "the pain gets so bad I feel like I'm crawling out

of my skin." What factors should the clinician consider in assessing whether opioids are effectively treating pain or merely suppressing withdrawal?

2. Mr. S, a 28-year-old man, underwent wisdom tooth extraction 2 weeks ago. He just completed a 10-day prescription for Vicodin® (acetaminophen/hydrocodone) provided by his oral surgeon. He is still having achiness in his jaw as well as recurrence of intermittent low back pain related to an occupational injury. He asks you (his primary care clinician) for a Vicodin® refill. How would you talk with Mr. S. about the risks and benefits of continuing opioids relative to other pain management alternatives?

3. Mrs. C comes to see you for the first time after becoming eligibile for Medicare. She has been taking diazepam 5 mg twice daily for many years for chronic anxiety and difficulty sleeping. You note that diazepam is on the "Beers list" of contraindicated medicines for older adults, and you are not enthusiastic about providing the refill. What factors should you consider in deciding whether and how fast to taper? How would you undertake the conversation?

4. In the study by Lesho et al., physicians frequently both underestimated and overestimated patients' suffering. What are the implications for prescribing of controlled substances?

5. In scenario 2 (Section 8.5), we observe the following dialog:

   Doctor: You can still stay on lower doses of pain meds, but we need to try to lower that and see how other things, a multidisciplinary approach—counselor, physical therapy, pain clinic—can help as well. Especially, physical therapy.

   Patient: Doc, I don't wanna do this. This meds are working. Nothing else is gonna work. I didn't wanna get on medication, but it worked.

   a. What is your emotional reaction to the dialog?
   b. What is your analysis of the dialog?
   c. How could the doctor have applied some of the principles of motivational interviewing to this scenario?

References:

1. Dowell D, Haegerich TM, Chou R. CDC Guideline for Prescribing Opioids for Chronic Pain--United States, 2016. *JAMA*. 2016;315(15):1624-1645.
2. Hughes A, Williams MR, Lipari RN, Bose J, Copello E, Kroutil LA. Prescription drug use and misuse in the United States: results from the 2015 National Survey on Drug Use and Health. Washington, DC: SAMHSA; 2016.
3. Olfson M, Wang S, Wall MM, Blanco C. Trends in opioid prescribing and self-reported pain among us adults. *Health Aff*. 2020;39(1):146-154.
4. Kravitz RL. Direct-to-consumer advertising of androgen replacement therapy. *JAMA*. 2017;317(11):1124-1125.
5. Pitcher MH, Von Korff M, Bushnell MC, Porter L. Prevalence and profile of high-impact chronic pain in the United States. *J Pain*. 2019;20(2):146-160.

6. Azevedo LF, Costa-Pereira A, Mendonca L, Dias CC, Castro-Lopes JM. Chronic pain and health services utilization: is there overuse of diagnostic tests and inequalities in nonpharmacologic treatment methods utilization? *Med Care*. 2013;51(10):859-869.

7. Gureje O, Von Korff M, Simon GE, Gater R. Persistent pain and well-being: a World Health Organization Study in Primary Care. *JAMA*. 1998;280(2):147-151.

8. Deyo RA, Mirza SK, Martin BI. Back pain prevalence and visit rates: estimates from U.S. national surveys, 2002. *Spine (Phila Pa 1976)*. 2006;31(23):2724-2727.

9. Henry SG, Eggly S. How much time do low-income patients and primary care physicians actually spend discussing pain? A direct observation study. *J Gen Intern Med*. 2012;27(7):787-793.

10. Tai-Seale M, Bolin J, Bao X, Street R. Management of chronic pain among older patients: Inside primary care in the US. *Eur J Pain*. 2011;15(10):1087. e1081-1087. e1088.

11. Levinson W, Stiles WB, Inui TS, Engle R. Physician frustration in communicating with patients. *Med Care*. 1993;31(4):285-295.

12. Matthias MS, Parpart AL, Nyland KA, et al. The patient-provider relationship in chronic pain care: providers' perspectives. *Pain Med*. 2010;11(11):1688-1697.

13. Upshur CC, Bacigalupe G, Luckmann R. "They don't want anything to do with you": patient views of primary care management of chronic pain. *Pain Med*. 2010;11(12):1791-1798.

14. Esquibel AY, Borkan J. Doctors and patients in pain: conflict and collaboration in opioid prescription in primary care. *PAIN*. 2014;155(12):2575-2582.

15. Street RLJr, Tancredi DJ, Slee C, et al. A pathway linking patient participation in cancer consultations to pain control. *Psychooncology*. 2014;23(10):1111-1117.

16. Henry SG, Matthias MS. Patient-clinician communication about pain: a conceptual model and narrative review. *Pain Med*. 2018;19(11):2154-2165.

17. Epstein RM, Street RL Jr. *Patient-centered communication in cancer care: promoting healing and reducing suffering*. Bethesda, MD, 2007. NIH Publication No. 07-6225.

18. Buchbinder M, Wilbur R, McLean S, Sleath B. "Is there any way I can get something for my pain?" Patient strategies for requesting analgesics. *Patient Educ Couns*. 2015;98(2):137-143.

19. Roberts F KJ. Medication and morality: Analysis of medical visits to address chronic pain. In: W-YS HHC, ed. *The Routledge handbook of language and health communication*. Routledge; 2014:477-489.

20. Matthias MS, Krebs EE, Bergman AA, Coffing JM, Bair MJ. Communicating about opioids for chronic pain: a qualitative study of patient attributions and the influence of the patient-physician relationship. *Eur J Pain*. 2014;18(6):835-843.

21. Hughes HK, Korthuis PT, Saha S, et al. A mixed methods study of patient-provider communication about opioid analgesics. *Patient Educ Couns*. 2015;98(4):453-461.

22. McCarthy DM, Engel KG, Cameron KA. Conversations about analgesics in the emergency department: A qualitative study. *Patient Educ Couns*. 2016;99(7):1130-1137.

23. Henry SG, Bell RA, Fenton JJ, Kravitz RL. Communication about chronic pain and opioids in primary care: impact on patient and physician visit experience. *Pain*. 2018;159(2):371-379.

24. Olsen Y, Sharfstein JM. Confronting the stigma of opioid use disorder--and its treatment. *JAMA*. 2014;311(14):1393-1394.

25. Burgess DJ, Nelson DB, Gravely AA, et al. Racial differences in prescription of opioid analgesics for chronic noncancer pain in a national sample of veterans. *J Pain*. 2014;15(4):447-455.

26. Eide H, Sibbern T, Egeland T, et al. Fibromyalgia patients' communication of cues and concerns: interaction analysis of pain clinic consultations. *Clin J Pain*. 2011;27(7):602-610.

27. Henry SG, Eggly S. The effect of discussing pain on patient-physician communication in a low-income, black, primary care patient population. *J Pain*. 2013;14(7):759-766.

28. Gallese V. The 'shared manifold' hypothesis. From mirror neurons to empathy. *J Conscious Stud*. 2001;8(5-6):33-50.

29. Halpern J. *From detached concern to empathy: humanizing medical practice*. Oxford University Press; 2001.

30. Mark TL, Parish W. Opioid medication discontinuation and risk of adverse opioid-related health care events. *J Subst Abuse Treat.* 2019;103:58-63.

31. Services UDoHaH. HHS guide for clinicians on the appropriate dosage reduction or discontinuation of long-term opioid analgesics. 2019. In:2019.

32. McKinlay JB, Trachtenberg F, Marceau LD, Katz JN, Fischer MA. Effects of patient medication requests on physician prescribing behavior: results of a factorial experiment. *Med Care.* 2014;52(4):294-299.

33. Findling RL, Connor DF, Wigal T, Eagan C, Onofrey MN. A linguistic analysis of in-office dialogue among psychiatrists, parents, and child and adolescent patients with ADHD. *J Atten Disord.* 2009;13(1):78-86.

34. Lensing MB, Zeiner P, Sandvik L, Opjordsmoen S. Adults with ADHD: use and misuse of stimulant medication as reported by patients and their primary care physicians. *Atten Defic Hyperact Disord.* 2013;5(4):369-376.

35. Colaneri N, Keim S, Adesman A. Adolescent patient education regarding ADHD stimulant diversion and misuse. *Patient Educ Couns.* 2017;100(2):289-296.

36. Rosen RC, Seftel AD, Ruff DD, Muram D. A pilot study using a web survey to identify characteristics that influence hypogonadal men to initiate testosterone replacement therapy. *Am J Mens Health.* 2018;12(3):567-574.

37. Gooren LJ, Behre HM, Saad F, Frank A, Schwerdt S. Diagnosing and treating testosterone deficiency in different parts of the world. Results from global market research. *Aging Male.* 2007;10(4):173-181.

38. Layton JB, Kim Y, Alexander GC, Emery SL. Association Between Direct-to-Consumer Advertising and Testosterone Testing and Initiation in the United States, 2009-2013. *JAMA.* 2017;317(11):1159-1166.

39. Baillargeon J, Urban RJ, Ottenbacher KJ, Pierson KS, Goodwin JS. Trends in androgen prescribing in the United States, 2001 to 2011. *JAMA Intern Med.* 2013;173(15):1465-1466.

40. Fink DS, Schleimer JP, Sarvet A, et al. Association between prescription drug monitoring programs and nonfatal and fatal drug overdoses: a systematic review. *Ann Intern Med.* 2018;168(11):783-790.

41. Meara E, Horwitz JR, Powell W, et al. State legal restrictions and prescription-opioid use among disabled adults. *New Engl J Med.* 2016;375(1):44-53.

42. Matthias MS, Johnson NL, Shields CG, et al. "I'm not gonna pull the rug out from under you": patient-provider communication about opioid tapering. *J Pain.* 2017;18(11):1365-1373.

43. Henry SG. Opioids. In: Feldman MD, Christensen JF, Satterfield JM, Laponis R, eds. *Behavioral medicine: a guide for clincal practice.* 5th ed. McGraw-Hill Education; 2020:251-268.

44. Beckman HB, Wendland M, Mooney C, et al. The impact of a program in mindful communication on primary care physicians. *Acad Med.* 2012;87(6):815-819.

45. Krasner MS, Epstein RM, Beckman H, et al. Association of an educational program in mindful communication with burnout, empathy, and attitudes among primary care physicians. *JAMA.* 2009;302(12):1284-1293.

46. Henry SG, Gosdin MM, White AEC, Kravitz RL. "It sometimes doesn't even work": patient opioid assessments as clues to therapeutic flexibility in primary care. *J Gen Intern Med.* 2019.

47. Fine DR, Herzberg D, Wakeman SE. Societal biases, institutional discrimination, and trends in opioid use in the USA. *J Gen Intern Med.* 2020:1-5.

48. Henry SG, Paterniti DA, Feng B, et al. Patients' experience with opioid tapering: A conceptual model with recommendations for clinicians. *J Pain.* 2019;20(2):181-191.

49. Laerum E, Indahl A, Skouen JS. What is "the good back-consultation"? A combined qualitative and quantitative study of chronic low back pain patients' interaction with and perceptions of consultations with specialists. *J Rehabil Med.* 2006;38(4):255-262.

50. Upshur CC, Bacigalupe G, Luckmann R. "They don't want anything to do with you": Patient views of primary care management of chronic pain. *Pain Med.* 2010;11(12):1791-1798.

51. Scott W, Yu L, Patel S, McCracken LM. Measuring stigma in chronic pain: preliminary investigation of instrument psychometrics, correlates, and magnitude of change in a prospective cohort attending interdisciplinary treatment. *J Pain*. 2019;20(10):1164-1175.

52. Lesho E, Foster L, Wang Z, et al. The accuracy of physicians' perceptions of patients' suffering: findings from two teaching hospitals. *Acad Med*. 2009;84(5):636-642.

53. Henry SG. Opioids. In: Feldman MD, Christensen J, ed. *Behavioral medicine: a guide for clinical practice*. McGraw Hill; 2020.

54. Colaneri N, Keim S, Adesman A. Adolescent patient education regarding adhd stimulant diversion and misuse. *Patient Educ Couns*. 2017;100(2):289-296.

55. Naik AD, Kallen MA, Walder A, Street RLJr. Improving hypertension control in diabetes mellitus: the effects of collaborative and proactive health communication. *Circulation*. 2008;117(11):1361-1368.

56. McCarberg B, Stanos S. Key patient assessment tools and treatment strategies for pain management. *Pain Pract*. 2008;8(6):423-432.

57. Street RLJr, Elwyn G, Epstein RM. Patient preferences and healthcare outcomes: an ecological perspective. *Expert Rev Pharmacoecon Outcomes Res*. 2012;12(2):167-180.

58. Silverstein W, Lass E, Born K, Morinville A, Levinson W, Tannenbaum C. A survey of primary care patients' readiness to engage in the de-adoption practices recommended by Choosing Wisely Canada. *BMC Res Notes*. 2016;9:301.

59. Atzmüller C, Steiner P. Experimental vignette studies in survey research. *Methodology (Gott)*. 2010;6(3):128-138.

60. Hannawa AF, Shigemoto Y, Little TD. Medical errors: Disclosure styles, interpersonal forgiveness, and outcomes. *Soc Sci Med*. 2016;156:29-38.

61. Medendorp NM, Visser LNC, Hillen MA, de Haes JCJM, Smets EMA. How oncologists' communication improves (analogue) patients' recall of information. A randomized video-vignettes study. *Patient Educ Couns*. 2017;100(7):1338-1344.

62. Boland SE, Street RLJr, Persky S. Weight-related genomic information and provider communication approach: looking through the lens of patient race. *Per Med*. 2019;16(5):387-397.

63. Graugaard PK, Finset A. Trait anxiety and reactions to patient-centered and doctor-centered styles of communication: an experimental study. *Psychosom Med*. 2000;62(1):33-39.

64. Mazor K, Roblin DW, Greene SM, Fouayzi H, Gallagher TH. Primary care physicians' willingness to disclose oncology errors involving multiple providers to patients. *BMJ Qual Saf*. 2016;25(10):787-795.

65. Dresselhaus TR, Peabody JW, Luck J, Bertenthal D. An evaluation of vignettes for predicting variation in the quality of preventive care. *J Gen Intern Med*. 2004;19(10):1013-1018.

66. Hannawa AF. Disclosing medical errors to patients: Effects of nonverbal involvement. *Patient Educ Couns*. 2014;94(3):310-313.

67. van Vliet LM, van der WE, Albada A, Spreeuwenberg PM, Verheul W, Bensing JM. The validity of using analogue patients in practitioner-patient communication research: systematic review and meta-analysis. *J Gen Intern Med*. 2012;27(11):1528-1543.

68. Gordon HS, Street RL. How physicians, patients, and observers compare on the use of qualitative and quantitative measures of physician-patient communication. *Eval Health Prof*. 2016;39(4):496-511.

69. Ayanian JZ, Udvarhelyi IS, Gatsonis CA, Pashos CL, Epstein AM. Racial differences in the use of revascularization procedures after coronary angiography. *JAMA*. 1993;269(20):2642-2646.

70. Capers IV Q, Sharalaya, Z. Racial disparities in cardiovascular care: A review of culprits and potential solutions. *J Racial Ethn Health Disparities*. 2014;1:171-180.

71. Schulman KA, Berlin JA, Harless W, et al. The effect of race and sex on physicians' recommendations for cardiac catheterization. *N Engl J Med*. 1999;340(8):618-626.

72. Hall WJ, Chapman MV, Lee KM, et al. Implicit racial/ethnic bias among health care professionals and its influence on health care outcomes: a systematic review. *Am J Public Health*. 2015;105(12):e60-76.

73. Dovidio JF, Fiske ST. Under the radar: how unexamined biases in decision-making processes in clinical interactions can contribute to health care disparities. *Am J Public Health*. 2012;102(5):945-952.

74. Phelan SM, Dovidio JF, Puhl RM, et al. Implicit and explicit weight bias in a national sample of 4,732 medical students: the medical student CHANGES study. *Obesity (Silver Spring)*. 2014;22(4):1201-1208.

75. Thornicroft G, Rose D, Kassam A. Discrimination in health care against people with mental illness. *Int Rev Psychiatry*. 2007;19(2):113-122.

76. Wilson TD, Lindsey S, Schooler TY. A model of dual attitudes. *Psychol Rev*. 2000;107(1):101-126.

77. Burgess DJ, van RM, Crowley-Matoka M, Malat J. Understanding the provider contribution to race/ethnicity disparities in pain treatment: insights from dual process models of stereotyping. *Pain Med*. 2006;7(2):119-134.

78. Chen I, Kurz J, Pasanen M, et al. Racial differences in opioid use for chronic nonmalignant pain. *J Gen Intern Med*. 2005;20(7):593-598.

79. Johnson RL, Roter D, Powe NR, Cooper LA. Patient race/ethnicity and quality of patient-physician communication during medical visits. *Am J Public Health*. 2004;94(12):2084-2090.

80. Penner LA, Dovidio JF, West TV, et al. Aversive racism and medical interactions with black patients: a field study. *J Exp Soc Psychol*. 2010;46(2):436-440.

81. van RM, Fu SS. Paved with good intentions: do public health and human service providers contribute to racial/ethnic disparities in health? *Am J Public Health*. 2003;93(2):248-255.

82. Maina IW, Belton TD, Ginzberg S, Singh A, Johnson TJ. A decade of studying implicit racial/ethnic bias in healthcare providers using the implicit association test. *Soc Sci Med*. 2018;199:219-229.

83. Burgess DJ, Crowley-Matoka M, Phelan S, et al. Patient race and physicians' decisions to prescribe opioids for chronic low back pain. *Soc Sci Med*. 2008;67(11):1852-1860.

84. Krupat E, Irish JT, Kasten LE, et al. Patient assertiveness and physician decision-making among older breast cancer patients. *Soc Sci Med*. 1999;49(4):449-457.

85. Gordon HS, Street RLJr, Sharf BF, Souchek J. Racial differences in doctors' information-giving and patients' participation. *Cancer*. 2006;107(6):1313-1320.

86. Gordon HS, Street RLJr, Kelly PA, Souchek J, Wray NP. Physician-patient communication following invasive procedures: an analysis of post-angiogram consultations. *Soc Sci Med*. 2005;61(5):1015-1025.

CHAPTER **9**

Negotiating with Hospitalized Patients and Their Families

Clinical Take-Aways

- The nature of the hospital setting (acute illness, compressed timelines, unfamiliar environment, involvement of family, increased power differential) makes clinical negotiation both more important and more difficult.
- Different issues for clinical negotiation tend to arise at the beginning, middle, and end of each hospital stay.
- Children, people with cognitive or communication disabilities, and patients with limited English proficiency need special attention in the negotiating process.
- Clinicians working in hospital inpatient settings should:
  - Apply principles of "etiquette-based medicine" (ask permission to enter, introduce self, sit down, explain role, ask how hospital stay is going).
  - When negotiating about admission decisions, show empathy; demonstrate interest; deflect, don't repel; and use substitution, contingency, and availability when possible, rather than direct confrontation or "scare tactics."
  - Recognize and respond to patients' attempts to manage uncertainty (e.g., "why won't anyone tell me what's going on?" "all you guys seem to be doing is putting me through more tests").
  - Discuss goals of care (including criteria for and expected timing of discharge) early and often.
  - Recognize that high-quality hospital care requires a team consisting of health care workers of all stripes as well as patients and their families.

SECTION 9.1: INTRODUCTION

When patients are hospitalized, they enter a very strange world. Not long after admission, patients are placed in isolation or roomed with strangers (who may be very sick or disruptive), their personal belongings are taken away, and their clothes are exchanged for a flimsy hospital gown which opens, immodestly, in the back. They surrender their autonomy, allowing the hospital staff to tell them whether and when to eat, sleep, get out of bed, have their bodies prodded, or have their veins poked. They are often separated from loved ones except during defined visiting hours. Even their sense of time is eroded, as alarms, early morning lab draws, and vital sign checks do battle against uninterrupted sleep.

This dim picture belies the range hospital of experiences. At one end are patients admitted overnight for elective procedures, a short course of intravenous antibiotics, or brief observation. As long as they are not subject to gross medical error or callousness, these patients are likely to emerge relatively unscathed. At the other end are patients with severe trauma, critical illness, or other medical, surgical, obstetrical, or neurological conditions, often complicated by tangled family situations; these patients are not only in for a prolonged and potentially rocky confinement, they are most at risk for posttraumatic stress disorder.[1-4] With patients in the first group, there may be little to negotiate. With those in the second, the clinician may need to be prepared to engage skillfully and proactively.

> *Zoe Murphy is a 19-year-old college student who is brought by a friend to the emergency department because of acute right lower quadrant abdominal pain, shown on CT to be acute appendicitis. She is admitted to the surgical service, undergoes uneventful appendectomy, and is discharged home to the care of her family within 36 hours.*
>
> *Ashley Taylor is a 39-year-old mother of two children presenting with acute abdominal pain after 2 months of vague abdominal bloating and discomfort. CT scan shows ovarian torsion with a possible mass. Frozen section of the mass is consistent with early-stage ovarian carcinoma. Salpingo-oophorectomy is performed but is complicated postoperatively by severe ileus. Discharge is delayed repeatedly; the patient finally returns home after 10 days.*

These two patients differ not only in medical complexity but also in the substrate for negotiation. In Zoe Murphy's case, the patient was admitted, treated, and sent home. The patient's mother, Brenda, was surprised at the timing of planned discharge and asked that the patient be permitted to stay over another night. But after brief a brief discussion with Dr. Baker, the attending surgeon, she seemed reassured and drove the patient home.

In Ashley Taylor's case, trouble was evident from the start. The patient herself was frantic, her defenses worn down by months of vague discomfort rapidly evolving into acute pain. Without family in the area, she needed to find care for her two children, ultimately relying on a neighbor. After being told that she was having surgery to "remove a twisted ovary," she awakened from anesthesia shocked to learn that she had cancer. There were ongoing conflicts with the doctors and nursing staff about pain control; the patient repeatedly asked for opioids, while the team's primary focus was the slow return of postoperative bowel function. Finally, there were ongoing debates about the best destination immediately post-discharge: the team felt that a short stay in a rehabilitation facility might be beneficial, whereas Ms. Taylor was eager to be home with her children.

Issues like these arise in the hospital every day. In this chapter, we will first address differences between inpatient and outpatient care that bear on the clinical negotiation. We will then review key touchpoints for negotiation between clinicians, hospitalized patients, and their families, focusing on the beginning, middle, and end of the hospital stay.

SECTION 9.2: IMPLICATIONS OF THE HOSPITAL SETTING FOR CLINICAL NEGOTIATION

In the outpatient setting, most primary care clinicians (PCCs) enjoy a continuing relationship with patients over time. If a health crisis arises, discussions ideally occur in the context of an established relationship. Contacts are brief and chronologically dispersed, and they occur face-to-face, by telephone, and increasingly through electronic health portals and secure email. The PCC and any consulting specialists rarely, if ever, see the patient on the same day, let alone together in the same room. PCCs expect to remain responsible for their patients' care even after the current episode of illness concludes.

Some PCCs, especially in rural areas, follow their patients into the hospital, thus ensuring continuity of care from the outpatient to inpatient setting and back again. However, in most parts of the United States, PCCs have largely ceded the role of inpatient management to a cadre of more than 50,000 hospitalists.[5] **The relationship between the hospitalist and the hospitalized patient is time-limited, intense, and focused on the issues that spurred admission. With no prior relationship to build on, and with critical decision-making often needed within the first few hours or days of the admission, there is no time for trust to evolve organically. It must be nurtured directly through the clinician's words and actions.**

A simple way for the hospital clinician to begin building trust is to practice "etiquette-based medicine," as proposed by Michael Kahn in a much-cited piece in the *New England Journal of Medicine*.[6] The six behaviors proposed by Kahn (Table 9-1) as the foundation of hospitalist-patient interaction seem obvious but in practice are followed inconsistently: in one study, *none* of the six behaviors were practiced in 30% of hospital encounters.[7]

Aside from the lack of a prior relationship, hospital-based physicians face many other challenges. Hospitalized patients are often scared and may be very sick. Some are unable to communicate effectively because of illness, language barriers, cognitive deficits, or problems with speech or hearing. Complicated family dynamics may be present in graphic relief.

Table 9-1 **Etiquette-Based Medicine**

1. Ask permission to enter the room; wait for an answer.

2. Introduce yourself, showing ID badge.

3. Shake hands (wear gloves if needed).

4. Sit down. Smile if appropriate.

5. Briefly explain your role on the team.

6. Ask the patient how he or she is feeling about being in the hospital.

Source: Data from Kahn MW. Etiquette-based medicine. *N Engl J Med.* 2008;358(19):1988-1989.

In a sense, hospital medicine is just like outpatient medicine, only more so. The rules of effective negotiation are also similar. Understand the request, understand the patient, and work towards flexible solutions that satisfy both the patient and standards of practice.

SECTION 9.3: BEGIN AT THE BEGINNING: CLINICAL NEGOTIATION NEAR THE TIME OF ADMISSION

Negotiating the Admission Decision

It is an axiom of health economics that patients decide when to seek medical care initially, while doctors determine the subsequent intensity of care.[8] Hospitalization is an exception, as the decision to admit to the hospital rests solely with the physician, at least as a matter of law. The responsible physician may be the patient's primary care or subspecialty outpatient provider; a surgeon or interventionist who has scheduled the patient for an elective procedure; a member of the emergency department medical staff; a nursing home physician; or a consultant called in by the emergency medicine team. In the majority of cases, alignment between the physician's medical judgment and the patient's preferences is good. In the two cases under discussion, both Zoe Murphy and Ashley Taylor experienced relief on learning that they would be admitted to the hospital. But concordance is not always guaranteed, and malalignment can swing both ways.

> Mrs. Fogarty, a 79-year-old woman with osteoporosis, saw her primary care physician Dr. Krasner because of acute mid-back pain. An x-ray in the office showed a fresh thoracic spinal compression fracture. Dr. Krasner prescribed an opioid-acetaminophen combination product and arranged for close follow-up (including a house call), but the patient and her daughter requested admission for better pain control. Dr. Krasner refused, explaining that hospitalization was not only unnecessary but could be harmful. Leaving the office disgruntled, the patient went to the emergency department where the family prevailed on the physician-in-charge to arrange admission. Subsequently, the family dropped Dr. Krasner as their primary care physician.

Mr. Cervantes, a 49-year-old man with long-standing type 1 diabetes complicated by nephropathy, neuropathy, and heart failure, sees Dr. Cleary because "my foot is swollen and draining something." Examination is consistent with a diabetic foot ulcer with surrounding cellulitis. Dr. Cleary urges admission via the emergency department, noting that "you need intravenous antibiotics and possibly some tests to make sure the bone isn't infected." Mr. Cervantes strongly prefers that he be treated as an outpatient. "You know that emergency room—they'll keep me waiting for days, and I'll probably end up leaving anyway." After prolonged negotiation, they agree to get an x-ray and some blood tests, start oral antibiotics, and return in 48 hours so Dr. Cleary can reassess. In the meantime, Dr. Cleary requests an urgent vascular surgery referral for debridement and further evaluation for possible osteomyelitis.

For patients like Mrs. Fogarty, insistence on admission in the absence of compelling medical indications is most likely a reflection of a) overwhelming symptoms; b) fear of rapid clinical deterioration; c) poor illness coping; d) prior treatment patterns; or e) an unsafe physical or social environment. In Mrs. Fogarty's specific case, multiple factors were likely at play. She had pain disproportionate to any outward physical signs. She was worried that the pain might get worse. Already lonely and depressed, she felt particularly vulnerable to the effects of her current illness. When she had a compression fracture five years ago, she was promptly hospitalized. And although afraid of being left alone, she was reluctant to impose on her daughter or grandchildren, all of whom "had their own lives."

Mr. Cervantes looked at the prospect of hospitalization very differently. Where Mrs. Fogarty saw the hospital as a place of refuge where she might take a few days to collect herself and recover, Mr. Cervantes sensed danger. He was a veteran of many emergency department visits, some of which entailed many hours of waiting, followed by admission and prolonged periods of imposed fasting (NPO), resulting in wild fluctuations in his blood sugar. His fixation on past tribulations distracted his attention from the seriousness of the current situation.

Could Drs. Krasner and Cleary have achieved different results? It is hard to know for sure. However, it is possible that use of the "strategies for negotiating over treatment" and "giving something to get something" (See Tables 7-5 and 7-7 in Chapter 7) might have tilted both encounters in a different direction. Table 9-2 suggests ways in which Krasner and Cleary might have been more effective clinical negotiators.

Negotiating Social Relations within the Hospital

Until the mid-2000s it was still common for patients admitted to community hospitals to be admitted by their own primary care or subspecialty physician. This scheme could be taxing for clinicians, who had to attend to hospitalized patients while also maintaining a busy outpatient practice. From the perspective of hospital administrators, this system of care was also inefficient, as outpatient physicians were not always immediately available to attend to urgent problems or to arrange prompt discharge when indicated. However, from the standpoint of clinical negotiation, this approach

Table 9-2 Sample Language for Advancing the Clinical Negotiation in Two Clinical Cases

Strategy	Krasner/Fogarty	Cleary/Cervantes
Show empathy or support	"I can see that you are in a lot of pain." "It must be scary to be so limited in your movements when you live alone."	"You must be pretty worried about your foot. I know you wouldn't come to the doctor if you weren't concerned." "I am very glad you came in."
Demonstrate interest in the problem	"It seems it might be very hard to take care of yourself without help."	"I'm worried too. I'd like to get this infection under control as quickly as we can."
Deflect, don't repel	"Admitting you to the hospital is definitely an option." "However, the hospital has its own problems, like disrupted sleep and risk of infection."	"We could try to take care of this as an outpatient. But I'm worried we might not be able to control the infection fast enough, and that could put your foot at risk."
Use sub-stitution, contingency, availability	"How about this? We send you home with pain medicine under the care of your daughter, who has already said she can take a day or two off from work. I'll stop by your apartment after I finish clinic tomorrow to see how you are doing. If you're still doing poorly, we'll admit you to the hospital for intravenous pain meds or a nerve block."	"I'm ok with trying oral antibiotics for a short while, as long as you agree that if your foot doesn't look better in 2-3 days, you'll come into the hospital. In the meantime, here's my cell number—if you feel like you're getting worse or your blood sugars go over 300 consistently, call me anytime up to 10 pm—and if it's later than that, call the clinic after hours number to speak with one of my colleagues on call."

had distinct advantages. Patients knew their physicians. Physicians (or other clinicians on the team) knew their patients. There was little need to establish trust, because in most cases trust was already established.

A version of the traditional approach is preserved in the case of elective surgery, where patients have often seen the attending surgeon at least once in the outpatient setting. However, as noted previously, many patients in community hospitals today are managed by hospitalists. Barring an encounter during a past hospitalization, these physicians have no preexisting relationship with the patient. Nevertheless, most patients under duress from acute illness just want to be taken care of, and they will enter the new relationship with an attitude of hope and expectancy. Hospitalists need to take care not to fracture this emerging bond. The simple rules of "etiquette-based medicine" (Table 9-1) are a good place to start. **Asking for permission to enter, introducing oneself, sitting down, asking what it has been like for the patient to be in the**

hospital so far, and sharing information about the medical team's initial impressions can go a long way to putting the patient at ease.

Among these interventions, making a proper introduction is paramount. Numerous surveys of hospitalized patients suggest that they are frequently ignorant of who is caring for them, what their roles are, and whether they can expect the same individual or team to continue to be involved for the duration of their hospital stay.[9] These issues are particularly acute in teaching hospitals, where even the primary medical team may consist of an attending physician, a resident, an intern, and one or more medical students. When consultants are included in the mix, a single patient may easily interact with 6-12 physicians every day. Keeping track of each provider's name, specialty, and position in the medical hierarchy would be challenging enough absent the stress of illness; being sick makes it worse. Some teaching hospitals have tried to address the problem by posting names (and sometimes pictures) of the attending physician and primary nurse by the patient's bedside. But even this may not be sufficient. Therefore, it is important that physicians caring for hospitalized patients introduce themselves repeatedly and be prepared to explain how they fit into the larger team. Some hospitals have created visual displays that clarify who is who (see Figure 9-1).

Deeper Dive: 9.1: Interventions to Improve Hospital Patients' Satisfaction—A Tale of Two Approaches

The Centers for Medicare & Medicaid Services (CMS) introduced Hospital Value-Based Purchasing as a means to reward health systems for improving quality of care. One dimension of health system quality is enhancing patients' experiences with care. A number of systems have invested in programs to improve patients' experiences, particularly as measured by the Hospital Consumer Assessment of Healthcare Providers and Systems measure (HCAHPS, for inpatient care) and the Clinician and Group Consumer Assessment of Healthcare Providers and Systems measure (CGCAHPS, for outpatient care).[41] In this Deeper Dive, we describe two such programs, one involving intensive communication training for physicians and another that relies on the power of pictures to help patients know their clinical team.

The Cleveland Clinic, a nonprofit, multispecialty academic medical center, has developed an 8-hour experiential communication training program called the REDE to Communicate® model (*Relationship: Establishment, Development and Engagement*).[42] The training is required for all staff physicians. The REDE model is grounded in the principles of relationship-centered care, the idea that effective communication is the foundation of establishing therapeutic clinician-patient relationships that enhance quality of care and patient well-being. The Relationship is developed in three phases: Establish (friendly greetings, introduce self and team, build rapport, elicit concerns, agenda setting), Develop (orient patient to history, elicit patient narrative, work toward shared understanding), and Engage (present diagnosis, goals setting, shared decision-making, agree on plan, confirm patient commitment). Trained facilitators conduct didactic teaching presentations, live or video demonstrations of communication skills, and small group practice and role playing. Together, these pedagogical practices have been shown to enhance clinician communication skill.[43]

To assess the effect of the training on patient satisfaction, Boissy et al.[44] assigned physicians to the REDE training or a control group. Two patient satisfaction measures (HCAHPS and CGCAHPS) were analyzed. Controlling for physician demographics, years of experience, specialty, and baseline scores, physicians in the intervention group had statistically significantly higher scores than the controls on the outpatient satisfaction (CGCAHPS) measure (mean = 92.9 vs. 91.9, p = 0.03). In particular, intervention physicians scored higher on the "conveyed clear information" and "knew patient's medical history" items. There were no other differences on the individual CGCAHPS items. There was no statistical difference between intervention and control on the combined inpatient measure (HCAHPS), although intervention physicians scored higher on the "show respect" item (91.08 vs. 88.79, p = 0.02).

By contrast, Northwestern Memorial Hospital, a large tertiary teaching hospital in Chicago, took a different approach to enhancing hospitalized patients' experiences with care.[45] Guided by the simple principle that hospitalized patients ought to know who is responsible for their care,[46] the investigators provided patients with "facecards" that had pictures of individual clinical team members as well as their role in the patient's care. The facecards were considered a simple way to foster relationship-building by helping hospitalized patients get to know the names and role of their doctors.

In their pilot study, Simons et al.[45] randomly assigned one of two similar hospitalist service units and one of two similar teaching-service units to implement the use of physician facecards. Comparable units were selected as controls. The facecards consisted of pictures and the role of each team member (facsimile recreated in Figure 9-1).

One of the team physicians delivered the cards to newly admitted patients during their initial introduction. The investigators then randomly selected patients for structured interviews on their second or third hospital day. Patients were asked (a) to name their physician(s), (b) describe the role of each doctor in their care, and rate their (c) satisfaction with care (HCAHPS items), (d) trust in their doctors, and (e) agreement with the doctor's explanations and plan for care.

UH UNIVERSITY HOSPITAL

Your hospital care team includes the physicians below. They will communicate and work with nurses, allied health professionals and even your primary care and specialist physicians to ensure you receive the best care possible.

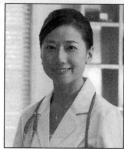

Attending Doctor
Dr. Julia Lee
The attending doctor is in charge of your care and oversees the other doctors on the team.

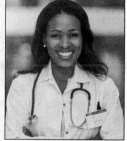

Resident Doctor
Dr. Annie Thomas
The resident doctor has at least one year of experience after medical school and helps lead the team.

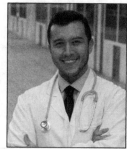

Intern Doctor
Dr. David Clark
The intern is the most junior doctor on the team and works under the supervision of the attending and resident.

Figure 9-1. Sample facecard.

Among 138 patients (66 intervention, 72 control), those who received the facecards were significantly more likely to correctly name one or more of their physicians (89% vs 51%) as well as correctly describe the role of the physician (67% vs. 16%). Patients who received facecards also tended to be more satisfied with their physicians, be more satisfied with the hospital, express greater trust, and have more agreement with their physicians than did patients not receiving facecards, although none of these differences were statistically significant.

What does this tale of two programs tell us? First, in both studies, patients reported high satisfaction regardless of group assignment. This is a problem for many studies of patient experience: if baseline ratings are too close to the highest possible value (something psychometricians call a "ceiling effect"), there's little room for improvement.

Second, in both studies there were few statistically significant, let alone clinically meaningful, differences. These findings are consistent with conclusions from systematic reviews that generally find that, with few exceptions, communication training and related interventions have minimal to modest effects on patient satisfaction.[41,47]

Third, the two interventions represent very different approaches to improving the hospital experience. The REDE model embraces the notion that the quality of patient satisfaction depends largely on the clinicians' and staff's effectiveness as communicators. As previously noted, the most successful health professional communication training programs are intensive, requiring hours (or days) of education; practice and role play; peer and expert feedback; self-reflection; and follow-up reinforcement.[43] On the other hand, the facecard intervention embraces the idea that patient experience can be improved if a key modifiable barrier or facilitator to satisfaction can be identified and targeted. In this case, it was simply addressing a question that for many hospitalized patients goes unanswered: "who are my doctors?"

So what's a hospital to do? Why choose? Both the comprehensive approach of the Cleveland Clinic initiative and the simple elegance of the Northwestern Memorial Hospital intervention are worth considering.

Another problem unique to teaching hospitals—and a matter that sometimes requires negotiation—is the involvement of specific members of the team. Most patients readily accept the implicit trade-off involved when seeking (or accepting) admission to a teaching hospital: more poking, prodding, and questioning by medical trainees in exchange for closer monitoring of their clinical situation and possibly higher quality of care.[10] Some, however, may resist trainee involvement.

> *Alan Goodman, a 78-year-old man with diabetes and marked lower urinary tract symptoms, is admitted to the hospital for transurethral resection of the prostate (TURP). Dr. Eng, a third-year urology resident, is sent to obtain consent for surgery. "No offense," Mr. Goodman says, "but I want only a board-certified urologist doing my surgery. I already talked to Dr. Walker about this."*

It would be easy for Dr. Eng to take offense at Mr. Goodman's blunt declaration. He could readily argue that trainees under Dr. Walker's supervision will augment patient care, not detract from it. Or he could mention that while experience and surgical volume are critical predictors of outcomes in complex operations, TURP is a relatively simple procedure. **But a better strategy would begin with understanding Mr. Goodman's concerns and attempting to address them.**

> *Dr. Eng: I understand. You want the best possible outcome from your surgery—anyone would! And Dr. Walker is truly an excellent surgeon.*
>
> *Mr. Goodman: Darn right! I checked around. That's why I don't want him turning over the job to someone else.*
>
> *Dr. Eng: So you are worried that having residents involved in the operation could create problems?*
>
> *Mr. Goodman: That's correct.*
>
> *Dr. Eng: Well, I am the resident who would be most involved, so maybe I could explain what my role would be. And if you still object, I'll talk with Dr. Walker about making you a private case.*
>
> *Mr. Goodman: (looking interested but skeptical) Ok, go ahead.*
>
> *Dr. Eng: (sitting down) Well, I would meet you in the pre-op area and help bring you into the OR. While the anesthesiologist performs the "spinal," I will scrub up with Dr. Walker. When you are fully anesthetized, I will insert the operating cystoscope, something I've done dozens of times. Your urethra and bladder will be shown on a large TV screen, so both Dr. Walker and I can view the operating field. Then, under Dr. Walker's supervision, I'll make some small cuts through the urethra into the prostate, removing excess tissue. Dr. Walker will be scrubbed in, giving me pointers, and ready to take over at any time. He will also confirm when sufficient tissue has been removed. We'll place a Foley catheter for purposes of irrigating the bladder. The whole thing should take less than 90 minutes. After that we'll take you to the recovery room and from there to your room upstairs. We'll monitor your blood sugars and urine flow overnight, and if all goes well you'll go home the next day.*
>
> *Mr. Goodman: No one ever explained things to me so thoroughly. I appreciate it! I guess it would be fine if you do things the way you just described. (Smiling) Just tell Dr. Walker he better be there too!*

Although Dr. Eng spends only a few moments hearing Mr. Goodman out, he quickly surmises that the problem may have two related components: lack of knowledge (of how responsibilities in teaching hospitals are divided) and lack of trust (that he will receive excellent care). Eng sits down, demonstrating an unhurried interest in connecting with the patient.

He reviews the steps of the operation one by one, something that no previous provider is likely to have done. He conveys his own competence ("...something I've done dozens of times") while underscoring the continued close involvement of the attending surgeon ("...ready to take over at any time"). By the end of the dialog, Mr. Goodman understands what is going to happen to him, realizes that his most acute fears are unfounded, and connects on an emotional level with the resident. Knowledge has been transmitted and trust restored.

To conduct this negotiation successfully, Dr. Eng needed to gain control of his own emotions. It was natural for him to feel somewhat flummoxed and even personally attacked by Mr. Goodman's resistance to resident involvement. But by taking a psychic "time-out" and putting himself in the patient's shoes, Dr. Eng navigated the discussion successfully. (The operation went well, too.)

But what if the conversation had gone sideways? This is not inconceivable. If Goodman had been more agitated, he might have interrupted Eng's efforts with an emphatic, "My insurance is paying Dr. Walker, and I want Dr. Walker to do the surgery. Period, end of story." If Eng had been more emotionally fragile (say, following a recent surgical misadventure or argument with his spouse), he might have abruptly departed the patient's room, saying, "I'm not sure what you were expecting. This is a teaching hospital! I'll talk to Dr. Walker and see what he says." In such situations, is there any room for compromise? Can the goal of delivering superb medical care while addressing patient preferences still be achieved?

Maybe. Perhaps Dr. Eng returns with Dr. Walker later that day. Dr. Walker explains the role of surgical residents at the medical center, emphasizes his confidence in Dr. Eng, and provides assurance that, as the attending surgeon, he will either perform or directly supervise every step of the operation—ready to take over at a moment's notice. But in the end, it is up to Mr. Goodman to decide.

By ceding power back to the patient ("I hope you allow us to proceed with Dr. Eng's involvement, but ultimately, it's up to you."), Dr. Walker not only acknowledges the ethical and legal imperative of patient autonomy, he quells Mr. Goodman's anger (which arose from a perception of powerlessness). It is very likely that the patient will now permit resident involvement in some form. But even if he doesn't, the decision now seems more fully informed, less driven by raw emotion, and more collaborative.

When Patient Preferences Conflict with Principles of Community, Diversity, and Inclusion

Patient preferences for the composition of their treatment team can extend beyond questions of training or seniority. For example, some patients may resist treatment by physicians of a particular race, ethnicity, gender, or sexual orientation.[11,12] Addressing these issues is complicated. Various algorithms have been proposed, most emphasizing consideration of patient acuity, presence of conditions that may alter decision-making capacity, and existence of "ethical" reasons for preferring one type of doctor over another.[13] From a practical standpoint, the admitting team must balance the interests of the patient against the interests of health care professionals and the organization in which they serve. **Patient interests are not necessarily equivalent to patient preferences; often, the best care will be provided by a team that includes the physician the patient is inclined, on the basis of discriminatory attitudes, to reject.** However, as articulated by Alfandre and Geppert,[14] clinicians are expected to evaluate patients' biases in the context of their commitment to the patient's welfare:

> *The fiduciary nature of the patient–provider relationship requires health care professionals to maintain a virtuous disposition. Society expects the professional to act with a humility, respect, and forbearance far beyond what is considered normative for many other professionals.*[14]

A related issue involves discriminatory or harassing comments by patients. In this instance, Alfandre and Geppert draw the line. For example, they suggest that when a female attending is told by a patient "You're very attractive," she should respond:

> "Your comments about my appearance make me uncomfortable. I wonder if you think you have to compliment me to get good care. For now, I want to focus on your healthcare. Please tell us how you're feeling and how we can help."

To us (full disclosure: two white men, privileged to have escaped many of the degrading and caustic remarks to which women and minorities are regularly subjected), this seems harsh. Except in egregious cases, we prefer deflection to confrontation, largely because we feel that patients in a state of vulnerability deserve the benefit of the doubt. The female attending might say, "Ok, but right now we need to focus on your health care. Can you tell us what most concerns you?" If an inappropriate comment is directed at a junior member of the team, the attending or senior resident can (and should) intervene: "Our team's primary concern right now is the illness that brought you into the hospital. Dr. Read is going to ask you some questions about that. Would that be ok?" Resolute body language and an assertive but respectful tone can communicate firmness while allowing the patient to avert humiliation and save face.

Humiliation is one of the four so-called self-conscious emotions (along with shame, embarrassment, and guilt) distinguished primarily by the exertion of power of one over another.[15] **Though it is tempting to push back at patients who have been rude, intrusive, or racist, humiliated patients are less likely to cooperate with treatment plans down the line. At the same time, members of the treatment team cannot be expected to endure repeated verbal assaults from patients.** The response should be measured, proportionate, and in consideration of the patient's intent. The goal of deflection is to maintain a sense of partnership with the patient while discouraging unwanted behavior. If deflection fails, stronger measures (chastisement, warning, even transfer to a different team or hospital) can be entertained.

Negotiating Over who will Speak for the Patient

In most Western countries, it is assumed that patients who have the capacity to make medical decisions should speak for themselves. In these cases, there is no negotiating over who is the ultimate "decider." **However, in hospital settings, an estimated 26% of older patients lack decision-making capacity and therefore require assistance from a surrogate.**[16] In these cases, practitioners are confronted by three questions: 1) Who is to speak for the patient? 2) What happens when multiple parties vie for the role? and 3) How can practitioners extract the most useful possible insights from the designated surrogate?

When a hospitalized patient lacks capacity to participate in medical decision-making, the physician can only hope that the patient has designated a surrogate through a durable power of attorney for health care (or the equivalent); the surrogate is available to fulfill his or her responsibilities (preferably in person, but sometimes remotely); and there is consensus among other interested family members and friends both in regard to the identity of the decision maker and the direction of the decisions themselves. Under such circumstances, little negotiating is required. However, when one or more of these elements are missing, several tactics may be helpful.

First, ask the family to designate a primary point of contact who can speak for the group. Second, arrange a family meeting without delay. In conducting such meetings, Fineberg et al. have emphasized the importance of *negotiation* (the process for reaching a decision and building consensus among participants around topics such as perspectives on the patient's situation, care goals, and discharge plans) and *personal stance* (application of interpersonal skills to convey empathy and a desire to find common ground among all participants).[17] Third, try to create an alliance with the designated surrogate. This can be achieved by setting aside 10-15 minutes early in the hospitalization to sit down with the surrogate, understand their relationship to the patient, and determine the extent to which the surrogate is familiar with the patient's values ("What do you think your mom would want were she able to express herself?"). The physician should affirm a commitment to keep the surrogate informed of key clinical developments, and then follow through on those commitments.

An even more difficult situation arises when the patient has no identifiable surrogate. These so-called "unbefriended patients" are increasingly common as society ages and disperses. Guidelines from the American Geriatrics Society are aimed at older adults but probably apply more broadly:

> The process of arriving at a treatment decision for an unbefriended older adult should be conducted according to standards of procedural fairness and include capacity assessment, a search for potentially unidentified surrogate decision makers (including non-traditional surrogates) and a team-based effort to ascertain the unbefriended older adult's preferences by synthesizing all available evidence.[18]

Deeper Dive 9.2: Clinical Negotiation in Accompanied Medical Encounters

Medical consultations often have others present in addition to a clinician and patient, and this is especially true with hospitalized patients. The presence of a third party (hereafter referred to as companion) can affect the communicative dynamics of clinical encounters in several ways. For example, in addition to one interaction between a clinician and patient, there are three other possible combinations when companions are present—clinician-companion, patient-companion, and clinician-patient-companion interactions. Moreover, the person present as a companion could be any number of people, including a spouse, adult child, friend, or neighbor.

Several studies have analyzed communication patterns in dyadic (patient-clinician) versus accompanied (clinician-patient-companion) encounters. In a study of lung cancer patients at a VHA facility, Street and colleagues[48] observed that physicians on average talked about 55-60% of the time in the consultations regardless of whether the patient was accompanied. The patient alone or patient plus companion accounted for the rest of the talk. This finding is comparable to what Shields et al.[49] and Wolff et al.[50] reported in investigations of clinician-patient-companion communication in geriatric and routine primary care visits, respectively.

However, the Street et al. investigation also analyzed different patterns of companion communication and found considerable variability across consultations. For example, in nearly half of the accompanied encounters the patient was the more active participant while the companion was relatively quiet. The reverse occurred in a third of the consultations—the companion was the active participant with the patient participating little. Finally, in only 17% of the consultations did the patient and companion interact as a "tag team" with each contributing roughly equally. From other research, we know that companions take a more active role when the patient is very sick, has cognitive deficits, or is sedated.[51]

The wide variability in companion communication in accompanied visits indicates that companions can serve a number of purposes in the interaction. Two recent reviews[52,53] on the communicative contributions of companions concluded that both patients and clinicians generally believed companions have a positive influence in the encounter, especially when asking clarifying questions, taking notes, providing missing information, and reinforcing the patient's understanding of important issues.[52,54] However, companions can also have a deleterious effect on consultations when they are demanding, nagging, and speaking "for" the patient even when the patient is capable of speaking for themselves.[55] When companions accompany patients with poorer mental health status, the interaction may produce more talk focused on biomedical issues (e.g., diagnosis, health status, treatment) and less on partnership-building and discussion of psychosocial issues.[56]

To optimize clinical negotiation in accompanied encounters, clinicians must be able to assess and manage the role of the companion which, as Laidsaar-Powell et al.[52] observe, can range from "active partner", to "welcome guest," to "intruder." These authors have published recommendations for how clinicians can facilitate collaborative interactions with family and companions[57] as well as strategies for managing more difficult encounters (e.g., involving anger, conflicts involving control, and family disagreements).[58] Here is a summary of some of these strategies that are particularly relevant for hospitalized patients.

- Welcome and involve companions in the conversation, as most patients believe their companion has a purpose for being there.
- Determine (if appropriate) why the companion has accompanied the patient to the visit, as companions accompany patients for a wide variety of reasons.
- Take opportunities to highlight helpful companion behaviors for the patient's care (e.g., informational, emotional, and tangible support).
- Assess and respect the patient's preferences for the companion's role in the consultation (patients and companions sometimes differ on what the companion's role should be).
- Create opportunities to privately discuss sensitive issues with the patient alone (patients may be uncomfortable discussing some personal issues such as sexuality, mental health, substance use, etc., with the companion present.)
- Be aware that companions often are very influential in decision-making discussion outside the consultation.
- Be mindful of one's own attitudes and behaviors toward the companion. Some patients report clinicians inappropriately or unintentionally ignore or discount what the companion has to say.

In quantum mechanics, the mathematics of "entanglement" between more than two particles becomes seriously complicated.[59] While communication in accompanied visits is nuanced and challenging, acknowledging and facilitating the positive role that companions can play while also affirming the primacy of the patient can help "untangle" some of these difficulties and support effective clinical negotiation.

What this means in practice is that the physician carefully determines whether the unbefriended patient has the capacity to engage in medical decision-making—recognizing that refusal to undergo a medically indicated procedure or the presence of major psychiatric illness does not by itself indicate incapacity. The clinician then engages relevant assistance (social work, discharge planning) to make all possible efforts to find a surrogate, including from nontraditional sources such as Alcoholics Anonymous, drug rehab, or the street. If the patient lacks capacity, efforts to find a surrogate fail, and the process of obtaining legal conservatorship is delayed, the clinician contemplating major decisions on the patient's behalf should seek consensus among colleagues or obtain the help of the hospital ethics committee.

SECTION 9.4: MUDDLING THROUGH THE MIDDLE: CLINICAL NEGOTIATION BETWEEN ADMISSION AND DISCHARGE

The admission process is complete. A history and physical examination have been performed, the diagnostic and treatment plan has been established, and initial orders have been written. Many subsequent clinical tasks are now the responsibility of other members of the team (nurses, respiratory therapists, physical therapists, pharmacists, etc.). At this point, the clinician may begin to relax. **However, for patients, the journey is just beginning.** At the same time that they are dealing with physical discomfort and emotional stress (perhaps the most severe of their adult lives), patients are also struggling to adapt to a wholly unfamiliar environment. During the postadmission phase of hospitalization, clinicians will be called upon to help patients navigate at least four additional hazards: dealing with uncertainty, adapting to daily life in the hospital, making major treatment decisions, and clarifying goals of care.

Dealing with Uncertainty

The hospital is rife with uncertainty for both clinicians and patients. For clinicians, questions abound about the accuracy of the history of present illness, the reliability and relevance of physical findings, the interpretation of diagnostic tests, the formulation of a working diagnosis, and the appropriateness of initial therapy. Making matters worse, these vagaries of clinical assessment are often clouded by inadequate or conflicting clinical evidence. Without minimizing the difficulties facing clinicians, patients face equal or greater uncertainties.

In Mishel's "middle-range theory," uncertainty is defined as difficulty finding meaning in the illness experience. At first glance, this seems like an oddly subjective interpretation of uncertainty. **Yet Mishel argues that illness is, for many patients, a descent into chaos. Finding meaning is key to restoring order.**

Mishel contends that uncertainty is *driven* by antecedents (such as symptoms and lack of familiarity with the hospital environment); *supported* by structures such as social networks or professional authority; *evaluated* as danger or opportunity; and *addressed* with problem-solving and emotional coping strategies leading, it is hoped, to adaptation.[19] Theories like this can be useful in understanding how patients process and react to the hospital experience, which in turn supports more effective clinical negotiation.

Patients admitted to the hospital wonder what is wrong (diagnosis) and how their illness will unfold (prognosis). In the first days following admission, they are unlikely to get definitive answers. The early hours of hospitalization, at least on general medical services, usually involve multiple brief bedside contacts by physicians, nurses, and other health care professionals; performance of diagnostic tests and imaging studies, some requiring transport to other parts of the hospital; initiation of new therapies, including drugs that may be accompanied by unfamiliar side effects; and usually, pitiably brief (and sometimes contradictory) explanations from different team members about what is happening and why. Naïve to the hospital and faced with new and potentially frightening symptoms, hospitalized patients are heavily dependent on support from family members, friends, and health professionals to help them interpret their own illness experience, develop coping strategies, and adapt to their new environment.

Patients will rarely ask directly for help with coping with uncertainty; more often, their requests arrive in more subtle form. For example:

- Can you tell me what's going on?
- All you guys seem to be doing is putting me through tests.
- I read that antibiotics are dangerous.
- I worry about how my daughter is taking this.
- When do I get something to eat?

Requests concerning seemingly trivial aspects of the hospital routine can be telling in two ways. **First, patients may be sharing legitimate concerns about avoidable physical discomfort.** In regard to fasting, this can be addressed by making sure that orders for "nothing by mouth" (NPO) are medically indicated, that the patient who requires an NPO order receives adequate intravenous hydration, and that the patient is provided with something to eat (even a light snack) once the medical contraindication to oral intake has lifted. Equally important, someone needs to explain to the patient why the NPO order is necessary, when it will be lifted, and (in the event) why the order needs to be extended.

Second, by focusing on the material and seemingly trivial, patients may simply be trying to exert control over one of the few aspects of their illness where control is still within reach. Therefore, such questions are best met with empathy, reflection, or concern, and not just raw information: "You have been without food or water now for almost 24 hours. I know how difficult that must be. It is very frustrating not to know the time of your surgery. I will go ask the nurse for an update and see if she knows anything."

Adapting to Daily Life in the Hospital

Entering the hospital is in some ways like visiting a foreign city. Like cities, hospitals have their own infrastructure, their own local ordinances, their own governance structures. Unlike a trip to Paris, however, hospital admission is rarely on anyone's wish list. The norms governing patient conduct within the hospital are aimed at beneficence but laced with authoritarianism. With few exceptions—and sometimes without a clear medical rationale—patients are given little choice in accommodation (often double-occupancy), dress (hospital gown), food (limited and often of dreadful quality), drink (restricted and decidedly nonalcoholic), and ability to associate with friends and family (strict visiting hours). Interestingly, pediatrics departments have done much better than medical and surgical ward administrators at trying to impart a sense of normalcy; for example, many have unlimited visiting hours, sleeping accommodations for parents, and "Child Life" programs that attend to children as people, not just persons who are ill.

> *Robert Bustamonte, a 55-year-old HIV-negative man who has sex with men (MSM), is admitted because of gradual onset of shortness of breath over the past month. Chest x-ray shows increased interstitial markings. Because tuberculosis is mentioned as one of many possibilities in the radiologist's report, the patient is placed in isolation per hospital policy. In the meantime, he is treated effectively for congestive heart failure. By hospital day 3, he is feeling better and asks to be discharged. However, because the County Department of Health was closed over the long holiday weekend, he is kept in isolation involuntarily for an additional 4 days. During this time, he has few visitors and feels depressed. He is also disgruntled because he did not get his usual glaucoma drops for 2 days, his food is served cold, and once after an episode of orthostatic hypotension, he had to crawl back into bed by himself as help was slow to arrive.*
>
> *Third-year medical student Hamda Moosani has been assigned to Mr. Bustamonte's case. When she sees him on the morning of hospital day 5, he lashes out. Recalling some of the cardinal principles of clinical negotiation she learned in her second-year medical communication class, Ms. Moosani tries to reach a compromise.*
>
> *Mr. Bustamonte: What am I still doing here? I want out.*
>
> *Ms. Moosani: (trying to convey empathy/concern) I can certainly understand that. You've been here 5 days, you're feeling much better, and there doesn't seem to be any good reason for being here.*
>
> *Mr. Bustamonte: Right. And things just keep getting worse. Yesterday I fell and no one bothered to help me up.*
>
> *Ms. Moosani (alarmed): You fell? I'm afraid I didn't hear about that. Did you lose consciousness? Hurt yourself?*
>
> *Mr. Bustamonte: No, nothing like that. I just got up too quickly, felt faint, and sort of allowed myself to drop to the floor.*
>
> *Ms. Moosani: Well (gesturing towards stethoscope), I'd like to check you out, if that's ok.*

[completes physical exam, sits down, and faces patient]

Ms. Moosani: (trying to find common ground): Well, your exam seems pretty normal; I'm relieved. Of course, some of the other doctors will be later to check my findings. But in the meantime I'd like to hear more about what this hospitalization has been like for you.

Mr. Bustamonte: I told you, it's been a mess. (looking sad) I think I'd be much better off at home. Please let me go home today.

Ms. Moosani: I can tell you're not very happy about any of this. That's understandable. (Pauses.) The good news is that you're looking and feeling so much better since you first arrived, now that we have taken some fluid off your lungs. Unfortunately, we're still waiting on your TB results.

Mr. Bustamante: In my mind, that's ridiculous. I don't have TB.

Ms. Moosani: We agree it's unlikely, it's just that the hospital has...these protocols. (Remembers substitution and availability strategies.) How about this? Let me see if I can arrange for someone to take you for a walk around the hospital grounds at least once a day, maybe twice. It doesn't get you home immediately like we'd like, but maybe you'd feel less cooped up. And in the meantime, I will call the County Health Officer myself and find out whether there's another way to handle this. Whether I get ahold of her or not, I'll stop by again later today to let you know.

Whether or not she succeeded in placating the patient, this student clearly paid attention in class. She conveyed empathy both verbally and nonverbally, showed interest in the patient's story by asking questions and performing a physical exam, and applied substitution and availability strategies to help reach a negotiated settlement.

Negotiating with Patients who are Reluctant to Proceed with Recommended Treatment

Hospital medicine is like outpatient medicine on steroids. Diagnoses are formed, treatment plans are implemented, progress is monitored, clinician-patient relationships are developed (and interrupted), patients get better (or worse)—all at an accelerated pace. **Also, in contrast to the outpatient setting, the most common negotiation challenge is not the patient who *requests* an equivocal or contraindicated procedure, but rather the patient who *resists* undergoing a recommended one.** Part of the reason these situations are so vexing is because of the economic pressures and logistical constraints that inform daily life in the hospital. Hospital administrators, under pressure from the federal government and other third-party payers to economize on length of stay, have implemented policies and "care pathways" in which every admission day represents a step towards discharge. Furthermore, radiology suite and operating room schedules are not infinitely flexible, so a patient who suddenly balks at a planned procedure may not have another turn for several more days. Thus, when patients resist undergoing a recommended procedure, there is often little time for the sort of deliberative shared decision-making espoused by experts.[20]

Some strategies for negotiating with inpatients who are reluctant to proceed with treatment are summarized here as a list of Do's and Don'ts and are further developed in Table 9-3.

DO:

1. Listen to the patient—their reluctance to proceed may conceal critical medical information or signal something important about their values.
2. Share information in small bites—after offering information on risks and benefits, stop and listen—the patient may give you important feedback (verbal or nonverbal) which informs your next step.
3. Try to get the whole team (especially other physicians and nurses) on the same page. The point is not to overwhelm the patient with a show of force but rather to ensure that the patient and family are receiving consistent information.
4. Seek opportunities for substitution (offering the next best treatment alternative) and contingency (obtaining agreement to proceed with the recommended therapy pending a trial of a less risky, but potentially less effective approach).

DON'T

1. Imagine that informed consent has been obtained simply because the patient has signed a form.
2. Overemphasize cognition at the expense of emotions—fear, powerlessness, lack of control, anger at perceived slights, and sometimes just pain and physical discomfort can overwhelm cognitive processes and make rational decision-making (based on the patient's values, not the clinician's) difficult. When the patient is feeling overwhelmed, ladling on facts will not help.
3. Contradict other members of the care team unless absolutely necessary. It is always best to resolve internecine disagreements among members of the medical staff before bringing a major recommendation to the patient. (See Chapter 10 for more on this topic.)
4. Assume that a patient's initial reluctance is the final word. Sometimes the patient needs time to process an extremely threatening situation and will be more amenable to negotiation later in the day.

Table 9-3 Strategies for Dealing with the Hospitalized Patient who is Reluctant to Accept Recommended Treatment

Strategy	Sample Language
Consider that the patient may be right.	*Well, you make a good point—given your previous reaction to intravenous contrast dye—which I'm very glad you just told me about—it is probably a bad idea to proceed without taking some additional precautions like using low-osmolality dye and pretreating you with Benadryl®*
Elicit patient concerns.	*Most anyone might be worried about the risks of [the proposed treatment or procedure]. Can you help me understand some of your specific concerns?*
Demonstrate empathy.	*No doubt procedures like the one we're proposing have risks—and some of those risks are scary. It would be natural to be…unnerved.* *The thought of losing even a part of your leg must bring up all kinds of feelings. You might even be wondering, how will I get along afterwards? Do you want to talk about that?*

(Continued)

Table 9-3 **Strategies for Dealing with the Hospitalized Patient who is Reluctant to Accept Recommended Treatment (Continued)**

Strategy	Sample Language
Establish patient values.	*Looking ahead to the future, what is most important to you?* *What were you hoping we would do for you during this hospitalization?*
Share information judiciously.	*Out of 100 people like you—an older man with a recent TIA and similar results on ultrasound, about 40 will have a stroke without operation. An operation can cut that risk about in half, but as you've already guessed, some of that risk comes on right away—about 5 of 100 patients will have a stroke on the table or soon thereafter. Now I know that's a lot to swallow. What do you make of that?*
Muster alliances.	*I know you and Dr. Kincaid have known each other for a long time. Would it help to get her opinion?* *Why don't we have a three-way conversation that involves your son in Wichita? You and I can meet in person and we'll get him on the phone.*
Seek opportunities for substitution and contingencies.	*While I don't think it's the best approach, we could try tacking down your retina with a laser first, and if that doesn't work we could do the sclera buckle a few days later.* *Why don't you try a single course of chemotherapy? If you tolerate it well, we can try a second course. But if you don't, you can stop at any time.*

Negotiating Goals of Care

The task of goal clarification has received the most attention in the context of severe illness and end-of-life care. However, eliciting and clarifying patients' goals is an essential step in the care of most patients hospitalized with complex illness. Best practices in discussing goals of care include sharing information about the likely course of illness, determining informational preferences, understanding what patients are most afraid of, considering trade-offs between life extension and quality of life, and soliciting preferences for family involvement. The American College of Physicians has developed model language that both inpatient and outpatient physicians can use in navigating these issues (Table 9-4).[21]

Focusing on goals of care is arguably more holistic, more humane, and more effective than talking narrowly about the patient's wishes regarding specific procedures such as cardiopulmonary resuscitation, intubation, or transfer to the intensive care unit.[22] Once goals are understood, it is easier to see which specific medical interventions are likely to advance those goals and which may actually interfere.

SECTION 9.5: CLINICAL NEGOTIATION NEAR THE TIME OF DISCHARGE

At some point during hospitalization, as the patient's illness improves or stabilizes, people will start talking about discharge. This happens sooner in the United

Table 9-4 American College of Physicians Model Language for Communicating About Serious Illness Care Goals

Topic	Suggested Language
Understanding	What is your understanding of where you are now with your illness?
Information preferences	How much information about what is likely to be ahead with your illness would you like from me?
Prognosis	Share prognosis, tailored to preferences, possibly employing a "best case, worst case" approach.
Goals	If your health situation worsens, what are your most important goals?
Fears/Worries	What are your biggest fears and worries about the future with your health?
Function	What abilities are so critical to your life that you can't imagine living without them?
Trade-offs	If you become sicker, how much are you willing to go through for the possibility of gaining more time?
Family	How much does your family know about your priorities and wishes?

Source: From Bernacki and Block, 2014.[21]

States than in other countries; mean hospital length of stay is 5.5 days in the United States versus 6.2 days for the median OECD country and 16.5 days in Japan.[23] These conversations tend to center on two intertwined issues: *when* the patient will be discharged and *where* they will go after leaving the acute care hospital.

Timing of Discharge

In the optimal scenario, patients and families are well-briefed on the likely hospital course, and there are no surprises. For example, in contemporary orthopedic practice, patients admitted for elective knee or hip surgery are advised that they will mobilize with physical therapy on the first postoperative day and go home 1-3 days later. Nurses, physical therapists, and discharge planners all know the drill and are likely to reinforce expectations for early discharge at multiple touch points. At the other extreme, patients with complex illness or who present as diagnostic dilemmas will inevitably receive ambiguous and often contradictory counsel. **Such mixed messages can readily confuse patients and families and lead to contentious discussions that will challenge physicians' skills as clinical negotiators.**

But it is not just lack of clarity in defining expectations for discharge that vex patients and families. Sometimes it is the timing of discharge itself.

Mrs. Timmons is 84-year-old widow with moderately severe COPD and mild dementia who is admitted because of a COPD exacerbation. Mrs. Timmons lives with her daughter Alice Baker, who is at her bedside for the better part of each day. On hospital day 5, the patient's condition has stabilized, although she is still using oxygen at 2 L/minute by nasal cannula. In addition, she is intermittently confused, sometimes not being sure where she is and occasionally mentioning visits by people who she hasn't seen in years (e.g., "Cousin Fred stopped by today."). A workup for reversible causes of delirium was unrevealing, and the team plans to send the patient home tomorrow. Dr. Quinones (the family medicine intern) delivers the news to Alice in the corridor just outside Mrs. Timmons' room.

Dr. Quinones: Hi, Mrs. Baker. I'm glad I found you here. Your mom is doing way better than on admission and we think she'll be ready to go home tomorrow.

Alice Baker: (looking worried) Oh? I don't think she's ready.

At this point it would be tempting for Dr. Quinones to build the case for discharge by listing the ways Alice's mother has improved (breathing better, less cough, less wheezing) and by issuing a warning about the medical dangers inherent in unnecessarily prolonged hospitalization (infection, iatrogenic injury, etc.). If things got heated, Dr. Quinones might even suggest that the patient could be financially liable for additional charges. By now, most readers will recognize this approach as a mistake. Instead, Dr. Quinones takes a breath and listens.

Dr. Quinones: Let's duck into this alcove over here (gesturing to a more private space). Tell me more about your concerns.

Alice Baker: Mom isn't herself. Today she's a little better, but last night she was very confused. Also, she's never had to be on oxygen before. Will she need to be on that forever?

In this statement, there are the words themselves and there are the thoughts and feelings that are carried on the words. Ms. Baker is concerned about her mother's cognitive function. She wonders what is the cause, whether mom is likely to get better, and—as her mother's primary caretaker—how she will cope. Her question about supplemental oxygen could signal uncertainty about the prognostic implications ("Is Mom going to get worse and die?") or pragmatic concerns about obtaining, setting up, and operating an oxygen delivery system at home. None of this is known to Dr. Quinones definitively. To explore what are now merely hunches, she must ask.

Dr. Quinones: Before we get to that, let's back up a bit. We know your mother is not herself. But it seems like she's on the right track; she was much more sharp this morning, for example, than either of the past 2 days. In addition, we've ruled out serious causes of mental status changes like infection and stroke. The hospital environment—with all the noises, alarms, unfamiliar routines—can really send older people into a tailspin. So she might actually do better at home.

Alice: Ok, but what if she doesn't improve. And what about the oxygen?

Dr. Quinones: (invoking the availability gambit) I will call your mom's primary care physician—I think we have the number up at the front desk—and make sure she's aware of what's happening and is ready to intervene if things don't improve as expected. As for the oxygen, we'll make sure you're set up with home health. Most likely, she'll be able to wean down on the oxygen and come off within the next couple of weeks.

Alice: That sounds ok. Thank you for explaining.

Dr. Quinones: Of course. We'll see your mom tomorrow on rounds and if there's any change for the worse we'll definitely re-evaluate.

As the dialog between Dr. Quinones and Alice Baker illustrates, patients and family concerns about the timing of discharge can reflect distinct anxieties. Often these are fueled by the perception that the patient has not returned to premorbid levels of function, and that the resources available at home (or in a subacute care facility) will be insufficient to provide good care. The truth is that acute care hospitals in the United States are in fact better staffed and better equipped than the typical home or skilled nursing facility. There is a very real and steep decline in human resources as one moves from ICU (nurse-to-patient ratios of 1:2) to floor (1:5) to SNF to home. Patients and families may justifiably worry about their ability to cope.

Physicians like Dr. Quinones can help by providing clear medical information and ensuring good communication among different members of the care team (including the primary care physician, if possible). However, physicians are not in this alone. They need support in the discharge process from nurses, pharmacists, physical and respiratory therapists, discharge planners, and sometimes social workers and other mental health professionals. If all these team members can work in a coordinated fashion, it is much easier to put concerns like those expressed by Alice Baker to rest. Often, the bedside or charge nurse is in a better position to coordinate these activities than the physician. **Even if medical teams do not routinely include nurses in rounds for most of the hospital stay, doing so near the time of discharge can pay off handsomely in enhanced coordination of care.**

Patients who Wish to Sign Out "Against Medical Advice"

Patient resistance to treatment achieves its apogee among those who leave the hospital "against medical advice" (AMA). These patients are so dissatisfied with their hospital care, or face such urgent life demands, that they insist upon immediate discharge, often against their own best medical interests. AMA discharges are uncommon (probably representing 1-2% of all admissions)[24] but tend to be seared in physicians' brains as among the most challenging clinical negotiations they have ever faced. Some of the difficulty arises from the confrontational mindset harkened by the AMA label itself. **As Alfandre et al. argue, the AMA designation (and accompanying documents for signature) is not legally required, nor is it likely to help as a liability defense.**[25,26] Instead, these patients should be approached as the quintessential opportunity for clinical negotiation.

Ronald Sprague is a 48-year-old unemployed construction worker with type 2 diabetes and intermittent methamphetamine use (smoked, snorted, and used intravenously) who is admitted for hyperglycemia and cellulitis. He recently fell behind in rent payments, resulting in eviction, and is currently "couch-surfing" with friends. He is treated with insulin and intravenous antibiotics. By hospital day 3 his cellulitis has significantly improved, but his finger stick glucose values remain above 300 mg/dL. When seen by the house staff in the morning he says he "has important business to take care of" and needs to leave. They advise him that would be unwise until his blood sugar is under better control. The patient becomes angry. The team replies that whether he leaves or not is up to him, but "you will have to sign out Against Medical Advice" and Medicaid may not pay for the admission, which could leave you with a significant bill."

"I'd like to see this f——ing hospital try to collect," says Mr. Sprague. "Give me the papers and let me out of here."

"Happens all the time with addicts," says the senior resident to his team. "He probably just wants a fix."

Clearly, this interaction was painful for all parties. What went wrong? The patient's judgment may have been altered by a variety of intrinsic and extrinsic factors, including medical illness, methamphetamine addiction, financial stress, housing insecurity, the regimentation inherent in hospitalization, disagreements with nurses about the timing of meals, and residual resentment from a prior hospitalization in which he felt "disrespected" by one of the younger doctors. There are nonetheless opportunities for improvement in the interaction itself.

1. The team could have explored more thoroughly the patient's reasons for requesting immediate discharge. ("Is this just about the business you need to take care of outside, or is there also something about your experience here in the hospital that makes you want to leave? Would you feel comfortable telling us more about that?")

2. The team failed to recognize that refusing medical treatment is the right of any adult with adequate decision-making capacity. In this light, the team's obligation is to make sure the patient understands the risks and benefits of their preferred choice (versus remaining in the hospital) and to formulate safe alternatives if possible. For example, they could have prescribed oral antibiotics and insulin, arranged for additional diabetic teaching that same day, and scheduled a follow-up visit with the patient's outpatient clinic (a local Federally Qualified Health Center) within 3-5 days.

3. The team confused signing a form with informed consent. The former is a legal ritual (which as mentioned, may have limited legal backing), whereas the latter is a discussion among the lines outlined in #2 above.

In summary, whether the issue is a hospital stay that is perceived to be too short or too long, the correct "dose" of hospitalization is a common source of contention. Clinicians can head off conflict by setting expectations for hospital length of stay on admission (when incomplete knowledge makes all prognostication vague) and regularly thereafter. As with most human affairs, understanding the other person's point of view will open the door to dialog, and with luck, effective resolution.

Place of Discharge

Timing of discharge is not the only potential locus of contention between hospital physicians, their patients, and their patients' families. Place matters too. In the

Distribution of Inpatient Hospital Stays by Discharge Status,* 2007

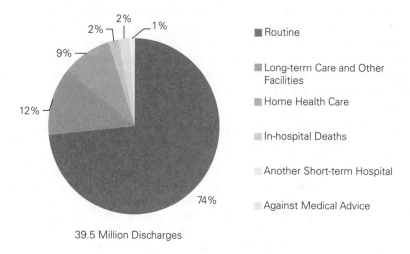

39.5 Million Discharges

*Excludes less than 9,000 discharges (0.01 percent) with missing discharge status.

Figure 9-2. Discharge destination for 39.5 million patients, 2007. *Source:* Reproduced with permission from Facts and Figures 2006. Healthcare Cost and Utilization Project (HCUP). September 2009. Agency for Healthcare Research and Quality, Rockville, MD. www.hcup-us.ahrq.gov/reports/factsandfigures/2007/exhibit1_4.jsp. https://www.hcup-us.ahrq.gov/reports/factsandfigures/2007/exhibit1_4.jsp.

United States, among 100 patients admitted to the hospital, 2 will die. Among the 98 survivors, 2 will be transferred to other acute care facilities, 84 will go home, and 12 will be discharged to a long-term care facility (Figure 9-2). (Practitioners in safety-net hospitals will recognize these statistics as incomplete, because for homeless individuals, "home" may mean the street or a temporary shelter.) While discussions concerning the site of care after hospital discharge are generally routine, disagreements can and do arise. Most often, the issue is whether the patient should return home (with or without support from family members, home health services, or paid caregivers) or transferred to a skilled nursing facility.

Patients and clinicians have somewhat predictable points of view. **Patients often lean towards familiarity and independence.** Most favor going home. **Health care providers privilege patient safety.** The patients they have nursed back from the brink during the acute hospital stay may be perceived as too sick, too frail, too cognitively impaired, or too socially isolated to stay safely at home. Without adequate help, they may fall, wander, fumble with their dressing changes, not take their medications. Patients' families can be the decisive swing vote, but their views run the gamut. Some families may be supportive of the patient's desire to return home and are willing to provide or arrange for the needed support. Others may balk, concerned that the patient is likely to need more help than the family is able to provide. This attitude may generate push-back from physicians, who hold the "often unsubstantiated belief that family members who face financial or care burdens will always put their own self-interest above that of the patient."[27] In fact, caregiver burden is an increasingly recognized public health problem, and some bioethicists have asked whether physicians should not embrace a more nuanced version of the Hippocratic commitment to the individual patient, attending more carefully to the needs of the family unit.[28]

> *Mrs. Collins is an 84-year-old widow who, after tripping on some steps at home and breaking her right hip, underwent a successful open reduction and internal fixation. She lives by herself, but receives some assistance from her daughter who visits weekly. Her hospital course was complicated by mild delirium, but by postoperative day #5, both the orthopedics team and physical therapy believe she is stable for transfer to a Skilled Nursing Facility (SNF) for further rehabilitation. Although the plan for SNF was presented to Mrs. Collins and her daughter the day before, the patient doesn't remember and is adamant that she wishes to return home, claiming that "my daughter can help me." However, in a sidebar conversation, the daughter confides that because of her own work and parental responsibilities, "I really can't get down there more than twice a week."*

This case raises three issues that are especially germane to older patients but also apply more broadly. First, many, if not most, older patients are slow to recognize or accept the loss of function that threatens their independence. Second, hospitalization may compromise cognition, which can in turn impair communication, alter decision-making, and force greater reliance on proxies. Third, patients and family members are not always in alignment.

To resolve an impasse like this, the skilled clinical negotiator first needs to make an accurate diagnosis. Does the patient have the capacity to be engaged in decision-making about the site of discharge? In other words, does the patient understand what is at stake, can she understand information about risks and benefits, and can she communicate her choice? If not, are there medical interventions that might hasten a return to baseline cognition? Once capacity is established, what is the patient's objection to SNF transfer? If the objection is based on a misconception (e.g., that a SNF stay will necessarily be prolonged), then correcting the error might suffice. Does the daughter's reluctance to take on what would admittedly be a huge burden of care reflect competing responsibilities, lack of interest, or lack of confidence? The physician can do little to address the first two elements but might (by connecting the daughter to training resources on how to care for patients with recent hip fractures) be able to address the third.

Reaching a negotiated agreement may require several brief conversations conducted separately with the patient and relevant family members. It is also important to communicate directly with others who may be sharing relevant information, including nurses, physical therapists, and discharge planners.

SECTION 9.6 NEGOTIATING WITH SPECIAL HOSPITALIZED POPULATIONS

Children

Hospitalization disrupts the lives of both children and their families. Parents naturally wish to be with their child in the hospital, to receive information about their child's care, and to be given practical and emotional support facilitating their participation in the child's care.[29] At the same time, the hospital experience is enervating, particularly for parents who take responsibility for monitoring treatment schedules, staying in contact with caregivers, and assisting with technical tasks such as administering medications or managing feeding tubes—not to mention fulfilling other work and childcare responsibilities. Parents' attitudes towards involvement in technical aspects of their children's illness care are variable: some may worry about making mistakes or antagonizing the nursing staff through overinvolvement,[30] whereas others may feel overburdened "because nurses expected or assumed they would do the majority of care for their child without negotiation."[29] The best way for ward staff to ascertain parents' expectations and preferences is also the most obvious: just ask.

Clinicians caring for children and their families know that the child's participation in the clinical negotiation depends on age, developmental stage, and psychological readiness. Reviewing age-appropriate communication strategies for dealing with toddlers, school-age children, and adolescents is beyond the scope of this book. **However, in general terms, practitioners in pediatric hospital settings should encourage parental participation in care and take a family-centered approach to decision-making.** As articulated by Kuo et al., principles of family-centered care include:[31]

- Open and objective information sharing;
- Mutual respect for family preferences, skills, and expertise, with sensitivity to cultural differences;
- Shared decision-making, taking into account varying preferences of family members for different levels of involvement;

In short, the principles of negotiating with children and their families during hospitalization are no different than those espoused for adults. But their application is trickier, if only because there are more parties (and therefore more needs, feelings, and interests) to account for.

People with Cognitive Disabilities or Communication Problems

Cognitive disabilities have many causes, are associated with a variety of comorbidities, and exist along a spectrum of severity. Consider the following three patients:

Mr. Fienstra is a 32-year-old man with Down syndrome who works in the cafeteria of the local academic medical center. He lives with his very supportive parents and younger sister. He reads and writes at the fourth-grade level.

Mr. Burgess is a 52-year-old veteran of the first Gulf War. While out on patrol, his armored personnel carrier ran over an improvised explosive device. He emerged from the vehicle dazed and confused, and was later diagnosed with traumatic brain injury. Following discharge and rehabilitation, he was able to obtain employment as a construction worker. However, he continues to suffer from headaches, episodes of mild confusion, occasional violent outbursts, and memory lapse.

Mrs. Applegate is an 84-year-old grandmother with severe dementia. She lives in a memory care facility and does not recognize her son or other caretakers. She becomes agitated with any change of environment.

All three of these patients are admitted to the hospital the same week with pneumococcal pneumonia. All three have cognitive disabilities. Yet the approach to the clinical negotiation in each case is different.

Mr. Fienstra retains the capacity to participate in all but the most complex or emergent medical decisions. His condition limits his ability to manipulate complex facts or to simultaneously imagine multiple depictions of the future, but he can more than adequately express his values and engage in shared decision-making together with his parents and his health care providers.

Mr. Burgess is similarly capable of participating in decisions about his own care. However, his emotional lability requires that discussions be timed to coincide with periods when he is relatively calm and collected.

Mrs. Applegate lacks capacity for medical decision-making and thus for clinical negotiation. With luck, she has designated a durable power of attorney for health care or other surrogate; expressed her values clearly; and perhaps completed a living will. Otherwise her clinicians will need to proceed based on their best understanding of the patient's wishes, consultation with family members and colleagues, and their own best medical judgment.

When negotiating with people living with cognitive disabilities, clinicians need to exercise flexibility as to when and how information is presented and who is included in the negotiation. **Amidst the pressures of a busy day in the hospital, clinicians may be tempted to deal solely with the surrogate, effectively cutting the patient out of the conversation. Except in cases of severe impairment or dire medical emergency, this is rarely justified.** But even if a fully triadic conversation (patient-surrogate-clinician) is the ideal, it is hard to realize in practice – even for pediatricians, who are nominally experienced in the art of the three-way interaction. Research suggests that even though pediatricians often begin triadic encounters by posing questions to the child, it is often the parent who answers.[32]

Should the patient be unable to participate in the negotiation, the biggest challenge is getting the surrogate to reflect the patient's values rather than their own. This can be achieved by asking the surrogate questions such as:

- What do you think [patient's name] would think (or say) in this situation, if s/he were able?

- Did you and [patient's name] ever have a chance to talk about what s/he might want in situations like this?
- What are some of the things that [patient's name] most values, that s/he finds most meaningful?

People with Speech, Hearing, or Communication Disorders

In contrast to many people with cognitive impairment, patients with speech, hearing, and communication disorders are usually intellectually intact. **Health care providers frequently make the mistake of both underaccommodating and overaccommodating such patients.**[33] For example, when meeting a patient with expressive aphasia due to a recent stroke, the physician may assume that effective communication is impossible and may simply ignore the patient's attempts. On the other hand, the clinician may raise his voice with a deaf person or speak slowly and loudly to a person with dysarthria from severe Bell's palsy—neither of which is useful. This mismatch is understandable, as few medical practitioners have received adequate training in speech, hearing and communication disorders.[34] Clinical negotiation in these cases requires patience, an understanding of a patient's specific deficits, and knowledge of appropriate accommodations such as those outlined in the FRAME protocol (Table 9-5).[33]

Patients with Limited English Proficiency

Any monolingual English-speaking American who has sought medical care in a non-English-speaking country knows the relief experienced when the doctor

Table 9-5 The FRAME Protocol for Accommodating Patients with Communication Disorders

	Key Principle	Example Strategies
F	Familiarize with how the patient communicates before starting medical interview	Find out whether patient already has a reliable and preferred communication method.
R	Reduce rate: Slow down!	Pause between phrases, one idea at a time, allow more time for patient to respond.
A	Assist with communication: Actively help the patient with communication	Ask questions in a different way to help patient understand (e.g., multiple choice; yes/no).
M	Mix communication methods: Show, do not tell	Keep a small white board/pad of paper handy to write key words or draw. Use pictures, alphabet boards, and gestures.
E	Engage the patient first: Respect each patient's abilities and autonomy	Communicate directly with the patient. Do not ignore patient and talk only to family/caregivers.

Source: Reproduced with permission from Burns MI, Baylor C, Dudgeon BJ, Starks H, Yorkston K. Health Care Provider Accommodations for Patients With Communication Disorders. Topics in Language Disorders. 2017;37(4):311–333.

walks into the exam room speaking good English. In contrast, attempting to communicate with doctors in Mexico about serious health concerns using high-school Spanish can be both frustrating and terrifying. These experiences can provide clinicians a sense of what it might be like for patients with limited English proficiency (LEP) who require hospitalization in the United States. Available data suggest the lived reality is not great. Patients and families who are not proficient in English receive less information and less support than their English-proficient peers.[35] **Despite good evidence that use of professional interpreters improves quality of care, many inpatient doctors (and most nurses) "get by" with use of family members or nonverbal gesturing.**[36–38]

Unfortunately, many hospitals are too small to have full-time interpreters on staff. In addition, the pace of care on many hospital wards precludes optimal use of professional interpreters even when they are theoretically available. It may be difficult, for example, to time ward rounds to coincide with interpreter and family availability. Increasingly, some of these problems are being addressed through use of telephonic- or video-interpretation services. However, in complex clinical situations (such as hospital discharge on an extensive medication regimen), remote interpretation has been deemed a poor substitute for the real thing (i.e., a live interpreter at bedside).[39]

In the absence of universal solutions, what is the clinician interested in fostering optimal clinical negotiation with hospitalized LEP patients to do?

- Make allowances in your schedule. Providing good care to LEP patients simply takes a little extra time.
- Use professional interpreters when possible, especially during critical intervals such as hospital admission, discharge, and when obtaining consent for significant procedures.
- If family members are used as interpreters, try to obtain the patient's permission, and postpone discussion of sensitive topics until a professional interpreter is available.
- Telephone and video-based interpretive services are increasingly available. There is some evidence that video may be more effective.[40]
- Be familiar with best practices for working with interpreters, such as those promulgated by the International Medical Interpreters Association (https://www.imiaweb.org/uploads/pages/380_5.pdf). It is particularly important to speak directly to the patient in short, clear sentences.

SUMMARY POINTS:

- Hospitalization, a stressful experience at best, furthers social distance and strains the balance of power between patients and clinicians.
- In preparing for clinical interaction with hospitalized patients, basic etiquette ("etiquette-based medicine") is a good place to start.

- Disagreement about the need for admission can work in two directions: the clinician advises admission and the patient expresses reluctance, or (less commonly) the patient desires admission but the clinician resists. In either case, it is important to understand *why* the patient feels as they do.
- Successful communication in the hospital will manage uncertainty, anticipate and address patient fears and insecurities, and clarify goals of care.
- Negotiation over the timing of discharge should connect with goals of care and begin near the time of admission.
- Clinical negotiations involving children, patients with cognitive or communication problems, or patients with limited English proficiency require special skills and often the assistance of other trained professionals such as speech therapists or medical interpreters.

QUESTIONS FOR DISCUSSION:

1. How do differences between the inpatient and outpatient settings influence the clinical negotiation?

2. Near the end of a visit focused on completing disability paperwork, Mr. Davos mentions recent exertional chest pain. On questioning, the most recent episode started this morning and he is currently having "a twinge." An electrocardiogram shows new T-wave inversions anterolaterally. You recommend admission, but Mr. Davos insists "I've had pain like this 100 times and it always goes away." In this instance, how does the patient's mental representation of illness differ from the clinician's? What could you say to help Mr. Davos make a medically safe decision?

3. In your opinion, does the hospital where you work help patients manage uncertainty effectively during the early days of hospitalization? How could the process be improved through actions of the patient and family, admitting physician, specialty consultants, nurses, and the hospital administration?

4. Mrs. Olson, a 73-year-old woman recovering from gallstone pancreatitis, has been in the hospital for 12 days. On day 8 she underwent cholecystectomy, and she is now eating, having bowel movements, and walking with assistance. After consulting with the surgeons, her hospitalist Dr. Khachaturian decides she is ready for discharge. On hearing this, Mrs. Olson clams up and says she is not ready to leave. Using your imagination, what are three possible medical reasons and three social reasons she may be reluctant to go? What would you say to better understand her reluctance?

5. As mentioned in the text, several studies have shown that when pediatricians address questions to school-aged children, in the majority of cases a parent will answer and then continue to dominate the conversation. In dealing with this situation in the hospital, what would you say to engage the child more directly?

6. Think back to the last time your interaction with a hospitalized patient could have benefited from the involvement of a professional interpreter, yet you proceeded alone. Why did you proceed as you did? How could your hospital or department better organize rounds so as to make professional interpreters more universally available?

References:

1. Bruggimann L, Annoni J, Staub F, Von Steinbüchel N, Van der Linden M, Bogousslavsky J. Chronic posttraumatic stress symptoms after nonsevere stroke. *Neurology*. 2006;66(4):513-516.
2. Zatzick DF, Rivara FP, Nathens AB, et al. A nationwide US study of post-traumatic stress after hospitalization for physical injury. *Psychol Med*. 2007;37(10):1469-1480.
3. Cuthbertson BH, Hull A, Strachan M, Scott J. Post-traumatic stress disorder after critical illness requiring general intensive care. *Intensive Care Med*. 2004;30(3):450-455.
4. Shalev AY, Schreiber S, Galai T, Melmed RN. Post-traumatic stress disorder following medical events. *Br J Clin Psychol*. 1993;32(2):247-253.
5. Wachter RM, Goldman L. Zero to 50,000-the 20th anniversary of the hospitalist. *N Engl J Med*. 2016;375(11):1009-1011.
6. Kahn MW. Etiquette-based medicine. *New Eng J Med*. 2008;358(19):1988-1989.
7. Tackett S, Tad-y D, Rios R, Kisuule F, Wright S. Appraising the practice of etiquette-based medicine in the inpatient setting. *J Gen Intern Med*. 2013;28(7):908-913.
8. Manning WG, Newhouse JP, Duan N, et al. Health insurance and the demand for medical care. *USA: The Rand Corporation (supported by flagrant from the US Department of Health and Human Services)*. 1988.
9. Olson DP, Windish DM. Communication discrepancies between physicians and hospitalized patients. *Arch Intern Med*. 2010;170(15):1302-1307.
10. Shahian DM, Nordberg P, Meyer GS, et al. Contemporary performance of US teaching and non-teaching hospitals. *Acad Med*. 2012;87(6):701-708.
11. Anstey K, Wright L. Responding to discriminatory requests for a different healthcare provider. *Nurs Ethics*. 2014;21(1):86-96.
12. Garcia JA, Paterniti DA, Romano PS, Kravitz RL. Patient preferences for physician characteristics in university-based primary care clinics. *Ethn Dis*. 2003;13(2):259-267.
13. Paul-Emile K, Smith AK, Lo B, Fernandez A. Dealing with racist patients. *N Engl J Med*. 2016;374(8):708-711.
14. Alfandre D, Geppert C. Discriminatory and sexually inappropriate remarks from patients and their challenge to professionalism. *Am J Med*. 2019;132(11):1251-1253.
15. Lazare A, Levy RS. Apologizing for humiliations in medical practice. *Chest*. 2011;139(4):746-751.
16. Sessums LL, Zembrzuska H, Jackson JL. Does this patient have medical decision-making capacity? *JAMA*. 2011;306(4):420-427.
17. Fineberg IC, Kawashima M, Asch SM. Communication with families facing life-threatening illness: a research-based model for family conferences. *J Palliat Med*. 2011;14(4):421-427.
18. Farrell TW, Widera E, Rosenberg L, et al. AGS position statement: making medical treatment decisions for unbefriended older adults. *J Am Geriatr Soc*. 2017;65(1):14-15(e11-e15).
19. Mishel MH, Clayton MF. Theories of uncertainty in illness. *Middle Range Theory for Nursing*. 2008;3:53-86.
20. Emanuel EJ, Emanuel LL. Four models of the physician-patient relationship. *JAMA*. 1992;267(16):2221-2226.

21. Bernacki RE, Block SD, American College of Physicians High Value Care Task F. Communication about serious illness care goals: a review and synthesis of best practices. *JAMA Intern Med.* 2014;174(12):1994-2003.
22. Kaldjian LC. Clarifying core content of goals of care discussions. *J Gen Intern Med.* 2020;35(3):913-915.
23. Anderson GF, Hussey P, Petrosyan V. It's still the prices, stupid: why the us spends so much on health care, and a tribute to uwe reinhardt. *Health Aff (Millwood).* 2019;38(1):87-95.
24. Kraut A, Fransoo R, Olafson K, Ramsey CD, Yogendran M, Garland A. A population-based analysis of leaving the hospital against medical advice: incidence and associated variables. *BMC Health Services Research.* 2013;13:415.
25. Alfandre D, Schumann JH. What is wrong with discharges against medical advice (and how to fix them). *JAMA.* 2013;310(22):2393-2394.
26. Alfandre D. Reconsidering against medical advice discharges: embracing patient-centeredness to promote high quality care and a renewed research agenda. *J Gen Intern Med.* 2013;28(12):1657-1662.
27. Levine C, Zuckerman C. The trouble with families: toward an ethic of accommodation. *Ann Intern Med.* 1999;130(2):148-152.
28. Hardwig J. What about the family? *Hastings Cent Rep.* 1990;20(2):5-10.
29. Power N, Franck L. Parent participation in the care of hospitalized children: a systematic review. *J Adv Nurs.* 2008;62(6):622-641.
30. Chapados C, Pineault R, Tourigny J, Vandal S. Perceptions of parents' participation in the care of their child undergoing day surgery: pilot-study. *Issues Compr Pediatr Nurs.* 2002;25(1):59-70.
31. Kuo DZ, Houtrow AJ, Arango P, Kuhlthau KA, Simmons JM, Neff JM. Family-centered care: current applications and future directions in pediatric health care. *Matern Child Health J.* 2012;16(2):297-305.
32. Tates K, Elbers E, Meeuwesen L, Bensing J. Doctor-parent-child relationships: a'pas de trois'. *Patient Educ Couns.* 2002;48(1):5.
33. Burns MI, Baylor C, Dudgeon BJ, Starks H, Yorkston K. Health care provider accommodations for patients with communication disorders. *Top Lang Disord.* 2017;37(4):311-333.
34. Burns MI, Baylor CR, Morris MA, McNalley TE, Yorkston KM. Training healthcare providers in patient–provider communication: What speech-language pathology and medical education can learn from one another. *Aphasiology.* 2012;26(5):673-688.
35. Thornton JD, Pham K, Engelberg RA, Jackson JC, Curtis JR. Families with limited English proficiency receive less information and support in interpreted ICU family conferences. *Crit Care Med.* 2009;37(1):89.
36. Flores G. The impact of medical interpreter services on the quality of health care: a systematic review. *Med Care Res Rev.* 2005;62(3):255-299.
37. Karliner LS, Jacobs EA, Chen AH, Mutha S. Do professional interpreters improve clinical care for patients with limited English proficiency? A systematic review of the literature. *Health Serv Res.* 2007;42(2):727-754.
38. Diamond LC, Schenker Y, Curry L, Bradley EH, Fernandez A. Getting by: underuse of interpreters by resident physicians. *J Gen Intern Med.* 2009;24(2):256-262.
39. Lee JS, Nápoles A, Mutha S, et al. Hospital discharge preparedness for patients with limited English proficiency: a mixed methods study of bedside interpreter-phones. *Patient Educ Couns.* 2018;101(1):25-32.
40. Lion KC, Brown JC, Ebel BE, et al. Effect of telephone vs video interpretation on parent comprehension, communication, and utilization in the pediatric emergency department: a randomized clinical trial. *JAMA Pediatr.* 2015;169(12):1117-1125.
41. Davidson KW, Shaffer J, Ye S, et al. Interventions to improve hospital patient satisfaction with healthcare providers and systems: a systematic review. *BMJ Qual Saf.* 2017;26(7):596-606.
42. Windover AK, Boissy A, Rice TW, Gilligan T, Velez VJ, Merlino J. The rede model of healthcare communication: optimizing relationship as a therapeutic agent. *J Patient Exp.* 2014;1(1):8-13.

43. Berkhof M, van Rijssen HJ, Schellart AJ, Anema JR, van der Beek AJ. Effective training strategies for teaching communication skills to physicians: an overview of systematic reviews. *Patient Educ Couns.* 2011;84(2):152-162.

44. Boissy A, Windover AK, Bokar D, et al. Communication skills training for physicians improves patient satisfaction. *J Gen Intern Med.* 2016;31(7):755-761.

45. Simons Y, Caprio T, Furiasse N, Kriss M, Williams MV, O'Leary KJ. The impact of facecards on patients' knowledge, satisfaction, trust, and agreement with hospital physicians: a pilot study. *J Hosp Med.* 2014;9(3):137-141.

46. Snow V, Beck D, Budnitz T, et al. Transitions of Care Consensus policy statement: American College of Physicians, Society of General Internal Medicine, Society of Hospital Medicine, American Geriatrics Society, American College Of Emergency Physicians, and Society for Academic Emergency Medicine. *J Hosp Med.* 2009;4(6):364-370.

47. Dwamena F, Holmes-Rovner M, Gaulden CM, et al. Interventions for providers to promote a patient-centred approach in clinical consultations. *Cochrane Database Syst Rev.* 2012;12:CD003267.

48. Street RL, Gordon HS. Companion participation in cancer consultations. *Psychooncology.* 2008;17(3):244-251.

49. Shields CG, Epstein RM, Fiscella K, et al. Influence of accompanied encounters on patient-centeredness with older patients. *J Am Board Fam Pract.* 2005;18(5):344-354.

50. Wolff JL, Clayman ML, Rabins P, Cook MA, Roter DL. An exploration of patient and family engagement in routine primary care visits. *Health Expect.* 2015;18(2):188-198.

51. Clayman ML, Roter D, Wissow LS, Bandeen-Roche K. Autonomy-related behaviors of patient companions and their effect on decision-making activity in geriatric primary care visits. *Soc Sci Med.* 2005;60(7):1583-1591.

52. Laidsaar-Powell RC, Butow PN, Bu S, et al. Physician-patient-companion communication and decision-making: a systematic review of triadic medical consultations. *Patient Educ Couns.* 2013;91(1):3-13.

53. Wolff JL, Roter DL. Family presence in routine medical visits: a meta-analytical review. *Soc Sci Med.* 2011;72(6):823-831.

54. Wolff JL, Roter DL. Hidden in plain sight: medical visit companions as a resource for vulnerable older adults. *Arch Intern Med.* 2008;168(13):1409-1415.

55. Mazer BL, Cameron RA, DeLuca JM, Mohile SG, Epstein RM. "Speaking-for" and "speaking-as": Pseudo-surrogacy in physician-patient-companion medical encounters about advanced cancer. *Patient Educ Couns.* 2014;96(1):36-42.

56. Wolff JL, Roter DL. Older adults' mental health function and patient-centered care: does the presence of a family companion help or hinder communication? *J Gen Intern Med.* 2012;27(6):661-668.

57. Laidsaar-Powell R, Butow P, Boyle F, Juraskova I. Facilitating collaborative and effective family involvement in the cancer setting: Guidelines for clinicians (TRIO Guidelines-1). *Patient Educ Couns.* 2018;101(6):970-982.

58. Laidsaar-Powell R, Butow P, Boyle F, Juraskova I. Managing challenging interactions with family caregivers in the cancer setting: Guidelines for clinicians (TRIO Guidelines-2). *Patient Educ Couns.* 2018;101(6):983-994.

59. Carroll S. Something *Deeply Hidden: Quantum Worlds and the Emergence of Spacetime.* Penguin Publishing Group; 2019.

CHAPTER 10

Negotiating with Physician Colleagues and Other Health Care Professionals

Clinical Take-Aways

- Conflict within and between health care teams is inevitable. The important thing is to successfully manage the conflicts that arise.
- The main objective for the clinician trying to manage conflict with fellow professionals is to prevent substantive conflict (over issues) from evolving into affective conflict (involving personalities and emotion).
- An "integrating" or problem-solving style is recommended as the best long-term strategy for addressing most conflicts.
- Clinicians should:
  - Try to separate people from the problem through active listening and empathizing;
  - Focus on interests, not positions, by framing the conflict as a problem to be solved collaboratively;
  - Generate options for mutual gain via brainstorming;
  - Decide on objective criteria by identifying shared principles.

SECTION 10.1: INTRODUCTION

This book is chiefly about negotiating with patients. A little over a half century ago, this might have been enough. In the community, most physicians were solo practitioners supported by a small, hand-picked staff; in the hospital the lines of power and authority were so clearly drawn that there was little doubt whose opinion actually mattered.

As health care developed in sophistication and complexity, however, the old models no longer sufficed. In the 21st century, health care is rarely delivered by a single individual acting alone. Most patients with complex illnesses are—at one time or another—cared for by *teams* of medical specialists; nurse practitioners and nurse anesthetists; physicians' assistants; nurses; medical assistants; pharmacists; physical, occupational, and respiratory therapists; imaging technicians; and phlebotomists, among others. Effective health care delivery often depends upon the coordinated functioning of multiple team members.

Although care coordination surely places technical and administrative demands on health care systems (e.g., IT infrastructure to support communication and manage population health; protocols for connecting worried parents with the on-call pediatrician at night), an additional critical requirement is effective conflict management. Without diminishing the importance of organizational climate, culture, and resources (e.g., a dedicated "ombuds" to help with disputes), most conflicts in health care settings are resolved by the parties themselves. In this chapter, we examine the nature and types of conflict *between* health care professionals and consider negotiation strategies they can adopt to resolve, attenuate, or manage conflicts in the interest of providing the best possible patient care.

SECTION 10.2: TYPES OF CONFLICT IN HEALTH CARE

Conflict is defined as a "process of social interaction involving a struggle over claims to resources, power and status, beliefs, and other preferences and desires."[1,2] **In essence, conflict involves competing interests or positions between individuals or groups in what appears to be a zero-sum situation—where gains on one side imply losses on the other.** Conflicts in health care can arise in almost any setting over almost any issue. However, not every disagreement is a "conflict." To qualify, a dispute must exceed a threshold sufficient for the individuals involved to experience the situation as problematic. This threshold is subjective. If both parties see the disagreement as trivial, it can be ignored. However, it is possible for one party to an evolving disagreement to experience the interaction as intensely salient and for the other to hardly notice.

This is not, however, the only sense in which conflict is subjective. Although it is easy to imagine situations where zero-sum framing is absolute (e.g., the classic Prisoner's Dilemma, in which the only rational choice is to "rat" on one's fellow prisoner), many real-world situations have alternative frames, in which mutual gains ("win-win") or minimal losses ("no lose-no lose") are realistic outcomes. In addition, conflict involves attribution of motive: the opposing party must be seen as thwarting one's aims (whether or not this is their actual intent).[2] Finally, because conflict is a process, arising in a background of pre-existing relationships, past transactions, cultural mores, and situational cues, the same set of behaviors may be interpreted as antagonistic, positive, or neutral depending on the context.

Classifying Conflict

Social scientists have advanced several different schemas for classifying conflict. Perhaps the most fundamental distinction is between substantive conflict and affective conflict. *Substantive conflict* involves intellectual opposition to ideas, such as an academic medical center's strategic commitment to research; the degree to which patient satisfaction scores should count in figuring physicians' annual bonuses; or whether a new antibiotic ought to be introduced to the hospital formulary.[3] Closely related is *process conflict*, in which the focus is on how a task is to be accomplished—addressing questions such as delegation (who?), timeliness (when?), and technique (how?).[2] In contrast, *affective conflict* is "a condition in which group members have interpersonal clashes characterized by anger, frustration, and other negative feelings."[4] **A certain amount of substantive or process conflict can—depending on how it is handled—be beneficial, whereas affective conflict is generally deleterious.** Additional examples of substantive, process, and affective conflict within health care settings are provided in Table 10-1.

Research outside of health care has established that *mild* levels of substantive conflict lead to positive outcomes: more information acquisition and greater innovation. However, more intense conflict may inhibit short-term goal attainment.[5,6] Research in health care settings has largely been restricted to operating rooms and rapid action teams, but it is easy to imagine that similar results might apply. For example, the intellectual give and take of "tumor boards" (interdisciplinary meetings of multiple oncologic professionals with a focus on management of individual cases) has been associated with alterations in treatment plans, resulting in benefits to patients.[7] If anything, the negative relationship between process conflict and team performance is even stronger than for substantive conflict.[8]

Substantive conflict has a narrow therapeutic window, and not only because high levels seem to impede aspects of performance and satisfaction. The other problem is that substantive conflict can readily spill into affective conflict. One can see this happening easily in the examples given in Table 10-1: the dispute over cancer treatment leads the medical oncologist to stop referring to the radiation oncologist, with resulting personal animus; the attending overrules the resident about the CT scan, leading the resident to accuse the attending of "micromanaging" on her evaluation form; the hospitalist sulks away from the encounter with the nurse supervisor who vetoed his transfer order, murmuring "guess who's going to get written up if the patient goes downhill."

The take-away message for health care teams is that a mild, controlled, and nonthreatening exchange of competing views on substantive issues such as patient management or hospital strategy is energizing and potentially beneficial in terms of improved team performance and quality of care. However, high levels of substantive conflict, more than modest levels of process conflict, and any level of affective conflict will tend to degrade performance.

Table 10-1 Substantive, Process, and Affective Conflict with Examples from Health Care Settings

Conflict Type	Examples
Substantive	*The radiation oncologist and medical oncologist disagree on whether a patient with follicular lymphoma should be treated first with radiation therapy or chemotherapy.* *The medical resident orders a CT angiogram on a patient with known deep venous thromboembolism (already on anticoagulants) and mild chronic kidney disease who becomes vaguely short of breath. The attending physician questions whether this will alter treatment enough to justify the cost and risk.* *The nursing supervisor informs the hospitalist that a patient with an asthma exacerbation may not be transferred to a telemetry ("step-down") bed because "she does not meet criteria."*
Process	*A patient who has been on the trauma surgery service for 45 days is awaiting placement. Transfer to the medical service is requested.* *The floor nurse pages the on-call resident at 2 a.m. because the oxygen saturation is 88%. After the resident jiggles the device to address a loose connection, the oxygen saturation reading is 95%.* *A family physician prepares to perform a pelvic examination, expecting to use the same disposable plastic speculum with attached light as she has used in the past. The MA hands her an unfamiliar speculum requiring use of an external headlamp.*
Affective	*The hospitalist has already fielded 7 admissions during the current shift. When the emergency room calls regarding a nursing home patient admitted for presumed urinary tract infection, the hospitalist characterizes the request as "completely inappropriate and a huge waste of resources."* *A nurse files an incident report after a consulting gastroenterologist fails to replace the bed railings for a geriatric patient who subsequently falls. The two individuals had dated in the past. Two weeks later, the gastroenterologist files an incident report after the same nurse neglects to give their mutual patient a single dose of medication.* *A general internist asks an endocrinologist for assistance with a patient who has difficult-to-manage diabetes. Over the next 6 months, the endocrinologist sees the patient four times (the internist only once). At one of the endocrine visits, the patient asks for "something to help with my neuropathy pain." The endocrinologist refuses, adding that "that's what your primary care physician is for." After finding out, the PCP fires off a nasty email to the endocrinologist with a copy to the clinic medical director.*

Therefore, optimal management of conflict between health care professionals requires:

- Accommodating (or otherwise effectively managing) low levels of substantive conflict
- Minimizing and managing process conflict
- Preventing the transformation of substantive or process conflict into affective conflict

Later in this chapter, we will address specific strategies for managing conflict with other health care professionals through clinical negotiation. But first, we review some of the most common conflict-laden situations health professionals are likely to face in both outpatient and inpatient settings.

SECTION 10.3: HOW CONFLICT UNFOLDS IN HEALTH CARE SETTINGS

The art is long, life is short, opportunity fleeting, experiment dangerous, judgment difficult.

As encapsulated by Hippocrates, medicine is an intensely gratifying yet highly demanding profession. The care of a complex patient demands hundreds of decisions and actions, large and small, every day. There is often little time for deliberation. The possibility of error looms everywhere. As the coronavirus pandemic of 2020 illustrates, risks to the health of clinicians and their families, while typically manageable, lurk in the background. And in the modern era, billing, documentation, and other third-party payer requirements sop up an increasing proportion of clinicians' time. It is no wonder, then, that burnout among health care professionals has generated sustained concern.[9]

In health care, one response to complexity has been the gradual transformation of medical practice from a solitary activity to a collective one. This is hardly a new phenomenon; physicians, nurses, and others have worked together for generations. But the rapid progress in medical science, the proliferation of treatments and procedures, and the promulgation of specialized treatment guidelines requiring multidisciplinary expertise, all lead in the same direction: health care delivered by groups of professionals, of varied background and training but connected by a common purpose.

Jenni Swanson is a 37-year-old middle manager, wife, and mother who has systemic lupus complicated by nephritis and stage III chronic kidney disease. Six months ago, she was hospitalized for induction therapy with pulse corticosteroids. Last week she saw her nephrologist for adjustment of her hypertension medicines and her rheumatologist to check labs and monitor the effects of low-dose corticosteroids and azathioprine. Next week she is scheduled to see an orthopedic surgeon about hip pain, which her primary care physician (PCP) fears might be caused by osteonecrosis. Meanwhile, she will continue with twice-weekly physical therapy. She will also check in with the nurse practitioner at the PCP's office about her most recent set of home glucose monitoring results.

Ms. Swanson's care team includes a primary care physician, nurse practitioner, nephrologist, rheumatologist, and physical therapist, not to mention the hospitalists, radiologists, pathologists, nurses, technicians, and other hospital staff who contributed during her last hospital stay. Some of these team members have worked together for decades, whereas others have met only a few times or not at all. Some will continue to care for Ms. Swanson for years to come, while others will contribute only briefly. The fluidity of health care teams is an important feature with consequences for both conflict management and clinical negotiation.

Organizational behaviorists have suggested that conflict can be analyzed at four levels: 1) intrapersonal; 2) interpersonal; 3) intragroup; and 4) inter-group.[2] Intrapersonal conflicts occur as a single individual grapples with competing demands and values. Interpersonal conflicts are dyadic: they involve a struggle between two persons, who may be part of the same group or different groups. Intragroup conflicts take place within a group, while intergroup conflicts take place between groups.

While this typology is fine as a point of departure, the boundaries between categories are amorphous. For example, Ms. Swanson's PCP may question the rheumatologist's continued use of prednisone in the face of possible osteonecrosis (with the PCP and rheumatologist each representing different specialty "groups"). This is an interpersonal conflict that could also be construed as within-group conflict (assuming the two physicians are both part of a team caring for Ms. Swanson) or as between-group conflict (with each physician representing their own specialty). Later on, the two doctors might unite in opposing their medical group's formulary committee in its decision not to stock belimumab.[10] In this case the PCP and rheumatologist represent one group (Ms. Swanson's care team), the formulary committee another.

With this broad (and imperfect) typology in mind, let us now examine some of the more common conflicts arising between health professionals. We first address conflicts between physicians, both within and between groups. We then consider conflicts between physicians and nurses. Conflicts among and between other health care professionals are taken up last.

SECTION 10.4: CONFLICT BETWEEN PHYSICIANS

Conflicts between Physicians within Groups or Team

Physicians may be no more conflict-prone than the average human, but they do frequently find themselves in conflict-prone situations. **Time pressure, high-stakes decision-making, and low tolerance for error fashion an environment that is often energizing but can also test the limits of resilience.** In a prior era, most physicians practiced solo, with a partner, or in small groups. While these practice models are still common in many parts of the country, they have been increasingly supplanted by larger single- and multispecialty group practices.[11] By definition, physicians in groups share facilities, staff, and income. Establishing fair, equitable, and efficient ways of distributing resources within group practices is the subject of entire books.[12] We will not delve extensively into conflicts arising from these business and administrative concerns, focusing our attention on three examples of within-group clinical conflict.

Example 1

Case: *Dr. Newton is part of a 12-physician primary care practice in a suburban area. The group typically assigns two physicians to provide coverage on nights and weekends. Dr. Newton receives a call from one of his partner's patients at 11 pm Thursday. Karen Holmes is a 32-year-old woman with migraine headaches. She developed a severe headache this afternoon that has not responded to repeated doses of sumatriptan. The patient requests Dilaudid® because "that's the only thing that works in these situations." Because of an Internet glitch, Dr. Newton is temporarily unable to access the patient's electronic health record (EHR), but she agrees to fax a written prescription to the patient's pharmacy for a short course of Dilaudid (hydromorphone). The next day, the partner confronts Dr. Newton, saying "I wish you wouldn't have prescribed Dilaudid to Ms. Holmes. She's a known drug-seeker."*

Analysis: **This is a dyadic conflict centered on clinical decision-making.** While it is true that Dr. Newton might have acted differently had she had immediate access to the EHR, it is not realistic to expect that she would have returned to the office to access the patient's record. Perhaps she could have questioned the patient more closely, conferred with her on-call partner (who may have had EHR access), or called her physician partner for counsel, but the hour was late and the decision to prescribe hydromorphone was, in the end, a judgment call. The goal here is to promote understanding of each physician's position without triggering defensiveness and spiraling into affective conflict. The partner, on learning of the prescribing decision, might have taken a few moments to reflect on why he found it so disconcerting— he has been working with this patient for months to reduce after-hours calls and emergency department visits and reduce intermittent opioid use. He could then ask Dr. Newton to sit down with him for a few moments, share his discomfort with the patient's situation, and brainstorm with her and perhaps other colleagues on how to help on-call doctors manage these situations.

Example 2

Case: *University Medical Associates (UMA) is an academically affiliated group practice of about 40 full-time family physicians, general internists, and family nurse practitioners. The group has several capitated contracts with managed care organizations. These contracts place UMA at full risk for outpatient and emergency care (including specialty consultation, diagnostic testing, and prescription* *medications). This means the group pays for these services out of funds it receives from the managed care plans for this purpose on a "per-member, per-month" basis. If the cost of caring for these managed care patients exceeds the capitated funds allocated, the group loses money.*

To maintain the group's financial health, UMA associate medical director Samantha Vierra convenes a weekly utilization review meeting, in which all of the group's referrals and "big-ticket" test requests are reviewed for medical appropriateness. Members of the group's utilization review committee attend regularly, with other group members attending on an ad hoc basis. Dr. Mansour knows that he has two referral requests pending this week, so he makes a special effort to attend the meeting.

Dr. Mansour's request for a neurology referral for a patient suspected of having Parkinson's disease is approved, but his request for a dermatology consult is denied. The majority of the doctors in attendance feel that empirical treatment of the rash, coupled with a skin biopsy, should suffice. One murmurs to a colleague, "I can't believe we're going through this again. Mansour needs to get with the program." Dr. Mansour objects, saying "Skin biopsies were not part of my training in internal medicine. Besides, I'm the only one in the room who actually saw the rash." After a brief discussion, Dr. Vierra calls for the group to move on to other cases. But Dr. Mansour is fuming.

Analysis: **This within-group conflict poses one against many and illustrates how disagreement over a specific issue can quickly devolve into destructive, ad hominem attacks**. On one level, disagreement about medical necessity for referral escalated rapidly to questioning of Dr. Mansour's clinical skills. While this may be an appropriate topic (depending on Dr. Mansour's overall clinical performance), it is best taken up in a one-on-one discussion between the group's medical director and Mansour himself. More broadly, the conflict can be seen as arising from external forces, including the capitated payment system itself, shortened clinic visits, and limited time for continuing medical education. Finally, the group's utilization review meetings are almost perfectly designed to engender interpersonal conflict that quickly descends into hurt feelings. To minimize this tendency, the group needs to establish clear ground rules for its meetings and pivot from asking "do we approve this request?" to "how do we deliver the best possible patient care, taking into account medical needs, patient preferences, and physician risk tolerance." Reframing the question allows for more constructive discussion and a collaborative, rather than competitive approach. With this altered focus, the group might have suggested several possible solutions. They could have approved the referral but used this case as a springboard to planning a CME program on common skin conditions in primary care. This approach would have both clinical and financial benefits in the long run. Or they could deny the external referral but offer to have the patient seen by another group member with a special interest in dermatology. As we will see later, a focus on "the issue, not the person" is a mainstay of effective conflict management.

Example 3

Case: *Marjorie Erikson, an 89-year-old retired bookkeeper lives with her 93-year-old husband in the house they have occupied for almost 50 years. Last week she woke up with difficulty moving her left arm and leg. Her husband called 911. She was admitted with an acute ischemic stroke and treated with alteplase.* [13] *By hospital day 5, she had recovered some function but was still having trouble transferring from bed to chair and back again. With the weekend approaching, the second-year neurology resident suggests that the patient is ready for discharge, but the chief resident resists, arguing that with a few more days of physical therapy the patient might be able to return home. The patient does make slow progress, but by the following Tuesday the second-year is frustrated: "We're not doing anything for her. I feel for her husband, but that's not a good reason to keep someone in the hospital." The chief replies, "Let's give it another day."*

Analysis: **This common scenario underscores the adage that "where you stand depends on where you sit."** Removed from the front lines, the chief resident can dispassionately weigh the needs of the patient, her elderly husband, the hospital, and the team. In contrast, the second-year resident, responsible for the day-to-day management of a growing patient list, may be feeling overwhelmed. He also understands that time devoted to a patient who no longer needs to be in the hospital is time taken away from other patients or from his own personal life. The chief resident needs to be careful in addressing this conflict. It would be easy to simply exert his power of authority. Or he could couch his decision in clinical terms ("The patient is making progress with PT, she would prefer to go home if possible, and I think she has a good chance of avoiding a nursing home stay if given a little more time"). However, this could readily be misinterpreted as an assault on the second-year resident's judgment. Instead, the chief might acknowledge the merits of the second-year's case and offer a compromise: "I see your point. We're not offering much in the way of acute care. But [the patient is making progress, etc.]. How about we talk with Ms. Erikson and her husband and explain that we're pleased with her progress and hope that she'll be ready to go home by this Thursday. But if she's not able to transfer independently by then, it might be better for her to have a short stay in a rehab facility, which we will arrange for Friday."

Conflicts between Physicians on Different Groups or Teams

For tens of thousands of years, human beings mostly associated with members of their own band, clan, or tribe. Contacts with outsiders were infrequent and often violent. From this anthropological perspective, strangers sitting together on the subway without attacking each other is remarkable.[14] Nevertheless, certain atavistic instincts persist. In addition, groups have material and ideological interests that incorporate but also transcend the interests of their individual members. In the heat of conflict, it is difficult to sort out these varied motives. When a surgical colleague says, "This patient could benefit from being on the internal medicine service," does she mean 1) the patient's medical condition is so medically complex that the likelihood of serious error would be lower on a medical service than a surgical service; 2) the patient is unlikely to require further surgery, and we need to make room on our service for patients who directly require our skills; or 3) we are weary of caring for this patient, who has many comorbid medical conditions and doesn't seem to be improving? Quite possibly, she is not fully aware herself. It will not surprise readers to learn that **the skilled clinical negotiator considers these motives without judgment and tries to keep the focus on the care of the patient**, to which everyone, regardless of their group allegiance, is presumably committed. The following examples illustrate some of the issues arising as part of between-group conflict in outpatient, emergency, and inpatient settings.

Example 1

Case: *For many years, the Department of Psychiatry at a major academic medical center has refused to take referrals (either internal or external) for patients covered by Medicaid, instead routing these patients to the County Mental Health Center (MHC). The department has always been transparent about the reason: "Medicaid reimbursement is simply too low." This practice has been particularly galling to the Department of Family and Community Medicine, which sees a large number of Medicaid patients and finds that referral to the County MHC involves long waits and spotty care. At a Family Medicine department meeting, several members propose that their group "boycott" the Department of Psychiatry (by refusing to send privately insured patients their way) and also consider hiring a part-time "in-house" psychiatrist to assist the practice with patients with complex or serious mental health conditions.*

Analysis: In *Exit, Voice, Loyalty*, Hirschman (1970) described the options available to disgruntled workers. Applying his framework here, this dispute has reached an advanced stage where one party (Family Medicine) has despaired of the efficacy of "voice" and is considering an abrupt "exit."[15] This may yet be needed as a last resort, but Family Medicine might be wise to first consider renewed attempts at issue-focused negotiation, best mediated by high-level administrators. The question is, in what seems like a zero-sum game, how can the interests of both departments be addressed while keeping the focus on patients? One approach is to form a task force comprising representatives from each department to develop options that would assure better patient access to mental health services, spread out the financial burden of caring for underresourced patients, seek creative cost-saving and revenue-augmentation schemes, and lobby government officials for fairer reimbursement policies.

Example 2

Case: *The hospitalist group at Mountainside Medical Center is fuming. Increasingly, patients admitted through the hospital's emergency department with fever seem to be started on empirical antibiotics before proper cultures have been obtained. While this pattern was marginally acceptable back in the day when nearly all community-acquired bacterial pathogens were susceptible to third-generation cephalosporins, the strategy seems untenable in a time of widespread antibiotic resistance. The current crisis came to a head when a 48-year-old man with quadriplegia and (rather clean appearing) decubitus ulcers was started empirically on ceftriaxone and vancomycin without cultures of blood or urine. The on-call hospitalist accepted the patient for admission but filed an incident report citing the emergency department as deficient. Two days later, the chief of emergency medicine called the chief of hospital medicine to complain about the lack of professionalism demonstrated by filing an incident report rather than discussing differences in clinical judgment face-to-face.*

Analysis: This is an intergroup conflict with some intrapersonal and dyadic elements. **Healthy organizations have ways for groups to discuss differences of opinion on a recurring basis, minimizing the need for measures (e.g., incident reporting) which may be perceived as punitive.** In the long run, the relationship between the hospital medicine and emergency medicine departments should be addressed through regular case conferences, QI brainstorming sessions, or joint management meetings. As for the current crisis, it is important for each side to clarify their interests (as opposed to positions). Hospital medicine can justly claim they have an interest in knowing the pathogen they are supposed to treat during the patient's hospital stay. Emergency medicine is concerned with rapid institution of broad-spectrum antibiotics to avert sepsis-related disasters. Often the most expeditious solution to intergroup conflicts of this sort is to develop a *provisional* policy that can be tested over a period of weeks to months. For example, the two groups might agree that in all cases of significant fever thought to require empiric antibiotics, the ED will routinely obtain blood and urine cultures. The groups might also agree to collaborate on a research project to determine whether antibiotic choices are altered based on culture results.

Example 3

Case. *Dr. Martinez is on call for the Parkland Hospitalist Group, which besides admitting adult patients to the medical floors, also provides perioperative consultation and co-management to Surgical Associates, a large group of general surgeons, cardiothoracic surgeons, orthopedists, proctologists, and urologists. By 1 am, Dr. Martinez has finished admissions for the night and is ready to settle down for sleep in the call room. He is jolted out of slumber by a call from the surgical nurse practitioner, who asks him to consult urgently on a 75-year-old woman with a tibial fracture. "We will probably take the patient to the operating room first thing in the morning." Dr. Martinez performs the consult (there are no barriers to immediate surgery), but in the morning the attending surgeon (who slept undisturbed) decides the patient can be treated nonoperatively. When Dr. Martinez mentions the situation to a colleague, she recalls several similar cases. They decide to bring up the issue for discussion at a Hospital Medicine departmental meeting.*

Analysis: From the standpoint of the hospitalists, physicians are being needlessly awakened to perform urgent perioperative consults on patients who have not been thoroughly evaluated by the primary service. On reflection, their grievance is multilayered: concerns about the effects of disturbed sleep on patient care and their own well-being, recognition of substantial hourly wage disparities between cognitive and procedural specialists,[16] and a feeling that they are not respected and are left to do the "scut work." The orthopedic surgeons are happy with the current arrangement, in which most night duties are delegated to a staff of nurse practitioners. Among other things, they believe with some justification that patient safety is enhanced by having well-rested surgeons in the operating room. Reconciliation will require some acknowledgement of the other group's interests and a sincere effort to find mutually satisfactory solutions. For example, questionable cases could be "held" until 5:30 or 6:00 am when they could be presented briefly at "phone rounds" involving both the consulting internist and the attending surgeon.

SECTION 10.5: CONFLICTS INVOLVING OTHER HEALTH CARE PROFESSIONALS

Conflicts Between Physicians and Nurses

In 1967, Stein described the "doctor-nurse game." The object of the game is that "the nurse is to be bold, have initiative, and be responsible for making significant recommendations, while at the same time she [sic] must appear passive. This must be done in such a manner as to make her recommendations appear to be initiated by the physician."[17] By 1990, Stein and colleagues noted, the game had been updated to reflect broad changes in civil rights, the women's movement, and nursing education, resulting in more autonomous nurses, less overt sexism, and more equal professional relationships. But keen observers know that elements of the game persist. Recently, attention has turned to interprofessional collaboration and education. The results of these efforts are, so far, indeterminate.[18]

Intensive care units (ICUs) have been attractive targets for study of interprofessional conflict. The reason is not necessarily that ICUs engender *more* conflicts than other settings like wards or clinics, just that such conflicts accumulate *faster*. Conflicts between physicians and nurses account for up to one-third of conflicts reported in ICUs.[19] In these high-stakes settings, the quality of relationships between physicians and nurses clearly affects patient outcomes.[20,21] However, **only a few studies have investigated the source of nurse-physician conflicts.** In conversations with ICU staff and administrators, researchers in Ontario, Canada[22] identified four broad categories:

- Failure to develop consistent goals of treatment among ICU staff (for example, nurses frustrated by lack of focus on symptom control or application of life-extending measures in terminal patients);
- Resource allocation issues, such as the intensivist wanting to admit patients even if nurse resources are short;
- Unanticipated alterations in care plans owing to shifting physician staffing (e.g., rotation of house staff); and
- Lack of communication, as when physicians do not update nurses on a patient's changing situation.

While this work is a useful starting point, we think a more generalizable (and arguably more practical) typology is to consider nurse-physician conflict in terms of who, what, when, and how. As depicted in Table 10-2, "who" concerns authority or responsibility, "what" concerns decision-making, "when" concerns pace or timing, and "how" concerns implementation.

Wrapping around each branch of this nurse-physician conflict typology is "communication." Although some investigators have called out communication as a separate category, gaps in communication contribute to most disputes in health care settings; nurse-physician conflicts are no exception. **In particular, abrasive or disruptive physician behaviors weigh heavily on nurses.** In one study, the

Table 10-2 **A Typology of Nurse-Physician Conflict**

Major Category	Focus	Examples
Who	Responsibility or authority	• Nurse sets up family meeting, informing physicians only in retrospect • Physician helps hospitalized patient take home meds without informing nurse
What	Clinical decision-making	• Nurse questions order for beta-blocker when patient's BP is 100/60 • Nurse tells physician to call Urology for placement of Foley catheter because patient has vague history of "urethral trauma" • Physician reluctant to order haloperidol for "chemical restraint" of a delirious older patient who is repeatedly pulling out IVs
When	Pace or timing of tasks	• Physician upset that order for "AFB x 3" has not been completed after 5 days in hospital • Nurse files incident report after resident fails to respond to urgent page within 10 minutes • Physician tells nurse that "patient pressed call button 3 times and no one came"
How	Implementation of tasks	• Nurse insists physician wear gown before talking with patient on "contact precautions" (even though physician plans no direct contact with patient or surroundings) • Physician speaks with nurses in "quiet zone" where they are supposed to prepare medications without interruption • Surgeon upset that circulating nurse doesn't keep operating room light focused on shifting surgical field

most frequent forms of physician disruptive behavior were yelling or raising the voice, disrespect, condescension, berating colleagues, berating patients, and use of abusive language.[23] In fact, perceived disrespect is an irksome common denominator reported by nurses as a major driver of job stress and dissatisfaction.[23]

The electronification of health records has both fostered and impeded communication between physicians and nurses. On the one hand, physicians can read nursing notes in the electronic health record (EHR) sequentially in far less time than it took formerly to track down handwritten notes on the ever-elusive "bedside" clipboard. On the other hand, the massive amounts of time spent by both nurses and physicians on clinical documentation reduce opportunities for direct discussion of clinical and ethical questions that are important to both groups.

Conflicts with and Among Other Health Professionals

Interprofessional conflicts can and do extend beyond the physician-nurse dyad. However, compared with nursing, most other health professions (pharmacy, social work, physical and occupational therapy) have only gradually started to defend their own autonomy, status, and power. Using French and Raven's taxonomy,[24] physicians maintain their relative dominance over these groups largely on the basis of legitimate, expert, and informational power coupled to a state-sanctioned monopoly on certain health care services (e.g., diagnosis and prescribing). This means that secure "top dog" status is based on who they are (credentialing), what they've achieved (education and training), and what they know (in terms of human health and disease). When conflicts arise, they are apt to arise from varying interpretations of institutional rules and guidelines ("Can ciprofloxacin still be used as first line for outpatient urinary tract infections?"), adverse decisions by third parties ("I know you ordered home health, but Medicare will not pay for it"), and occasionally, ethical dilemmas tinged by moral distress ("I know you want me to push harder on Mr. Ganz's postoperative rehabilitation, but he seems to be having a lot of pain.") And while physicians ostensibly have the last word, there are many ways that members of other health professions can advance different (and sometimes better) care strategies. One of the aims of conflict management is to identify, clarify, and resolve disagreements before they interfere with patient care.

SECTION 10.6: STRATEGIES FOR MANAGING CONFLICT

As discussed in previously in this chapter, mixed evidence suggests that mild substantive (task) conflict can spur creative discovery and better problem solving. However, excessive levels of substantive conflict -or any conflict that is not well managed and degenerates into an emotional tug-of-war -can be deleterious.[2] In health care settings, the goal is to constrain substantive conflict to levels that sustain participants' energy without engendering animosity. The question is how.

Some features of health care settings make conflict management challenging. With a few exceptions (e.g., solo and small group private practices), the composition of teams changes often, sometimes by the hour. The variety of possible conflicts is nearly endless. And the stakes are often high. But one advantage health care has over other industries is that all parties can be assumed to share (at least in part) a common goal: doing what is best for the patient. This is not to say that other priorities (personal, group, institutional) are irrelevant. Nevertheless, the astute clinical negotiator is wise to remember that the person or group he is fighting probably shares a similar commitment to patient welfare. It's just that such commitments are often expressed in very different ways.

Conflict Management Styles

In reviewing research on taxonomies of conflict resolution, Rahim (2011, p. 33) describes a "five-factor" model of conflict management that includes 1) avoiding, 2) accommodating, 3) dominating, 4) integrating, and 5) compromising.

Table 10-3 Four-Factor Model for Handling Interpersonal Conflict

Style	Description	Relative Advantages/Disadvantages
Avoiding	Suppressing, dodging, or otherwise not acknowledging disagreement	Most efficient strategy when disagreement is trivial or transient, but can allow problems to fester.
Accommodating	Giving up something to oblige the other party	Useful when one party seems to care more about the issue than the other; can generate chagrin (buyer's regret) if too much is relinquished.
Dominating	Imposing one's will in pursuit of winning a point	Leads to a quick win for party in position of strength; can sap team spirit in long run.
Integrating	Problem solving (maximize winnings or minimize losses for each party)	Best long-term strategy, but initial investment of time and patience can be large.

Source: Based on Rahim, 2011.[2]

However, viewing compromise as a form of *accommodation* in which each side gives up something in order to capture some benefit, we find a **four-factor model** both comprehensive and parsimonious. Some of the advantages and disadvantages of each style are given in Table 10-3.

Avoiding means not acknowledging, ducking from, or withdrawing from the conflict. This is one of the more common conflict management styles deployed by health care professionals.[25] It is easy to see why. Many issues are simply not worth contesting. Avoidance is efficient in the short term but may foster anger, resentment, or disillusionment over time.

Accommodating means giving up something to reach agreement with the other party in an effort to preserve the relationship. When accommodation is one-sided, one party is effectively sacrificing their own interests to resolve the conflict. When accommodation is more balanced, parties reach a compromise.

Dominating occurs when one party exerts his or her will or power to force a resolution. This represents a victory for self and a defeat for the other. It is a tempting strategy for the more powerful party to a conflict; it is efficient in the short term; and it is sometimes necessary to preserve order and preserve confidence in organizational leadership. However, when used to excess, a dominating strategy can fuel resentment and subterfuge.

Finally, *integrating* or problem solving (sometimes called *collaborating*) is an approach in which there is open communication about the disagreement and the interests of both parties can be advanced. While recommended by many conflict management experts as optimal, this strategy entails risk. One rarely knows in advance how the other party will react. Integrating also demands considerable creativity. It is not always easy to generate solutions that advance mutual interests *and* maximally benefit the patient, particularly in situations (like medical emergencies or urgencies) that call for rapid action. And indeed, problem solving can be exhausting. Nevertheless, in many situations an integrating strategy will result in the best long-term outcomes.

The four approaches should not be viewed as mutually exclusive. In fact, two or more approaches can be deployed simultaneously or sequentially to address different sub-elements of the conflict.

> *Dr. Alison Brown is called to the emergency department to admit a 66-year-old woman with heart failure and preserved ejection fraction to the hospitalist service. Over the past 5 days, the patient has noted difficulty putting on her shoes, dyspnea on exertion, and orthopnea. Physical examination shows BP 150/94, mild jugular venous distension, rales about ¼ of the way up the posterior lung fields, and bilateral 3+ edema to the mid-shins. Chest radiograph and brain natriuretic peptide levels are consistent with volume overload. Dr. Brown agrees with the admitting diagnosis of heart failure but learns that the patient ran out of her usual medication several days before symptoms began. She notes that other than having a heparin lock established, the patient has received no treatment for volume overload in the emergency room. Dr. Brown is skeptical that the patient requires admission, and she voices her opinion to the emergency medicine specialist, Dr. Kirk.*

> Dr. Brown: *I agree with your diagnosis, but what about a trial of Lasix in the emergency room?*

> Dr. Kirk: *She's got florid heart failure. She'll never turn around that quickly. Tune her up and she'll be out in a few days. Trust me.*

Here Dr. Kirk uses flippant humor to steer Dr. Brown towards admitting the patient immediately, suggesting she is either clinically naïve or trying to avoid work. Either way, he makes assumptions that may not be justified.

> Dr. Brown: *I could certainly admit her, but we'll never know how she's going to respond unless we try. How about we give her 40 mg of IV furosemide and see what happens? If she feels better, she can probably go home with a fresh prescription for Lasix.*

> Dr. Kirk: *She already has CKD-II, her potassium is 3.7, and we don't really have the staff to properly monitor her. That's what the wards are for.*

If it weren't clear before, Dr. Kirk is attempting to resolve the conflict through dominance. At this point, Dr. Brown can fight back (attempt counter-dominance), back down (accommodate), or try to engage Dr. Kirk in problem solving.

> Dr. Brown: *Well, let's lay out our options here. I think we both agree we want to deal with the patient's volume overload in the safest, most expeditious way possible. We could give her a one-time trial of Lasix, we could admit her, we could call her PCP Dr. Savoy for advice, or...*

> Dr. Kirk: *Or I suppose we could check with the observation unit and see if there's a bed available.*

Here Dr. Brown has identified the interest she and Dr. Kirk share in getting the patient better in the least disruptive way possible.[26] She then coopts Dr. Kirk into problem solving.

> Dr. Brown: *While you're checking, I'll place an order for furosemide 40 mg and call Dr. Savoy to get her thoughts. Let's circle back in 20 minutes to make a plan.*

The conflict isn't yet resolved, but the tone has changed. As it happens, no observation bed is available. The PCP Dr. Savoy is comfortable with discharge and offers to see the patient for a follow-up visit in 2 days. In the meantime, the patient is starting to diurese. To allay some of Dr. Kirk's concerns, Dr. Brown offers to "admit" the patient [a form of accommodation] but then discharge her from the ED. Dr. Kirk agrees with this plan.

In this scenario, the protagonists enlist three of four conflict resolution styles (domination, accommodation, integration), eschewing only "avoidance." It would have been relatively easy for Dr. Brown simply "suck it up." However, had Dr. Brown chosen to duck around the nearest corner rather than defend her position, the patient would have been subjected to a potentially unnecessary hospital stay, In addition, such grudging accommodation might have permanently colored Dr. Brown's view of Dr. Kirk, which could distort their future working relationship. While conflict avoidance may temporarily avert some discomfort, in the long run this approach has been associated with increased levels of work stress, higher turnover, and even worsened patient outcomes.[27,28]

Roger Fisher, *Getting to Yes*, and Some General Principles of Negotiation

In the course of a long and influential career, Harvard law professor Roger Fisher worked with colleagues to develop a grounded and practical approach to conflict management.[29] As summarized in the best-selling book, *Getting to Yes*,[30] Fisher stressed four principles:

- Separate people from the problem
- Focus on interests, not positions
- Invent options for mutual gain
- Insist on objective criteria

Let's unpack these principles, then examine how they might apply to conflicts among health care professionals.

Separating people from the problem means looking at the conflict as an opportunity for joint problem solving and trying not to ascribe dark or ulterior motives to the opposing party. This can be difficult. All relationships are colored by history. The gynecology attending who was curt in her interaction with the infectious disease fellow 3 weeks ago may have long forgotten that encounter, only to be puzzled by the fellow's delayed response to her telephone pages today. Similarly, the psychiatry chair who sustained his department's policy to reject consults from the Primary Care Center may wonder why Primary Care is suddenly closed to new patients coming from psychiatry. **Nevertheless, to the extent that clinicians can frame the current conflict as a puzzle to be solved rather a war to be waged, they will likely reach a more mutually satisfactory and amicable resolution.**

One of Fisher's more astute contributions was urging negotiators to consider not just their own decision-making but the other party's decisions as well. **A critical tool for undertaking this analysis is the "best alternative to a negotiated agreement" (BATNA) for oneself and for the opposition.** The BATNA is simply the set of options both you and fellow participants in a conflict have to fall back on, should negotiations stall or break down. For example, the aforementioned Primary Care Center might not have been so quick to lock out psychiatric patients had they realized that Psychiatry was ready to sign a new agreement with the nearby Federally Qualified Health Clinic, which was eager to arrange for mental health coverage from a prestigious medical school department.

Parties to conflict often get fixated on positions or demands (what one *chooses to ask* of the other party) rather than interests (the underlying motivation behind the negotiation). Interests include but are not limited to material concerns. It may very well be more important to many physicians to maintain their self-image as competent, caring doctors than to generate additional income, have more time off, or hold down the department's utilization statistics. In other words, positions are about *what*, interests about *why*.

Positions can be far apart even when interests overlap. For example, a primary care group demands protected time to respond to the increasing volume of patient messages being received through the health system's secure patient portal. Concerned that patient access to timely appointments is already tenuous, the administration refuses. However, frank discussion leads to a 3-month experimental trial where protected time is provided in the hope that demand for in-person visits decreases, in turn decreasing wait times, which the administration considered a growing cause for concern. Both sides agree to evaluate wait times after 3 months before determining whether to expand, modify, or disband the experiment.

In this example of conflict over resources for managing patient messages, primary care clinicians and administrators not only focused on the problem and avoided posturing, they also invoked the other two principles of getting to yes: inventing options for mutual gain (the protected time experiment) and insisting on objective criteria (decreased appointment wait times). Proposing a "therapeutic trial" is a useful strategy for breaking deadlocked negotiations, but it is not the only way. The key ingredients are 1) a willingness to brainstorm and 2) a commitment to rely on facts, evidence, precedent, or principles that both parties accept as fair standards.

Brainstorming can be conducted both within one's own group and between groups. The main rules of brainstorming are to generate as many ideas as possible; strive to make the ideas as wild as possible; improve or combine ideas already suggested; and not be critical.[31] Brainstorming is far from a no-brainer, however. In fact, a large body of fascinating experimental evidence suggests that groups generate fewer unique ideas than they would if the individuals constituting those groups were kept apart and left to think on their own.[31,32] If the goal were merely to produce lots of ideas, then isolating individuals to cogitate separately might make sense. **The reason Fisher and other negotiation scholars endorse brainstorming within and between groups is that negotiation is essentially a social process. Ideas that are developed and vetted internally are more likely to be accepted than ideas imported or imposed from without.**

Deeper Dive 10.1: From Cockpits to Operating Rooms: Using Crew Resource Management for Patient Safety

High-stakes environments such as cockpits, nuclear power plants, operating rooms, emergency departments, and intensive care units have at least one thing in common—mistakes can be deadly. In fact, preventable medical errors are a major contributor to death and suffering in the United States.[36] Although team effectiveness depends in large part on how the team's collective expertise matches up with the task at hand, it is also important to identify specific communication tools, or "levers," that best align team processes to specific task requirements.[37] One such application to health care teams is Crew Resource Management.

Crew Resource Management (CRM) is a communication intervention developed in the aviation industry to prevent airline disasters. CRM is designed to overcome barriers to effective decision-making and performance that result from poor interpersonal communication, inadequate information exchange, poor judgment, inefficiencies, and lack of leadership.[38] In an effort to reduce medical errors, some health care organizations have embraced the principles of CRM, which are well suited for high-risk, complex medical units where errors in communication, judgment, and technique—as well as failure to notice and appropriately react to signs of imminent physiologic decline (sometimes called "failure to rescue")—put patients' lives at risk.[39]

What is unique about CRM relative to other group communication tools is that CRM practices are focused on one primary goal—patient safety. While there may be secondary benefits to CRM practices (e.g., greater team cohesion, increased provider satisfaction, enhanced culture of safety),[40] its primary goal is help the team efficiently and effectively accomplish their task (e.g., a surgical procedure or cardiopulmonary resuscitation). Although there are a number of adaptations of CRM, the key components[41,42] include:

- Leadership
- Monitoring
- Situational awareness
- Interpersonal communication
- Conflict management
- Decision-making

At first glance, these elements have an almost bland, generic quality, and indeed, they are integral to a wide range of group interactions. In the high-stakes situations for which CRM was developed, however, these components are mobilized to advance the goal of safe care within specific clinical contexts. Consider a cardiac surgery team. *Leadership* calls for the attending surgeon to emphasize, through words and actions, the responsibility of each and every member of the team to contribute to patient safety. *Monitoring* requires each team member to be alert for signals of impediments to individual performance (in self and others) such as fatigue, multitasking, and distraction. For example, a medical student might be the first to notice that a graft site is bleeding while the surgeon's attention is otherwise consumed by the primary operation. *Situational awareness* refers to team members' being primed to recognize threats (e.g., sudden drop in blood pressure, cardiac arrhythmias) and instigating error-mitigation strategies (e.g., exploration of the surgical site for "bleeders," administration of vasopressors, defibrillation). *Interpersonal communication* refers to communication practices such as respect for team members, briefing the team before beginning surgery, verifying patient identification and surgical site, and being assertive (e.g., speaking up when suspecting something is not right). *Conflict management* is not only speaking up but also understanding that challenging a higher-ranking team member should not be construed as insubordination but rather as a valued contribution to patient care and safety.[42] For example, if a nurse questioned whether two sutures were too far apart, the surgeon would check to verify. Finally, effective *decision-making* under pressure can be facilitated through checklists, decision support tools, and other procedural protocols.

A systematic review of interventions aimed at improving health care team effectiveness found evidence that CRM-based interventions led to improved team behavior, more favorable attitudes toward teamwork, improved assessments of institutional support, fewer medical errors, and reduced time to decision.[39] Other studies suggest that CRM can reduce both adverse events and health care costs. For example, a 2010 CRM program at the Ohio State University Wexner Medical Center[40] was associated with a 26% reduction in observed relative to expected adverse events and cost savings of at least $12.6 million.

In 2003, a CRM program was implemented in an obstetrics unit within the Yale–New Haven Hospital system.[43] CRM training was coupled with other safety-oriented interventions such as an enlisting an outside team to review risk assessment and management, hiring an obstetrics safety nurse, implementing protocols and guidelines, and creating an anonymous reporting system where any member of the hospital staff could report adverse events, near-misses, or medical errors. During the 3 years of evaluation, the composite rate of adverse events such as maternal death, maternal ICU admission, uterine rupture, and fetal traumatic birth injury was reduced by roughly 50%.

Finally, there is evidence CRM also contributes to a culture of patient safety.[44] For example, prior to CRM training, the Wexner Medical Center (described above) sent the Hospital Survey on Patient Safety Culture (HSOPS) to all employees. The HSOPS assesses employees' perceptions of the safety culture across 12 dimensions, including teamwork within units, promotion of safety by supervisors, communication openness, and nonpunitive responses to errors. The survey was readministered following CRM training. Compared to the baseline assessment, there were significant improvements across 10 of the 12 indicators.[45]

"To err is human, to forgive is..." hard to do when patients and families experience a significant medical error, especially one that was preventable.[46] CRM represents an approach to teamwork that has had success in reducing errors and adverse events because the *team's* responsibility, respect, protocols, checklists, and goals are stressed over and above an *individual's* rank, status, and ego.

Deeper Dive 10.2: Towards a Meeting of Minds: Conventional versus Nominal Groups

Meetings are a fundamental feature of organizations. In health care, meetings take many forms, including hospital committees, tumor boards, department meetings, ethics boards, and pre-clinic "huddles." The common thread is that members of the organization gather to discuss matters important to the organization's goals and purposes (e.g., patient care, quality improvement, education). But how should these team discussions unfold? Consider two very different approaches to group brainstorming and decision-making.[47]

The first and most familiar is the *conventional group* (CG) meeting. This approach begins with the statement of a problem followed by a free flowing, unstructured discussion in which group members share information, ideas, and solutions in order to reach agreement on the best plan of action. By contrast, the *nominal group* (NG) technique employs a moderator or group facilitator who presents a problem to the team and asks each member to silently reflect on it and generate ideas. After a short pause, team members present their ideas in a round robin fashion. These are summarized and recorded by the group facilitator. After everyone's ideas have been presented (or after a pre-established time limit has been reached), there is discussion focused on clarification and evaluation. The meeting concludes when a decision is reached by a vote or a move toward consensus.

The advantages of the CG approach emerge from the unrestricted discussion of the problem. If done well, group members generate a diverse set of ideas, build upon the ideas by others, identify and resolve differences of opinion, and achieve consensus, while at the same time fostering group solidarity and cohesion. However, the relative formlessness of the CG approach may also have downsides: the discussion is dominated by higher-status individuals with some members not speaking up, the discussion can go off-kilter, and conflict may be unresolved, leading to escalation of interpersonal tensions. Conventional groups may also be prone to *groupthink*[48] where the group fails to critically analyze the problem due to arrogance or a sense of invulnerability, failure to get outside information, or because group members value conformity over expressing differences. Groupthink produces poor decisions which, in the context of health care, can lead to medical error and adverse events.[49]

In contrast, the advantages of NGs are that they ensure equal participation by all group members, are more time efficient than CGs, give each group member equal influence on the decision, and minimize pressure to conform to the power dynamics in the group. The disadvantages of NGs are that they restrict group interaction, which in turn may preclude in-depth discussion of complicated problems and can restrict opportunities to build group solidarity.

Given that CGs are currently the default meeting arrangement in most health care organizations, when might NGs be employed to greatest effect? That will depend on the task, the power hierarchy, and the interpersonal climate of the group or team. For example, the conventional group works best when the team is informed, capable of communicating openly and equitably, is governed by mutual respect, is comfortable with disagreement, and works toward consensus. In health care, as in most other social settings, these conditions do not uniformly apply.[50] While the highly structured NG approach may not be universally applicable in health care settings, CGs can still use communication practices that focus on the group "process" in addition to the "task" at hand.[51] This includes asking for the opinions of less participatory members, making more dominant participants temporarily pause, bringing the group back on task when veering off target, and defusing unproductive conflict.

However, there are some types of group tasks where nominal groups could be very effective. First, NGs have been used in *quality improvement*. For example, Pena et al.[52] gathered a group of 27 health workers (nurses, physicians, technicians, and unit clerks) to address suboptimal pain control among hospitalized patients. Using the NG technique, the group generated a list of obstacles to pain control that included system factors (inadequate pain assessment, communication delays within the team, low priority), human factors (provider bias, lack of knowledge about pain management, patient reluctance to take medications), and system-human interface factors (lack of standardized policies and practices) that needed to be addressed to improve pain management of hospitalized patients.

Second, NG can be used in *teaching rounds*, where students or residents hear a case presentation and generate a differential diagnosis. In contrast to the typical approach (in which the attending physician or other group leader questions team members), each member of the group writes down their diagnostic hypotheses in order of probability, severity, or both. Then in round robin fashion, everyone's ideas are written on the board and discussed.

Finally, NGs can be used in developing *recommendations for clinical practice.* For example, Rubin et al.[53] used NGT with a group of general practitioners in Europe to generate criteria for diagnosing irritable bowel syndrome (IBS) in primary care. Shaw et al.[54] assembled representatives from diverse stakeholder groups (patients, clinicians, policy makers, academics, technology experts) to make policy recommendations for patient-centered virtual care in Ontario, Canada.

The proverb, "All roads lead to Rome," refers to the notion that there are various ways to reach a single destination. In the academic parlance of group communication, this idea is referred to as *equifinality*—there are multiple pathways to reaching good group decisions.

Both CGs and NGs can lead to good group decisions. The key requirement is that the group interaction successfully accomplishes the key *functions* of effective decision-making—analyzing the problem, generating ideas, establishing criteria the decision must meet, evaluating options, and agreeing on the final decision.[51] In other words, whether through conventional, nominal, or other group communication methods, the key to group decision-making success is less about how it was done and more about what "work" the communication accomplished.

Relying on objective criteria is the *sine qua non* of Fisher's method, but in defining objectivity he casts a wide net to include material, scientific, and moral standards. Material criteria include market value, costs, and efficiency. Scientific criteria include clinical evidence, scientific judgment, and professional standards. Moral criteria include beneficence, autonomy, fairness, reciprocity, and tradition or precedent. Should we be deterred by the subjectivity of these so-called objective criteria? Fisher would say no, because the main thing is for all parties to the negotiation to accept a common standard. Consider this scenario involving a patient with suspected sepsis.

Intensivist: *I'm sorry, but we can't accept your patient for transfer to the ICU.*

Hospitalist: *Why not?*

Intensivist: *His blood pressure is 110 systolic, his oxygen saturation is fine on 4 liters, and he looks comfortable.*

Hospitalist: *What about his mental status?*

Intensivist: *You haven't worked him up for that. Has he even had a CT scan?*

From the hospitalist's perspective, this discussion is going nowhere. On the one hand, he is worried about his patient's trajectory (he seems to be getting sicker by the hour, even though current vital signs don't look that bad) and he is getting pressure from the floor nurses to get the transfer done. On the other, he is the object of serious push-back from the intensivist, who seems to be missing the point but in the end controls access to the ICU.

Hospitalist: *This is ridiculous. You're looking at this wrong. You need to take this patient. He's going downhill, and the nurses are starting to complain that they can't keep up.*

Intensivist: *I'm sure the patient will be fine. Just keep the fluids and antibiotics going and call if anything changes.*

In this exchange, the hospitalist violates all four principles for "getting to yes." He attacks the intensivist's judgment, he emphasizes position over interest, he doesn't try to generate new options, and he doesn't offer any objective criteria to advance the negotiation. But with a little creativity the conversation might have gone differently:

Hospitalist: *A head CT would be reasonable, if we can arrange for a nurse to go down with him and provide sedation if needed. But I'd like to go over exactly what concerns us. This is a pretty frail older guy with diabetes and hypertension who developed a fever and pyuria yesterday. He seemed to respond to antibiotics initially but today his fever is back, his heart rate has climbed from 70 to 105, and his blood pressure has fallen from 160-170 (his usual range) to the low 100s despite 3 liters of fluid over the past 12 hours. Plus he's ordinarily sharp as a tack.*

Intensivist: *I wasn't aware of all that. I can see why you're concerned.*

Hospitalist: *Would you agree that it's sometimes reasonable to admit to the ICU for intensive monitoring, even if the patient doesn't need lifesaving care immediately?*

Intensivist: *Ordinarily, yes, but we are pretty full right now.*

Hospitalist: *What if you take the patient overnight, and if he starts to turn around we'll take him back at 10 am tomorrow?*

Intensivist: *That works for us. If you write a brief transfer note I'll take care of the admitting orders. And don't worry about the CT scan—we'll take care of it.*

In this redo, the hospitalist offers up a common set of facts, suggests a principle (patient trajectory) to guide the decision, and generates an option that addresses one of the intensivist's stated interests: to keep ICU beds available for the sickest patients. This quickly leads to a satisfactory resolution of the substantive (task) conflict while laying the groundwork for a sound future working relationship.

Developing a Personal Toolkit for Conflict Resolution

In an influential piece in *JAMA* over a decade ago, Arnold and Back enumerated a set of specific communication tools or skills which could be applied in addressing conflicts arising while caring for the seriously ill.[33] In Table 10-4, we organize these tools according to Fisher's "getting to yes" framework. The tools are specific skills that facilitate the enactment of Fisher's principles. For example, separating

Table 10-4 Aligning Fisher's Principles with Arnold and Back's Communication Tools*

Fisher Principle	Communication Tools	Description	Examples
Separate the people from the problem	Self-awareness/ self-disclosure	Understand and reveal to listener some aspect of your own psychological state, without casting blame.	"To be honest, the patient's failure to improve has unnerved all of us."
	Empathizing	Show listener that you are sensitive to his or her emotions	"Your team has been through a lot with this patient and his family."
Focus on interests not positions	Active listening	Turn full attention to speaker rather than rehearsing own arguments; don't interrupt; show that concerns are being heard	"It sounds like you are concerned that this patient might spiral down even further if she is not transferred to a higher level of care—whether that be the medical ICU or somewhere else."
	Reframing	Describe situation as a mutual problem to be solved collaboratively	"I wonder if we could look at the issue of further chemotherapy as not just 'How likely is it to work?' but 'How does this fit into the big picture?'"
	Explaining	Tell listener which aspects of the problem you are most concerned about	"I am concerned that a general medicine ward team will have difficulty dealing with the patient's complex wound care needs."
Invent options for mutual gain	Brainstorming	Generate potential solutions that advance interests of both parties to the conflict	"I suppose we could transfer to the ICU, perform a trial of noninvasive ventilation on the floor, or treat the dyspnea with morphine."
Insist on objective standards	Upholding shared foundations	Seek mutually agreed upon principles (based on clinical evidence, pathophysiological reasoning, community standards or expert consensus)	"Both of us want to achieve better control of the patient's pain." "What does the ACC say about stenting in two-vessel disease in a patient like this?"

*Middle two columns are taken with minor changes from Arnold and Back, 2005.

people from the problem is difficult unless clinicians are prepared to closely examine their own emotional reactions to the conflict and to selectively disclose those reactions to the other party. A moment of deep breathing and silent acknowledgement of one's own discomfort can sometimes be enough to quell the most reactive impulses and salvage the negotiation. Provided that care is taken not to cast blame, measured self-disclosure can also encourage more honest communication and lead to more complete mutual understanding. Empathetic statements, sincerely delivered, are also generally appreciated and can turn down the emotional volume enough to let problem solving begin.

To focus on interests rather than positions, clinicians can invoke active listening, reframing, and explaining. *Active listening* involves offering one's full attention and demonstrating understanding of the other person's point of view. The clinician showing interest in what the other party has to say is less likely to provoke defensiveness. *Reframing* can be used to convert a conflict from a contest of wills to an exercise in problem solving. *Explaining* goes beyond information transfer: the idea is not so much to persuade as to give the other party insight into one's concerns and priorities. Clinicians who deploy these tools are more likely to identify common ground and less likely to derail the negotiation before it even gets started.

Finally, *brainstorming* and *upholding shared foundations* align directly with "inventing options for mutual gain" and "insisting on objective standards," respectively. Brainstorming does not require a conference room and a whiteboard. The psychological hurdle most clinicians face is not generating viable solutions to complex problems; they do that every day with patients. The challenge is thinking of a conflict as a problem to be solved in the first place. The solution will most likely involve dealing with both the rational and emotional aspects of the conflict. Upholding shared foundations means finding a common point of reference in professional values, standards, scientific evidence, tradition, or precedent. In so doing, the expert negotiator avoids the temptation to invoke ethical principles or scientific facts to gain advantage over the other party; a solid foundation is established only through mutual assent.

Dr. Steven Kantor is the intern on a busy medical service at the VA. Earlier in the day his resident performed a diagnostic thoracentesis on an elderly male smoker with a left-sided pleural effusion. The nurse calls him to the bedside because the patient is acutely short of breath. Vitals are stable except for moderate tachypnea. Breath sounds seem diminished on the left side but are difficult to interpret because of the known effusion. Dr. Kantor orders a stat chest x-ray. The x-ray is performed, but when Dr. Kantor appears at the radiology department to retrieve and read the film (the department has not yet converted to digital imaging), he finds a sign: "Radiology Film Library Hours 8 am-5 pm." It is currently 4:55 pm. The walk-up service window is closed and locked, but Dr. Kantor spots the radiology file clerk packing up his things. "Hey," he says. "Can I get an x-ray?" "Done for the day," the clerk responds.

How could Dr. Kantor respond? He is sorely tempted to yell at the clerk and write him up for gross patient endangerment. In a fit of pique, he also briefly

Table 10-5 **Behaviors to Avoid**

Traps to Avoid	Example Scenario
Ignoring attendant emotions	Resident physician on consulting service is repeatedly asked to see non-emergent cases in early hours of morning; says nothing; later erupts in anger.
Assuming the context or that you understand the other party's intentions	Attending upbraids resident for ignoring multiple secure clinical text messages; later learns that resident's cellular phone network does not reliably transmit these messages.
Attempting to convince the other party by relying on logic alone	Pediatrician suspects appendicitis in 9-year-old boy despite negative CT scan and presses for admission based on posterior probability of >20%; surgeon unmoved.
Questioning the ethics or moral compass of another party	Patient requests refills of chronic medications. Covering physician says, "you should get all your refills from your PCP." Learning of this, PCP sends staff message saying, "if I didn't know better, I'd think you were lazy." PCP and covering physician do not speak for weeks.
Expecting another party to take responsibility for resolving the problem	In shared office space, Nurse Practitioner A asks Nurse Practitioner B to please "clean up your mess when you eat." Nurse Practitioner B responds, weakly, "I will try, but I guess if it really bothers you maybe you could just toss things in the trash."

Source: Adapted from Arnold RM, Back AL. Dealing With Conflict in Caring for the Seriously III. *JAMA.* 2005;293:1374–1381.

considers calling the chief of medicine at home. But that wouldn't help the patient's situation. Instead, he extends empathy ("I realize this must be the end of a long day for you"); engages in mild self-disclosure ("I'm really worried about this patient"); and considers the clerk's interests ("If you grab the film I'll take a picture of it with my phone and get out of your way within minutes"). If this fails, he needs to consider his BATNA, which might include paging the radiology resident on call, asking the senior resident for advice, or requesting a pulmonary consult.

Arnold and Back also identified some behaviors to avoid when handling conflict;[33] these are captured in Table 10-5. Some of these behaviors are mirror images of the positive tools the authors encourage. For example, clinicians who are self-aware are unlikely to deny conflict or suppress negative emotions (which is usually a vain exercise). Those who listen actively are unlikely to assume they know the context or fully understand the other party's intentions. Other pitfalls may seem self-evident but are nonetheless encountered frequently in practice. Disruptive behavior, gratuitous criticism, and use of loaded terms are clearly unproductive.[34,35]

Word choice matters. An easy way to derail any incipient negotiation is to declare that "this admission [or discharge] is inappropriate," "that behavior is unprofessional," or "if you do that, I wouldn't blame the patient for suing." There are several problems with statements of this sort. First, they imply definitive judgment where none is really possible. Second, they are guaranteed to provoke resentment or a stern counter-reaction. Third, they shut down conversations when what really needs to happen is more talk.

In summary, conflict between health care professionals is ubiquitous and likely inevitable. There are always three parties to any conflict: the two contestants plus the patient whose well-being is directly or indirectly at stake. **By assuming that both parties are interested in seeking a resolution that advances the patients' needs, avoiding hardened positions, demonstrating cognitive and emotional flexibility, and hewing to mutually embraced principles, clinicians can not only solve today's conflicts but lay the ground for better, more productive, and more patient-centered relationships tomorrow.**

SUMMARY POINTS:

- Health care takes place increasingly in teams.
- In health care, conflicts are seen within individuals, between individuals, within groups, and between groups. However, the boundaries separating these categories are porous.
- Three categories of conflict are substantive conflict, process conflict, and affective conflict. Substantive and process conflict can (to a point) benefit performance. Affective conflict is often destructive and needs to be managed.
- Conflicts between clinicians practicing within the same group or setting can arise because of disagreements over clinical practice, distribution of resources, or practice organization.
- Conflicts between clinicians belonging to different teams or groups are often difficult to analyze because the underlying motivations of the opposing parties are not necessarily obvious.
- Physician-nurse conflict has evolved since Stein's 1967 depiction of the "physician-nurse game" but persists as a threat to high-quality patient care.
- Most physician-nurse conflicts involve disputes about *who* (which individual has responsibility or authority), *what* (the specific clinical care decision), *when* (timing of a task), or *how* (implementation of a task).
- Abrasive or disruptive behavior never helps, and in the modern era, often leads to disciplinary action.
- Four styles for managing conflict between and among clinicians are avoiding, accommodating, dominating, and integrating.
- Fisher's strategies for "getting to yes" can be readily applied to health care situations:
  - Separate people from the problem

- Focus on interests, not positions
- Invent options for mutual gain
- Insist on objective criteria
- Things to avoid when negotiating with colleagues are assuming you know the whole story behind their position and repeatedly trying to convince the other party rather than probing further to understand their needs and motives.

QUESTIONS FOR DISCUSSION:

1. Distinguish between intrapersonal, interpersonal, intragroup, and intergroup conflict.

2. How might mild levels of substantive conflict improve clinical decision making and quality of care? Why does substantive conflict slide so easily into affective conflict? How can you try to head off this tendency in your own interactions with colleagues?

3. Dr. Minor (Chief, General Internal Medicine) and Dr. Liang (Chair, Psychiatry) are at a planning meeting to discuss expansion of the medical center's geriatrics program. Dr. Minor cites some examples of excellent geriatrics programs at other medical centers throughout the country. Dr. Liang, who happens to focus on geriatric psychiatry in her own practice, responds, "I would say you are thinking much too narrowly. What about nursing, family medicine, social work, and psychiatry." Dr. Minor is deeply offended because he believes clinical geriatricians trained in internal medicine are at the core of any solid geriatrics program. But he only nods in response and says nothing. The meeting chair moves on to the next agenda item.

   a. What conflict resolution "style" (avoiding, accommodating, dominating, integrating) do Drs. Minor and Liang apply?

   b. If Dr. Minor's goal is to help the medical center establish the best possible geriatrics program, how did his conflict resolution style fall short? What could he have done instead?

4. What is the "doctor-nurse game"? In what ways has the game changed, and in what ways has it persisted, since Stein's original description in 1967? In your opinion, is the relationship between female physicians and (largely female) nurses healthier than between male physicians and nurses?

5. Micro-aggressions are the "everyday slights, indignities, put-downs and insults that people of color, women, LGBT populations, or those who are marginalized experience in their day-to-day interactions with people" (Derald W. Sue as quoted in Vox: https://www.vox.com/2015/2/16/8031073/what-are-microaggressions). What are some examples of micro-aggressions have you have witnessed (or been the victim of) within health care settings? How might these behaviors impair effective negotiation between colleagues?

6. What does Fisher mean when he says separate people from the problem; focus on interests, not positions; invent options for mutual gain; and insist on objective criteria? How can each of these principles be applied in health care settings?

References:

1. Rogers DA, Lingard L. Surgeons managing conflict: a framework for understanding the challenge. *J Am Coll Surg*. 2006;203(4):568-574.
2. Rahim MA. *Managing conflict in organizations*. Routledge; 2011.
3. Jehn KA. Qualitative analysis of conflict types and dimensions in organizational groups. *Admin Sci Quart*. 1997;42(3):530-557.
4. Pelled LH, Eisenhardt KM, Xin KR. Exploring the black box: An analysis of work group diversity, conflict, and performance. *Admin Sci Quart*. 1999;44(1):1-28.
5. De Dreu CK. When too little or too much hurts: Evidence for a curvilinear relationship between task conflict and innovation in teams. *J Manag*. 2006;32(1):83-107.
6. Todorova G, Bear JB, Weingart LR. Can conflict be energizing? A study of task conflict, positive emotions, and job satisfaction. *J Appl Psychol*. 2014;99(3):451.
7. Wheless SA, McKinney KA, Zanation AM. A prospective study of the clinical impact of a multidisciplinary head and neck tumor board. *Otolaryngol Head Neck Surg*. 2010;143(5):650-654.
8. O'Neill TA, Allen NJ, Hastings SE. Examining the "pros" and "cons" of team conflict: a team-level meta-analysis of task, relationship, and process conflict. *Hum Perform*. 2013;26(3):236-260.
9. Rotenstein LS, Torre M, Ramos MA, et al. Prevalence of burnout among physicians: a systematic review. *JAMA*. 2018;320(11):1131-1150.
10. Postal M, Costallat LT, Appenzeller S. Biological therapy in systemic lupus erythematosus. *Int J Rheumatol*. 2012;578641.
11. Muhlestein DB, Smith NJ. Physician consolidation: rapid movement from small to large group practices, 2013–15. *Health Aff*. 2016;35(9):1638-1642.
12. Wolper LF. *Physician practice management*. Jones & Bartlett Publishers; 2012.
13. Campbell BC, Ma H, Ringleb PA, et al. Extending thrombolysis to 4· 5–9 h and wake-up stroke using perfusion imaging: a systematic review and meta-analysis of individual patient data. *Lancet*. 2019;394(10193):139-147.
14. Pinker S. Violence vanquished. *Wall Street Journal*. September 24, 2011.
15. Hirschman AO. *Exit, voice, and loyalty: responses to decline in firms, organizations, and states*. Harvard University Press; 1970.
16. Leigh JP, Tancredi D, Jerant A, Kravitz RL. Physician wages across specialties: informing the physician reimbursement debate. *Arch Intern Med*. 2010;170(19):1728-1734.
17. Stein LI. The doctor-nurse game. *Arch Gen Psychiatry*. 1967;16(6):699-703.
18. Reeves S, Perrier L, Goldman J, Freeth D, Zwarenstein M. Interprofessional education: effects on professional practice and healthcare outcomes. *Cochrane Database Syst Rev*. 2013(3).
19. Azoulay E, Timsit J-F, Sprung CL, et al. Prevalence and factors of intensive care unit conflicts: the conflicus study. *Am J Respir Crit Care Med*. 2009;180(9):853-860.
20. Baggs JG, Schmitt MH, Mushlin AI, et al. Association between nurse-physician collaboration and patient outcomes in three intensive care units. *Crit Care Med*. 1999;27(9):1991-1998.
21. Knaus WA, Draper EA, Wagner DP, Zimmerman JE. An evaluation of outcome from intensive care in major medical centers. *Ann Intern Med*. 1986;104(3):410-418.
22. Meth ND, Lawless B, Hawryluck L. Conflicts in the ICU: perspectives of administrators and clinicians. *Intensive Care Med*. 2009;35(12):2068.
23. Rosenstein AH. Nurse-physician relationships: impact on nurse satisfaction and retention. *Am J Nurs*. 2002;102(6):26-34.
24. Raven BH. The bases of power: Origins and recent developments. *J Soc Issues*. 1993;49(4):227-251.
25. Akel DT, Elazeem HA. Nurses and physicians point of view regarding causes of conflict between them and resolution strategies used. *Clin Nurs Studies*. 2015;3(4):112.
26. May C, Montori VM, Mair FS. We need minimally disruptive medicine. *BMJ*. 2009;339:b2803.
27. Tabak N, Orit K. Relationship between how nurses resolve their conflicts with doctors, their stress and job satisfaction. *J Nurs Manag*. 2007;15(3):321-331.

28. Nelson HW. Dysfunctional health service conflict: causes and accelerants. *Health Care Manag.* 2012;31(2):178-191.

29. Sebenius JK. What Roger Fisher Got Profoundly Right. *Negotiation Journal.* 2013;29(2): 159–170.

30. Fisher R, Ury WL, Patton B. *Getting to yes: Negotiating agreement without giving*; Penguin; 2011.

31. Diehl M, Stroebe W. Productivity loss in brainstorming groups: toward the solution of a riddle. *J Pers Soc Psychol.* 1987;53(3):497.

32. Taylor DW, Berry PC, Block CH. Does group participation when using brainstorming facilitate or inhibit creative thinking? *Admin Sci Quart.* 1958:23-47.

33. Arnold RM, Back AL. Dealing with conflict in caring for the seriously III. *JAMA.* 2005;293:1374-1381.

34. Clark PG, Cott C, Drinka TJ. Theory and practice in interprofessional ethics: A framework for understanding ethical issues in health care teams. *J Interprof Care.* 2007;21(6):591-603.

35. Leape LL, Shore MF, Dienstag JL, et al. Perspective: a culture of respect, part 1: the nature and causes of disrespectful behavior by physicians. *Acad Med.* 2012;87(7):845-852.

36. Makary MA, Daniel M. Medical error-the third leading cause of death in the US. *BMJ.* 2016;353:i2139.

37. Koslowski SWJ, Ilgen, D.R. Enhancing the effectiveness of work groups and teams. *Psychol. Sci. Public Interest.* 2006;7(3):77-124.

38. Hughes KM, Benenson RS, Krichten AE, Clancy KD, Ryan JP, Hammond C. A crew resource management program tailored to trauma resuscitation improves team behavior and communication. *J Am Coll Surg.* 2014;219(3):545-551.

39. Buljac-Samardzic M, Dekker-van Doorn CM, van Wijngaarden JD, van Wijk KP. Interventions to improve team effectiveness: a systematic review. *Health Policy.* 2010;94(3):183-195.

40. Moffatt-Bruce SD, Hefner JL, Mekhjian H, et al. What is the return on investment for implementation of a crew resource management program at an academic medical center? *Am J Med Qual.* 2019;34(5):502-508.

41. Taylor CR, Hepworth JT, Buerhaus PI, Dittus R, Speroff T. Effect of crew resource management on diabetes care and patient outcomes in an inner-city primary care clinic. *Qual Saf Health Care.* 2007;16(4):244-247.

42. Sundar E, Sundar S, Pawlowski J, Blum R, Feinstein D, Pratt S. Crew resource management and team training. *Anesthesiol Clin.* 2007;25(2):283-300.

43. Pettker CM, Thung SF, Norwitz ER, et al. Impact of a comprehensive patient safety strategy on obstetric adverse events. *Am J Obstet Gynecol.* 2009;200(5):492 e491-498.

44. Singer S, Lin S, Falwell A, Gaba D, Baker L. Relationship of safety climate and safety performance in hospitals. *Health Serv Res.* 2009;44(2 Pt 1):399-421.

45. Hefner JL, Hilligoss B, Knupp A, et al. Cultural transformation after implementation of crew resource management: is it really possible? *Am J Med Qual.* 2017;32(4):384-390.

46. Institute of Medicine Committee on Quality of Health Care in America. In: Kohn LT, Corrigan JM, Donaldson MS, eds. *To err is human: building a safer health system.* Washington, DC: National Academies Press; 2000.

47. van de Ven A, Delbecq, A. The effectiveness of nominal, delphi, and interacting group decision-making processes. *Acad Manag J.* 1974;17:147-178.

48. Janis I. *Victims of groupthink.* Houghton Mifflin; 1972.

49. Kaba A, Wishart I, Fraser K, Coderre S, McLaughlin K. Are we at risk of groupthink in our approach to teamwork interventions in health care? *Med Educ.* 2016;50(4):400-408.

50. Brown J, Lewis L, Ellis K, Stewart M, Freeman TR, Kasperski MJ. Conflict on interprofessional primary health care teams--can it be resolved? *J Interprof Care.* 2011;25(1):4-10.

51. Gouran DS, Hirokawa RY, Julian KM, Leatham GB. The evolution and current status of the functional perspective on communication in decision-making and problem-solving groups. *Ann Intern Commun Assoc.* 1993;16(1):573-600.

52. Pena A, Estrada CA, Soniat D, Taylor B, Burton M. Nominal group technique: a brainstorming tool for identifying areas to improve pain management in hospitalized patients. *J Hosp Med.* 2012;7(5):416-420.

53. Rubin G, De Wit N, Meineche-Schmidt V, Seifert B, Hall N, Hungin P. The diagnosis of IBS in primary care: consensus development using nominal group technique. *Fam Pract.* 2006;23(6):687-692.

54. Shaw J, Jamieson T, Agarwal P, Griffin B, Wong I, Bhatia RS. Virtual care policy recommendations for patient-centred primary care: findings of a consensus policy dialogue using a nominal group technique. *J Telemed Telecare.* 2018;24(9):608-615.

Epilogue

FINAL THOUGHTS: HOW AND WHY CLINICAL NEGOTIATION MATTERS

Like politics, clinical negotiation is the art of the possible. However, in contrast to politics (where some would say the driving force is money), the essence of clinical negotiation is good communication. When patients and clinicians are struggling to find common ground, effective communication is how clinicians help patients understand their health states and treatment options, uncover what patients think and what's important to them, foster caring and compassionate relationships, work out differences of opinion, and collaborate to reach decisions based on the evidence and consistent with patient values. In this framework, communication is integral to safe, effective, efficient, patient-centered, timely, and equitable health care.[1-3] Our goal in writing this book was to provide in-depth analysis and guidance for clinicians striving to accomplish these goals as they seek to find common ground with patients.

And yet, some may still question whether communication skills are too soft, too ethereal, or too remote from real medicine to count for much. This view is encapsulated in the challenge offered by some of our colleagues over the years: would you rather have a surgeon with a great bedside manner and a 3% surgical mortality rate or one with the personality of cardboard and a 1% mortality rate?

We reject that Hobson's choice. We want good technical quality of care *and* good communication. In fact we would argue that they are related to one another. In this concluding section, we offer a glimpse of the evidence demonstrating how and why communication matters, especially as it concerns the clinical negotiation.

COMMUNICATION AND QUALITY OF HEALTH CARE

Patient satisfaction with health care, adherence to treatment regimens, and shared understanding are important indicators of health care quality. Patients typically report greater satisfaction with their care when physicians are perceived

343

as good listeners, are interested in what patients have to say, provide understandable explanations of complex medical information, address patient's questions and concerns, treat patients with respect, and include patients as active participants in health care decision-making.[4] Shared decision-making, an important component of effective clinical negotiation, often leads to greater patient understanding and less decision regret.[5]

Other research has investigated the relationship between clinician-patient communication, adherence to medical recommendations, and health outcomes. A 2009 systematic review[6] of research on the relationship between adherence and three aspects of physician communication found a 19% higher risk of poor adherence among patients seeing physicians who provided scant information, neglected psychosocial concerns, and failed to build trust and rapport. Moreover, the odds of patient adherence were significantly higher when physicians received training in communication skills. In related research, adherence tended to be higher when patients (especially those belonging to racial and ethnic minority groups)[7,8] believed they and the clinician were "working together."[9,10]

A major theme of this book is the centrality of shared understanding (of goals, values, beliefs, and expectations) for effective clinical negotiation. Although receiving less empirical attention than patient satisfaction and adherence, shared understanding has been linked to several features of clinician-patient communication. For example, clinicians who support and encourage patients to be active participants in the consultation process (e.g., by asking questions, sharing concerns, and expressing feelings) can more accurately predict patients' health beliefs and priorities.[11] Patients and clinicians are more likely to be in agreement about the patient's health status, needs, and treatment approaches when physicians use more partnership-building (i.e., actively encourage patient involvement) and patients are more participatory.[12,13]

Effective medication management is a fundamental component of high-quality primary care. Misunderstandings about a medication's purpose are less likely when patients are more involved in the interaction[14] and when clinicians emphasize important information, check for patient comprehension, and review key take-home points at the end of the visit.[15,16]

COMMUNICATION AND HEALTH OUTCOMES

The most intriguing evidence in support of the belief that communication matters is found in research examining the relationship between clinician-patient communication and health outcomes. Vast research suggests that communication measures, however assessed, frequently predict quality of health care delivery (process of care) but not health outcomes—at least not directly.[5,17,18] While vexing, this finding should not be surprising: health outcomes (survival, biomarkers of disease status, and quality of life) are affected by multiple factors through multiple causal pathways. However, there is a substantial body of evidence that effective clinician-patient communication can *indirectly* contribute to improved outcomes.[19] If, for example, effective clinician-patient communication supports greater patient satisfaction with care, mutual understanding between clinician and patient, mutually agreed upon decisions, greater trust, and patient confidence in following a treatment plan, then patients may in turn gain greater commitment to the treatment plan, better access to needed care, more self-care skills, healthier lifestyles, and better emotion management. Each of these could in turn be part of a mechanism leading to better health outcomes. *Communication* is the catalyst that activates the pathway needed to produce the outcomes of interest.

In a study with which we are deeply familiar, cancer patients with pain cancer patients with pain were randomized to a communication coaching intervention (in which they were "coached" to negotiate for better pain treatment) or usual care.[20] Patients receiving the coaching intervention expressed more concerns, made more requests, and asked more questions about pain management.[21] Neither receiving the intervention itself nor communication about pain predicted better pain control. But patients who talked more about their pain-related concerns were more likely to have their analgesic regimen changed.[22] Analgesic intensification in turn predicted better pain control.[23] In short, the intervention activated a communication pathway that helped patients discuss their pain concerns, which in turn prompted clinicians to make needed analgesic adjustments leading to improved pain outcomes.

Another indirect pathway connecting communication to health outcomes involves patient satisfaction. Although an element of controversy exists,[24] several high-quality studies support links between communication and patient satisfaction,[25] and between patient satisfaction (or the related concept of patient experience) and health outcomes.[26]

Previous research has also supplied evidence linking communication to biomedical outcomes, often mediated through adherence. In one seminal study conducted in primary care, more information sharing and more patient involvement in care were associated with better blood pressure and glucose control, at least in the short term.[27] In another, glaucoma patients whose clinicians emphasized the importance of ocular medication therapy and who solicited patients' input achieved better intraocular pressure control.[28] Finally, in a longitudinal study of patients with diabetes, Parchman et al.[29] found support for a pathway by which physicians' encouragement of patient involvement prompted more active patient participation in the consultation. Active participation in turn was associated with medication adherence, and medication adherence predicted subsequent improvement in blood pressure and glucose control.

Finally, although clinician-patient communication rarely has *direct* effects on health outcomes, a clinician's words and deeds (including nonverbal behaviors) can alleviate patients' emotional distress. In a study of cancer patients, by saying "I know this is tough for you," "let me know if I say something confusing," and "I'm with you every step of the way," oncologists eased patients' anxiety during shared decision-making about chemotherapy.[30] Even in less life-threatening and emotion-laden situations, saying the right words, in the right way, can make a difference that patients will remember for a long time.

Still, in clinical negotiation, as in all human endeavors, we will never get it right every time. Becoming a better participant in the clinical negotiation through the cultivation of communication skills is a lifelong endeavor. UCLA Hall of Fame Basketball coach John Wooden was a stickler for coaching his players on the fundamentals of basketball—dribbling, passing, movement, defense, shooting. He once said, "It's the little details that are vital. Little things make big things happen." In many ways, communication skills are the "little things" that enable clinicians to achieve "great things" as health care professionals. We hope this book helps you achieve ever greater things in your careers as healers.

References:

1. Langberg EM, Dyhr L, Davidsen AS. Development of the concept of patient-centredness - A systematic review. *Patient Educ Couns*. 2019;102(7):1228-36.
2. Epstein RM, Street RL Jr. *Patient-centered communication in cancer care: promoting healing and reducing suffering*. Report No.: NIH Publication No. 07-6225.
3. Committee on Quality Health Care in America IoM. Crossing the quality chasm: a new health system for the 21st century: Washington, D.C.: National Academy Press; 2001.
4. Boquiren VM, Hack TF, Beaver K, Williamson S. What do measures of patient satisfaction with the doctor tell us? *Patient Educ Couns*. 2015.
5. Shay LA, Lafata JE. Where is the evidence? A systematic review of shared decision making and patient outcomes. *Med Decis Making*. 2015;35(1):114-31.
6. Zolnierek KB, DiMatteo MR. Physician communication and patient adherence to treatment: a meta-analysis. *Med Care*. 2009;47(8):826-34.
7. Schoenthaler A, Chaplin WF, Allegrante JP, Fernandez S, az-Gloster M, Tobin JN, et al. Provider communication effects medication adherence in hypertensive African Americans. *Patient Educ Couns*. 2009;75(2):185-91.
8. Beach MC, Roter DL, Saha S, Korthuis PT, Eggly S, Cohn J, et al. Impact of a brief patient and provider intervention to improve the quality of communication about medication adherence among HIV patients. *Patient Educ Couns*. 2015;98(9):1078-83.
9. Wilson SR, Strub P, Buist AS, Knowles SB, Lavori PW, Lapidus J, et al. Shared treatment decision making improves adherence and outcomes in poorly controlled asthma. *Am J Respir Crit Care Med*. 2010;181(6):566-77.
10. Bauer AM, Parker MM, Schillinger D, Katon W, Adler N, Adams AS, et al. Associations between antidepressant adherence and shared decision-making, patient-provider trust, and communication among adults with diabetes: Diabetes Study of Northern California (DISTANCE). *J Gen Intern Med*. 2014;29(8):1139–47.
11. Street RL Jr, Haidet P. How well do doctors know their patients? Factors affecting physician understanding of patients' health beliefs. *J Gen Intern Med*. 2011;26(1):21-7.
12. Street RL Jr, Richardson MN, Cox V, Suarez-Almazor ME. (Mis)understanding in patient-health care provider communication about total knee replacement. *Arthritis Rheum*. 2009;61(1):100-7.
13. Heisler M, Vijan S, Anderson RM, Ubel PA, Bernstein SJ, Hofer TP. When do patients and their physicians agree on diabetes treatment goals and strategies, and what difference does it make? *J Gen Intern Med*. 2003;18(11):893-902.
14. Britten N, Stevenson FA, Barry CA, Barber N, Bradley CP. Misunderstandings in prescribing decisions in general practice: qualitative study. *BMJ*. 2000;320(7233):484-8.

15. Jansen J, Butow PN, van Weert JC, van Dulmen S, Devine RJ, Heeren TJ, et al. Does age really matter? Recall of information presented to newly referred patients with cancer. *J Clin Oncol.* 2008;26(33):5450-7.

16. McCarthy DM, Waite KR, Curtis LM, Engel KG, Baker DW, Wolf MS. What did the doctor say? Health literacy and recall of medical instructions. *Med Care.* 2012;50(4):277-82.

17. Rathert C, Wyrwich MD, Boren SA. Patient-centered care and outcomes: a systematic review of the literature. *Med Care Res Rev.* 2013;70(4):351-79.

18. Street RL Jr. How clinician-patient communication contributes to health improvement: Modeling pathways from talk to outcome. *Patient Educ Couns.* 2013;92(3):286-91.

19. Street RL Jr, Makoul G, Arora NK, Epstein RM. How does communication heal? Pathways linking clinician-patient communication to health outcomes. *Patient Educ Couns.* 2009;74(3):295-301.

20. Kravitz RL, Tancredi DJ, Grennan T, Kalauokalani D, Street RL Jr, Slee CK, et al. Cancer Health Empowerment for Living without Pain (Ca-HELP): effects of a tailored education and coaching intervention on pain and impairment. *Pain.* 2011;152(7):1572-82.

21. Street RL Jr, Slee C, Kalauokalani DK, Dean DE, Tancredi DJ, Kravitz RL. Improving physician-patient communication about cancer pain with a tailored education-coaching intervention. *Patient Educ Couns.* 2010;80(1):42-7.

22. Kravitz RL, Tancredi DJ, Jerant A, Saito N, Street RL, Grennan T, et al. Influence of patient coaching on analgesic treatment adjustment: secondary analysis of a randomized controlled trial. *J Pain Symptom Manage.* 2012;43(5):874-84.

23. Street RL Jr, Tancredi DJ, Slee C, Kalauokalani DK, Dean DE, Franks P, et al. A pathway linking patient participation in cancer consultations to pain control. *Psychooncology.* 2014;23(10):1111-7.

24. Jerant A, Fenton JJ, Kravitz RL, Tancredi DJ, Magnan E, Bertakis KD, et al. Association of clinician denial of patient requests with patient satisfaction. *JAMA Intern Med.* 2018;178(1):85-91.

25. McMillan SS, Kendall E, Sav A, King MA, Whitty JA, Kelly F, et al. Patient-centered approaches to health care: a systematic review of randomized controlled trials. *Med Care Res Rev.* 2013;70(6):567-96.

26. Doyle C, Lennox L, Bell D. A systematic review of evidence on the links between patient experience and clinical safety and effectiveness. *BMJ Open.* 2013;3(1):e001570.

27. Kaplan SH, Greenfield S, Ware JE Jr. Assessing the effects of physician-patient interactions on the outcomes of chronic disease. *Med Care.* 1989;27(3 Suppl):S110-S27.

28. The cascade effect in the clinical care of patients. *N Engl J Med.* 1986;315(5):319-20.

29. Parchman ML, Zeber JE, Palmer RF. Participatory decision making, patient activation, medication adherence, and intermediate clinical outcomes in type 2 diabetes: a STARNet study. *Ann Fam Med.* 2010;8(5):410-7.

30. Fogarty LA, Curbow BA, Wingard JR, McDonnell K, Somerfield MR. Can 40 seconds of compassion reduce patient anxiety? *J Clin Oncol.* 1999;17(1):371-9.

Index

Page numbers followed by f and t indicate figures and tables